# Clinical Practice of Alternative Medicine

# Clinical Practice of Alternative Medicine

Editor: Tanner Perry

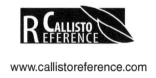

www.callistoreference.com

**Callisto Reference,**
118-35 Queens Blvd., Suite 400,
Forest Hills, NY 11375, USA

Visit us on the World Wide Web at:
www.callistoreference.com

ISBN: 978-1-63239-882-6 (Hardback)

The publisher's policy is to use permanent paper from mills that operate a sustainable forestry policy. Furthermore, the publisher ensures that the text paper and cover boards used have met acceptable environmental accreditation standards.

**Trademark Notice:** Registered trademark of products or corporate names are used only for explanation and identification without intent to infringe.

Printed in the United States of America.

### Cataloging-in-Publication Data

Clinical practice of alternative medicine / edited by Tanner Perry.
    p. cm.
Includes bibliographical references and index.
ISBN 978-1-63239-882-6
1. Clinical medicine. 2. Alternative medicine. I. Perry, Tanner.
RC46 .C55 2017
616--dc23

# Table of Contents

# Preface

Alternative medicine is defined as a set of medical treatments and therapies that provide healing and well-being. This book on clinical practice of alternative medicine deals with interventional and physiotherapeutic techniques of this field. Alternative medicine diagnoses disease through an assessment of various bodily processes and psycho-physiological conditions. Interventional ability of alternative medicine is one of the key areas where considerable progress has been made. This book is a valuable compilation of topics, ranging from the basic to the most complex advancements in the field of alternative medicine. Students, researchers, experts and all associated with this field will benefit alike from this book.

The researches compiled throughout the book are authentic and of high quality, combining several disciplines and from very diverse regions from around the world. Drawing on the contributions of many researchers from diverse countries, the book's objective is to provide the readers with the latest achievements in the area of research. This book will surely be a source of knowledge to all interested and researching the field.

In the end, I would like to express my deep sense of gratitude to all the authors for meeting the set deadlines in completing and submitting their research chapters. I would also like to thank the publisher for the support offered to us throughout the course of the book. Finally, I extend my sincere thanks to my family for being a constant source of inspiration and encouragement.

**Editor**

# Prior to Conception: The Role of an Acupuncture Protocol in Improving Women's Reproductive Functioning Assessed by a Pilot Pragmatic Randomised Controlled Trial

Suzanne Cochrane,[1] Caroline A. Smith,[2] Alphia Possamai-Inesedy,[3] and Alan Bensoussan[2]

[1]School of Science & Health, Western Sydney University, Locked Bag 1797, Penrith, NSW 2751, Australia
[2]National Institute of Complementary Medicine, Western Sydney University, Locked Bag 1797, Penrith, NSW 2751, Australia
[3]School of Social Science & Psychology, Western Sydney University, Locked Bag 1797, Penrith, NSW 2751, Australia

Correspondence should be addressed to Suzanne Cochrane; s.cochrane@westernsydney.edu.au

Academic Editor: Kieran Cooley

The global average of couples with fertility problems is 9%. Assisted reproductive technologies are often inaccessible. Evidence points to acupuncture offering an opportunity to promote natural fertility. This study asked whether providing a multiphasic fertility acupuncture protocol to women with sub/infertility would increase their awareness of fertility and achieve normalisation of their menstrual cycle compared with a lifestyle control. In a pragmatic randomised controlled trial sub/infertile women were offered an intervention of acupuncture and lifestyle modification or lifestyle modification only. There was a statistically significant increase in fertility awareness in the acupuncture group (86.4%, 19) compared to 40% ($n = 8$) of the lifestyle only participants (Relative Risk (RR) 2.38, 95% confidence interval (CI) of 1.25, 4.50), with an adjusted $p$ value of 0.011. Changes in menstrual regularity were not statistically significant. There was no statistical difference in the pregnancy rate with seven women (adjusted $p = 0.992$) achieving pregnancy during the course of the study intervention. Those receiving the acupuncture conceived within an average of 5.5 weeks compared to 10.67 weeks for the lifestyle only group ($p = 0.422$). The acupuncture protocol tested influenced women who received it compared to women who used lifestyle modification alone: their fertility awareness and wellbeing increased, and those who conceived did so in half the time.

## 1. Introduction

Fertility problems have become a major presenting condition in gynaecological clinics. Estimates of the number of couples encountering fertility problems vary from one in six to one in ten, with 9% currently cited as the probable global average [1]. As the biomedical response to infertility IVF remains "absent, inaccessible, or unaffordable for the majority of the world's infertile couples" [1, page 2], populations may utilise their traditional medical health systems. Chinese medicine has been used to treat female fertility problems using a range of methods throughout its history. In Western settings acupuncture is used as a primary intervention for fertility problems [2, 3]. Acupuncture is increasingly used as an adjunct to assisted reproductive technologies [4] and more widely in the complementary health care system.

Outside the context of assisted reproductive technologies (ART) clinics, there has been little research that supports the role of acupuncture in promoting women's reproductive health. Research of Chinese medicine's supportive contribution to fertility largely consists of case reports. In a survey of Australian and New Zealand acupuncturists [5] it was found that general fertility health treatments were the most common treatments administered to women. This emphasis in clinical practice has also been reported in the UK [6].

Clinical case reports support the value of acupuncture in the lead up to conception, although no clinical trial has been reported to date that either supports or contradicts this case-based evidence [7–10]. A prospective consecutive case series study of a course of 3 months of acupuncture for amenorrheic women with premature ovarian failure has found, compared to baseline, serum follicle stimulating hormone (FSH) and luteinising hormone (LH) were decreased ($Z = 4.68$, $p = 0.001$) and estradiol (E2) was increased ($Z = 4.48$, $p = 0.001$). Within the 3-month intervention approximately 20 percent of trial participants resumed their menstruation [11]. Chinese medicine texts and case history books, for example, frequently cite the use of acupuncture to induce ovulation. Early research reported that electroacupuncture induced ovulation in six out of 13 anovulatory cycles as well as higher hand skin temperature and lower blood radioimmunoreactive [beta]-endorphin concentrations in acupuncture induced ovulation cycles [12]. Gerhard and Postneek [13] found that infertile women with hormonal disturbances and anovulation treated with auricular acupuncture had similar pregnancy rates when compared with those treated with hormones.

The absence of previous research on applying acupuncture in the period of periconception for women who are having difficulty conceiving is identified as a research gap. This study sought to explore the potential contribution of an acupuncture protocol to enhancing female fertility.

## 2. Materials and Methods

The pilot study objective was to provide preliminary data to explore whether women with subfertility undergoing a course of acupuncture and lifestyle modification compared with an active control of lifestyle modification alone would demonstrate improved reproductive outcomes, improved menstrual cycles, and increased fertility awareness.

The study hypothesised that providing acupuncture to women with sub/infertility would increase their awareness of their fertility and achieve normalisation of their menstrual cycle compared with lifestyle as a control.

Secondary hypotheses were that acupuncture compared with lifestyle control would demonstrate reduced time from study entry to conception; increased clinical pregnancy rates; improved quality of life changes; and increased lifestyle change.

*2.1. Participants and Recruitment.* Participants were recruited from the community in Sydney, Australia between October 2009 and December 2011. Participants were initially recruited from existing contact lists within the research centre. Further recruitment sources were via media and social network advertising, such as local paper and Facebook and other internet sites. Also posters and pamphlets were distributed, within the university campuses and to other likely referral sources such as medical centres, chemists, and community centres. Women who made early contact also suggested further avenues for recruitment, their main suggestion being accessing the forums on fertility-specific websites. Several web forums agreed to include a statement about the trial and a request for women to contact the researcher for further information. A letter requesting referrals to the study was forwarded to women's health centres, medical centres, TCM clinics, and fertility centres in the target area of Western Sydney.

Ethics approval for this study was obtained from the Human Research Ethics Committee of University of Western Sydney: H7588. The trial was registered with the Australian and New Zealand Clinical Trial Registry as ACTRN12610000631000.

*2.2. Inclusion/Exclusion Criteria.* The inclusion criteria were women of reproductive age (18–44 years old) who had been actively trying to conceive (unprotected sex) without success (including miscarriage) for at least 12 months; who had a gynaecological diagnosis of the causes of their infertility; who are not planning to use acupuncture during the trial intervention; and who are able to attend at least 7 of 9 treatment sessions.

Gynaecological assessments and diagnoses were provided by participants based on their previous biomedical examinations prior to the study and were not reassessed at screening. Women were excluded if they met the criteria of having nonpatent fallopian tubes; absence of uterus; primary anovulation; or partner sperm defect (and not enrolled in IVF to use intracytoplasmic sperm injection (ICSI) to counter defect).

The randomisation sequence was computer generated by a researcher independent of the study based at the University of Western Sydney. The random allocation was sealed in opaque numbered envelopes held in sequential order and accessed by the acupuncturist in sequential order. Random allocation of participants was to either an acupuncture plus lifestyle intervention or lifestyle modification alone. As this was a pragmatic design there was no blinding of patient or acupuncturist. Data entry and analysis were undertaken blind to group allocation.

*2.3. Intervention and Follow-Up.* The intervention was administered over three months. The control of lifestyle support comprising diet and exercise is the most common first-stage intervention offered in general preconceptual care and is an appropriate base from which to assess fertility changes from an acupuncture intervention [15, 16]. Although lifestyle advice is a standard component of Chinese medicine care [17] a specifically targeted lifestyle intervention, focused on diet and exercise, provides a viable active comparator to an acupuncture intervention.

The diet was based on the CSIRO Total Wellbeing Diet [18] and is supported by research evidence that the diet optimises fertility treatment outcomes [15, 19]. The CSIRO Total Wellbeing Diet has been tested both in research and in the marketplace. It offers an explanation of a recommended diet and exercise regimen, detailed recipes, and a long-term maintenance plan. As this research project lacked the resources for individualised assessment and program design the CSIRO diet was adopted as it is considered nutritionally balanced. In its presentation the diet is accessible and sufficiently applicable to a range of women and has a health, rather than just a weight loss, focus. All participants were also asked to develop an exercise program within the guidelines offered by Noakes and Clifton to incorporate within their daily schedule. Those participants with already heavily weighted active exercise regime were asked to include softer exercise routines like meditation, yoga, Tai Chi, or walking and to reduce the amount of heavy exercise during their menses and ovulation. Those with little active exercise were encouraged to increase this, especially outside the times of menstruation and ovulation. Those who smoked cigarettes and/or drank alcohol or caffeine regularly were encouraged to develop a plan to reduce or remove them from their daily lives. Each participant was contacted by phone or email at least fortnightly or an attempt was made to have such contact by the study investigator to assess compliance with the lifestyle intervention.

In addition to the same lifestyle advice all participants randomised the acupuncture intervention received a Chinese medicine assessment. This was undertaken by the lead researcher who allocated each participant a TCM diagnosis and treatment strategy. The allocated diagnoses were forwarded to the treating acupuncturist. Acupuncture was administered using a manualised treatment protocol [20], predominantly within a TCM paradigm. The collective development of the protocol began from the foundation work of Lyttleton from Table 4.11 in the 2004 edition of her book ([14]: 158-9). Treatment was administered over three months with weekly acupuncture; acupuncture treatment was tailored and based on their TCM diagnosis, the phase of their menstrual cycle, an assessment of their spirit or emotional state, and biomedical condition. Their TCM diagnosis and phase of their menstrual cycle were given greatest priority followed by their presenting emotional state, their biomedical diagnosis, and specific presenting signs and symptoms, such as a headache.

Acupuncture points were needled bilaterally on body channels except for unilateral needling on channels that bisect along the midline (Ren and Du channels). Needle insertion was at a location and to tissue depth as defined by recognised acupuncture text [21], and the needling sensation known as "Deqi," a sensation experienced by patient and acupuncturist as successful contact between the needle and the correct point [22], was sought on each point, and needles were retained for 20–30 minutes each session. Needles used on all treatments were Vinco brand sterile acupuncture needles in guide tubes (sizes 0.22 × 25 mm, 0.25 × 40 mm, and 0.25 × 75 mm). Additional TCM modalities were included in the treatment and individualised; these included heat applied as appropriate by Teding Diancibo Pu (TDP) Infrared Heat Lamp or smokeless moxibustion. At each session, details of participant signs and symptoms and treatment given were recorded. This included pulse and tongue presentation, changes to basal body temperature (BBT), compliance with exercise and diet, and acupuncture points needled. The acupuncturists included the lead researcher who was TCM trained with 23-year clinical experience and TCM trained practitioners based in Sydney and trained in the study protocols who had a minimum of 3-year clinical experience.

All subjects were free to withdraw from the study at any stage. When participants in either group reported pregnancy, their treatment intervention was terminated. They were asked to confirm pregnancy by blood test.

2.4. Outcome Measures. The primary study endpoints were assessed by reported variation in self-knowledge about fertility and ovulation and knowledge of fertile period at 3 months; regularity of menstrual cycle at 3 months displayed on BBT; and reduced menstrual symptoms at 3 months recorded on menstrual record.

Secondary study endpoints included the time from study entry to conception; biochemical pregnancy demonstrated by blood test at six weeks; quality of life changes as measured by MYMOP at three months; and lifestyle change demonstrated by body mass index (BMI) at three months.

Increased awareness of fertility was measured by comparing self-knowledge about fertility and ovulation at intake and exit at three months, and a self-report question of whether their knowledge of when they were fertile had improved and in which way. Menstrual normalisation was documented on a BBT chart issued to participants and they were asked to record their temperature daily prior to rising using the same temperature each day. The chart had an addendum to document menstrual changes, including menses onset and duration, level of pain, menstrual flow, and incidence of clotting, which were also recorded by participating acupuncturists. The incidence of pregnancy was measured by self-report and record of human chorionic gonadotropin (hCG) blood test. The time from study entry to conception was assessed from the date of recruitment to the report of first missed period that resulted in pregnancy. BMI was assessed before and after the intervention.

Measure Your Medical Outcome Profile 2 (MYMOP) [23] was used to measure the quality of life outcomes that the patient considered the most important, including symptoms and desired activities. For the MYMOP2 questionnaire participants are asked prior to intervention to "choose one or two symptoms (physical or mental) which bother you most." The participants were also asked to "choose one activity (physical, social, or mental) that is important to you and that your problem makes difficult or prevents you doing."

An adverse event was defined as one that endangers an existing pregnancy, future fertility or the health, and wellbeing of participants. All adverse events (serious and nonserious) were reported to the primary researcher. They were recorded firstly on the treatment record, a copy lodged in a separate adverse event record and analysed and reported.

2.5. Sample Size of Pilot Study. Given the lack of research in this area it was difficult to estimate the effect of acupuncture compared to control on changes in lifestyle and pregnancy. Previous research into acupuncture's action in regulating menstrual characteristics suggested a moderate effect size [24]. We expected to detect an absolute improvement in menstrual regularity of 40% from baseline between groups, from 40% in the control group to 80% in the intervention group at the end of the intervention ($p < 0.05$, 80% power). A trial of 56 women was required, 28 women per group, with 80% power at the 5% significance level.

2.6. Data Analysis. Quantitative data analysis was undertaken using software program IBM SPSS 20 (IBM SPSS Statistics Version 20). Descriptive analyses including mean, standard deviation, and frequency were undertaken describing the baseline characteristics of participants.

An "intention to treat" analysis was performed. Comparisons were made of primary and secondary outcomes by means of analysis of variance and measures of effect size using relative risks and 95% confidence interval. $p < 0.05$ has been considered statistically significant. An adjusted analysis or covariance was undertaken to assess unexplained or error variance using the variables that were unequal between the two groups, namely, age, duration of fertility problems, and diagnosis of PCOS. For categorical variables a chi-square measure was used and a binary logistic regression undertaken. For continuous variables ANOVA and ANCOVA were used to analyse covariants.

## 3. Results

Over 12 months 160 inquiries were received with 56 women randomised to the study. Of those who met the inclusion criteria and refused to join the study a significant proportion were not willing to undergo randomisation and risk delaying the receipt of an acupuncture intervention for 3 months. As represented in Table 1 the retention rate of participants over the full 3 months in each intervention group was 82% in the acupuncture + lifestyle intervention and 71% in the lifestyle only group. Several potential or actual participants reported moving house or city and it is assumed that at least some of the 21 (37.5% of the total) women lost to follow-up may also have undergone changes, as they were no longer accessible via their work and home contact details. All data collected to the point of exit from the study was analysed.

Baseline characteristics of women are reported in Figure 1. Of the women recruited the average duration of their fertility problems was 4.85 (SD 4.1) years. Twenty-six (46.4%) women had fertility problems solely sourced in female factors; for 24 (42.9%) women their fertility difficulties were unexplained and the balance of six women had combined female-male factors that were being addressed through techniques such as intracytoplasmic sperm injection (ICSI). Nine women were currently enrolled in IVF and further nine reported having tried IVF in the past, 21 had taken clomiphene citrate to stimulate ovulation, and 25 women (44.6%) of the study sample had used no other biomedical treatment prior to the study. Twenty-five women (44.6% of the total group) reported previous use of acupuncture.

Thirty-three women (58.9%) were of English speaking background and the remaining 23 (41.1%) identified themselves as from non-English speaking backgrounds.

The awareness of fertility through identifying ovulation was 28 (50%) indicating that they knew when they ovulated. Of these 13 (46.4%) recognised ovulation by their fertile mucus, seven (25%) by abdominal pain, seven (25%) based on other factors and two (7.2%) by monitoring temperature changes. Twenty-six women (46.4%) monitored their mucus discharge, nine (16.1%) monitored their BBT, and 13 (23.2%) recorded other changes to assist in identifying their fertile period.

In response to the MYMOP questionnaire there was remarkable consistency in the symptoms nominated with a clear dominance of weight loss and tiredness. Surprising, given the purpose of the clinical trial, was the small percentage of these women who nominated infertility and pregnancy failure as their primary concern at that time. Perhaps the women did not perceive fertility as impacting on their wellbeing. It was poignant to read "*I just want to feel good in my body*

*without continuous pain – like I used to be*" on a form which did not encourage lengthy contributions. Several women wrote "depression," "jealousy," "anger," "being emotionally vulnerable," and "anxiety," testifying to the difficulty of their lives at that time.

Of the respondents, 37.5% nominated getting more exercise or getting up and moving as their major desired activity.

There was an imbalance between the two study groups for two variables at baseline: the duration of infertility and biomedical diagnosis; these were adjusted for in the analysis.

## 4. Primary Study Endpoints

As indicated in Table 2 there was a statistically significant increase in fertility awareness in the group of women who received acupuncture (86.4%, 19) compared to 40% ($n = 8$) of the lifestyle only participants, (Relative Risk (RR) 2.38, 95% confidence interval (CI) of 1.25, 4.50), with an adjusted $p$ value of 0.011 (Table 5).

There was no significant change in menstrual regularity over time between the two groups; however, the participants receiving acupuncture trended toward retaining regularity over 3 cycles (of 71.4%) whereas the lifestyle only group lost regularity (71.4% to 50%). The low numbers of responses of 3rd-cycle data limit the value of interpreting this trend. There were no statistically significant differences in the length of the follicular and ovulatory phases of the menstrual cycle over three months between groups.

## 5. Reduced Menstrual Symptoms

There were no statistically significant differences between groups in other menstrual characteristics including length of cycle [Table 3], presence of menstrual clots, and menstrual pain.

There was no statistical difference in the pregnancy rate between groups with seven women (adjusted $p = 0.992$) achieving a pregnancy during the course of the study intervention. Those receiving the acupuncture conceived within an average of 5.5 weeks compared to 10.67 weeks for the lifestyle only group ($p = 0.422$). For those who received acupuncture this is effectively half the time to conception. There is a trend in the follow-up data indicating a difference in the numbers of pregnancies in the 12 months following trial completion: 10 women in total in the acupuncture group became pregnant and 5 in the lifestyle only group, with the number of live births also varying to 80% in the acupuncture group and 60% in the lifestyle only group ($p = 0.176$).

Quality of life improved for women receiving acupuncture [Table 4]. In relation to changes in desired activity the acupuncture intervention participants recorded a change of 1.80 (1.2) compared to the lifestyle only group of 0.94 (1.2). This represented a statistically significant adjusted $p$ value of 0.047. The MYMOP measure of changes in wellbeing also showed significant differences between the two groups: 0.95 (1.4) in the acupuncture group and 0.05 (1.4) in the lifestyle only group. This represented a statistically significant adjusted $p$ value of 0.042.

TABLE 1: Extract of guidelines issued to trial acupuncturists.

| | | | | |
|---|---|---|---|---|
| Frequency | Weekly | | | |
| Number of treatments | 9 | | | |
| Timing | 1 hour [include front (anterior) and back (posterior) treatment per session] | | | |
| Point location | As per Deadman's *A Manual of Acupuncture* | | | |
| Needle depth | As per Deadman's *A Manual of Acupuncture* | | | |
| Manipulation | Achieve deqi on insertion and renew qi sensation 10–15 minutes after insertion | | | |
| Retention time | 20–30 minutes | | | |
| Needling | Bilateral unless on Ren and Du channels | | | |
| Needles | Use needles supplied by Helio Supply Co., that is, AcuGlide and Vinco | | | |
| Heat | If heat is necessary, apply using TDP lamp or smokeless moxa | | | |
| Differential diagnosis relating to phase of menstrual cycle | Phase 1 during period | Phase 2 after period | Phase 3 during ovulation | Phase 4 after ovulation |
| Core points [14] | Sp 10, 6, 8 LI 4 St 28Ki 14 | Ren 4, 7 Ki 3, 4, 5, 6, 8, 13 St 27, 30, 36 Bl 23, 32 Liv 3 Sp 4, 6, 10 | Liv 3, 5 Ki 13, 14, 8, 5, 4 Sp 13, 8, 6, 5 Pc 6, 5 Ht 7, 5 Yintang Zigong GB 26 | (A) [boost yang by supplementing yin] Ren 2, 4, 5, 7, 15 Ki 3, 6 Bl 23 (B) [boost yang promoting qi] Ren 4, 5, 6, 12 St 25, 36 Sp 6 Ki 3 Bl 20, 23 (C) [boost yang by nourishing blood] Ren 4, 12 St 36 Sp 6, 10 Ki 5 Bl 17 |
| Examples of other commonly used acupoints | *Shen* (emotional) disorders | GV 20, Yintang, Ht 7, Pc 6, Kidney chest pts: Ki 23, 24, 25 | | |
| | Ovulation failure | St 29, Ren 4, 3 Zigong, LI 4, Sp 6 | | |
| | Biomedical diagnosis, PCOS | Sp 6, Zigong, Ren 3, 4, Bl 20, 23, 18 | | |
| Termination of treatment | On pregnancy For 2 weeks after embryo transfer or on negative pregnancy test | | | |

There was no significant difference in BMI in conclusion of the intervention for women in the lifestyle only group compared with the acupuncture group.

Analysis of attendance for acupuncture shows that only 67% received the full course of 9 treatments with a mean of 7.62 and standard deviation of 2.5. Four trial participants randomised to receive acupuncture completed either part or all treatments and then failed to agree to an exit interview. Of the 28 women one was excluded because she fell pregnant prior to receiving any acupuncture; 3 withdrew after receiving less than the prescribed 9 acupuncture treatments (2 of these were lost to follow-up because they moved outside the area); 2 women completed their acupuncture (administered by acupuncturists other than the researcher) but would not respond to requests for an exit interview and they also became lost to follow-up. This represents 6 women (21%) either not completing the intervention or leaving the trial reporting requirements incomplete.

Two women randomised to the lifestyle only intervention telephoned within a few days of recruitment to withdraw from the study. In all, 8 women (28.6%) were lost to follow-up in the lifestyle only group although some partial data from some of these women were able to be included in the analysis. Of the women who completed the acupuncture intervention none expressed dissatisfaction with the intervention despite some not complying with data collection measures.

The average number of days in treatment was 64.74 (SD 24.1). In actuality only 4 (14.3%) women received treatment over 84 days or more (being equivalent to 3 menstrual cycles assuming an average length of menstrual cycle of 28 days).

Eighteen women (nearly 82 percent) reported no side effects during the acupuncture intervention. Three women (13.6%) reported side effects which were nominated as "*slight bruising on some points,*" "*headaches in the first three sessions which decreased in severity, felt very emotional (more than usual),*" "*awareness of old buried feelings,*" and "*a little pain*

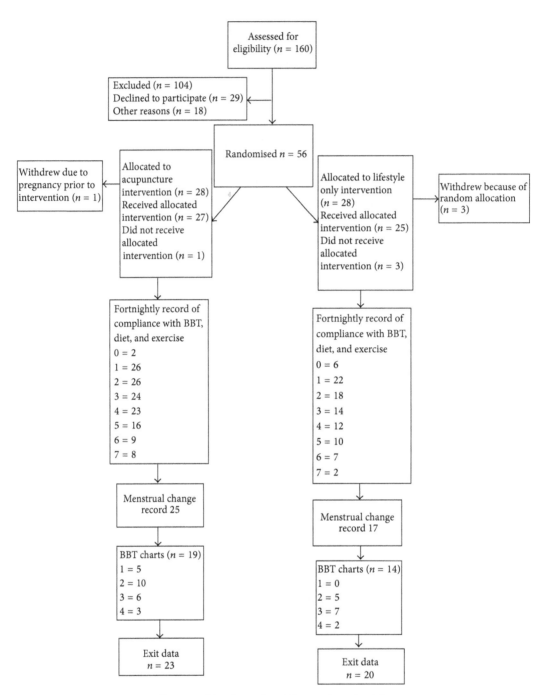

FIGURE 1: Flowchart of participants through trial.

*and occasional bruising."* There were no reported adverse events from the lifestyle only participants.

## 6. Discussion

The main findings were that this acupuncture intervention, compared to lifestyle only, resulted in significant increases in fertility awareness and quality of life measures in relation to wellbeing; it increased the ability of the recipients to engage in desired activities, such as exercise or rest, and it shortened the time to conception by half. The findings provide preliminary

evidence that the acupuncture intervention is acceptable and is not inert and that acupuncture dose may have a significant influence on outcomes. It was also apparent that the lifestyle only intervention was less acceptable to this population and as a comparator to acupuncture. The measurement tools to identify physiological changes, particularly menstrual change, require greater refinement to make adherence easier for the participant and to improve the researcher's capacity to analyse the data.

Estimating the treatment effect in this pilot study was difficult due to small numbers in the sample and the study

TABLE 2: Baseline characteristics of women at trial entry to allocated treatment group.

| | Acupuncture intervention $n = 28$ | Lifestyle only intervention $n = 28$ | p value |
|---|---|---|---|
| Age (years) | 33.14 (5.4) | 33.93 (5.0) | 0.572 |
| Fertility history | | | |
|   Gravida = 0 $n$ (%) | 11 (39.3) | 7 (25) | 0.252 |
|   Parity = 1 or >1 $n$ (%) | 8 (28.6) | 7 (32.1) | 0.771 |
|   Duration of infertility | | | |
|     Mean (SD) | 3.9 (3.4) | 5.8 (4.6) | 0.080* |
| Reasons for infertility | | | |
|   Female factor $n$ (%) | 15 (53.6) | 11 (39.3) | |
|   Unexplained | 10 (35.7) | 13 (26.4) | |
|   Unknown, combined + male factor | 3 (10.7) | 4 (14.3) | |
| Biomedical fertility diagnosis | | | |
|   PCOS $n$ (%) | 12 (42.9) | 9 (32.1) | 0.408 |
|   Unknown $n$ (%) | 10 (35.7) | 14 (50) | |
|   Other $n$ (%) | 6 (21.4) | 5 (17.9) | |
| BMI | | | |
|   Combined mean (SD) | 30.0 (9.8) | 30.3 (7.4) | 0.893 |
| Previous use of acupuncture $n$ (%) | 13 (46.4) | 12 (42.9) | 0.788 |
| Demographic details | | | |
|   Employment $n$ (%) | | | |
|     Working full time | 17 (60.7) | 16 (57.1) | 0.528 |
|     Working part time | 8 (28.6) | 6 (21.4) | |
|     Unemployed/home duties | 2 (7.1) | 6 (17.9) | |
|   Education status $n$ (%) | | | |
|     School incompletion | 0 | 2 (7.1) | |
|     School/TAFE completion | 16 (57.1) | 13 (46.4) | 0.309 |
|     Tertiary completion | 12 (42.9) | 13 (46.4) | |
|   Racial origin $n$ (%) | | | |
|     Caucasian | 16 (57.1) | 19 (67.9) | 0.408 |
|     English speaking background (ESB) | 15 | 18 | 0.415 |
|     NESB | 13 | 10 | 0.275 |
|   Marital status $n$ (%) | | | |
|     Married | 25 (89.3) | 22 (78.6) | |
|     De facto | 3 (10.7) | 6 (21.4) | |

* indicates possible significance, for example, $p < 0.05$.

being underpowered. Calculated against the measure that meant most to the participants, pregnancy, the power of the study was 3%. Analysing poststudy pregnancy rates the achieved power was 33% (calculated on the G*Power program). Several effects were evident in the study, specifically in awareness, wellbeing, capacity to undertake desired activity, and time to conception. Changes in menstrual indicators were not significant; however, this may have resulted from both poor record keeping and reporting by participants and an inadequate dose of acupuncture that did not cover at least 3 menstrual cycles. This also may have been influenced by the high proportion of women with PCOS.

A more fully powered study is justified on the basis of results, including trends and indications, displayed by this underpowered feasibility study. On the measure of pregnancy a fully powered study would require a sample size of 189 (calculated on the dropout rate of 12.5% in this study added to 168 participants to achieve full power) (G*Power). The clear benefits to the women involved of increased awareness of their fertility, their improved sense of wellbeing, and being able to engage in desired activities may flow on to improved fertility outcomes. There are trends that indicate this may be the case: reduced time to conception, reduced incidence of menstrual clotting, reduced length of pain and intensity of pain, normalisation of the length of the menstrual cycle, and the increased heaviness of menstrual flow in the acupuncture intervention participants. Cai et al. [25] that undertook a prospective analysis of cases using a standard acupuncture

TABLE 3: Primary study endpoints by treatment group.

| | Acupuncture intervention N = 28 | Lifestyle only intervention N = 28 | p value | Adjusted analysis | RR/CI (CI 95%) |
|---|---|---|---|---|---|
| Increase in fertility awareness (%) | 19 (86.4) | 8 (40) | 0.002* | 0.011* | 2.38 (1.25, 4.50) |
| Regularity of cycle n (%) | | | | | |
| At entry (%) n = 56 | 20 (71.4) | 20 (71.4) | | | |
| M1 n = 43 | 16 (61.5) | 12 (70.6) | 0.543 | 0.823 | 0.87 (0.57, 1.34) |
| M2 n = 31 | 12 (60) | 5 (45.5) | 0.436 | 0.262 | 1.32 (0.63, 2.77) |
| M3 n = 15 | 5 (71.4) | 4 (50) | 0.398 | 0.252 | 1.43 (0.65, 3.30) |
| Menstrual details (mean/SD) | | | | | |
| Length of period | | | | | |
| M entry n = 56 | 4.86 (2.3) | 4.85 (1.5) | 0.984 | | |
| M1 n = 36 | 5.39 (2.5) | 5.08 (1.1) | 0.671 | 0.383 | 0.31 (−1.18, 1.8) |
| M2 n = 30 | 5.11 (2.0) | 4.33 (1.4) | 0.255 | 0.631 | 0.78 (−0.77, 2.33) |
| M3 n = 18 | 5.11 (1.3) | 4.67 (1.3) | 0.478 | 0.452 | 0.44 (−0.85, 1.73) |
| M exit n = 39 | 4.52 (2.2) | 4.72 (2.2) | 0.783 | 0.764 | −0.2 (−1.65, 1.25) |
| Length of cycle | | | | | |
| M entry n = 56 | 34.64 (18.3) | 35.43 (18.4) | 0.873 | | |
| M1 n = 34 | 32.52 (13.9) | 31.00 (6.2) | 0.713 | 0.360 | 1.52 (−6.8, 9.84) |
| M2 n = 29 | 29.12 (4.0) | 29.25 (8.9) | 0.957 | 0.802 | −0.13 (−5.15, 4.89) |
| M3 n = 16 | 29.43 (2.6) | 26.78 (3.1) | 0.091 | 0.996 | 2.65 (−0.48, 5.78) |
| M exit n = 37 | 29.05 (11.9) | 30.65 (6.4) | 0.624 | 0.285 | −1.6 (−8.15, 4.95) |
| Nature of menstrual flow (%) | | | | | |
| Heavy | | | | | |
| M entry n = 56 | 11 (39.3) | 12 (42.9) | | | 0.92 (0.49, 1.72) |
| M1 n = 41 | 11 (44) | 2 (12.5) | | | 3.52 (0.89, 13.85) |
| M2 n = 29 | 11 (55) | 1 (11.1) | | | 4.95 (0.75, 32.76) |
| M3 n = 14 | 2 (28.6) | 2 (28.6) | | | 1 (0.19, 5.25) |
| Moderate | | | | | |
| M entry n = 56 | 9 (32.1) | 11 (39.3) | | | 0.82 (0.4, 1.66) |
| M1 n = 41 | 10 (40) | 8 (50) | *Chi-square* | | 0.8 (0.4, 1.59) |
| M2 n = 29 | 6 (30) | 3 (33.3) | M entry 0.716 M1 0.077 | | 0.9 (0.29, 2.82) |
| M3 n = 14 | 3 (42.9) | 2 (28.6) | M2 0.009* | | 1.5 (0.35, 6.4) |
| Light | | | | M3 0.819 | |
| M entry n = 56 | 5 (17.9) | 4 (14.3) | | | 1.25 (0.37, 4.17) |
| M1 n = 41 | 4 (16) | 6 (37.5) | | | 0.43 (0.14, 1.28) |
| M2 n = 29 | 1 (5) | 5 (55.6) | | | 0.09 (0.01, 0.66) |
| M3 n = 14 | 2 (28.6) | 3 (42.9) | | | 0.67 (0.16, 2.84) |
| Inconsistent | | | | | |
| M entry n = 56 | 3 (10.7) | 1 (3.6) | | | 3 (0.33, 27.12) |
| M1 n = 41 | 0 | 0 | | | |
| M2 n = 29 | 2 (10) | 0 | | | |
| M3 n = 14 | 0 | 0 | | | |

* indicates possible statistical significance, for example, $p < 0.05$.

TABLE 4: Primary study endpoints by treatment group (C).

| | Acupuncture intervention N = 28 | Lifestyle only intervention N = 28 | p value | Adjusted analysis | RR/CI (CI 95%) |
|---|---|---|---|---|---|
| Incidence of menstrual clots (%) | | | | | |
| None | | | | | |
| M entry n = 56 | 10 (35.7) | 9 (32.1) | M entry 0.556 | | 1.11 (0.53, 2.31) |
| M1 n = 39 | 11 (45.8) | 11 (73.3) | M1 0.221 | | 0.63 (0.37, 1.06) |
| M2 n = 28 | 9 (47.4) | 7 (77.8) | M2 0.287 | | 0.61 (0.34, 1.1) |
| M3 n = 13 | 6 (85.7) | 4 (66.7) | M3 0.188 | | 2.14 (0.95, 4.85) |
| Small | | | | | |
| M entry n = 56 | 12 (42.9) | 9 (32.1) | | | 1.33 (0.67, 2.65) |
| M1 n = 39 | 8 (33.3) | 3 (20) | | | 1.67 (0.52, 5.31) |
| M2 n = 28 | 7 (36.8) | 1 (11.1) | | | 3.32 (0.48, 23.06) |
| M3 n = 13 | 1 (14.3) | 0 | | | |
| Large | | | | | |
| M entry n = 56 | 6 (21.4) | 9 (32.1) | | | 0.67 (0.27, 1.62) |
| M1 n = 39 | 5 (20.8) | 1 (6.7) | | | 3.13 (0.4, 24.22) |
| M2 n = 28 | 3 (15.8) | 1 (11.1) | | | 1.42 (0.17, 11.83) |
| M3 n = 13 | 0 | 2 (33.3) | | | |
| Variable | | | | | |
| M entry n = 56 | 0 | 1 (3.6) | | | |
| Incidence of menstrual pain | | | | | |
| M entry n = 56 | 23 (82.1) | 20 (71.4) | 0.342 | | 1.15 (0.86, 1.54) |
| M1 n = 40 | 17 (68) | 5 (33.3) | 0.033* | 0.056 | 2.04 (0.95, 4.38) |
| M2 n = 30 | 10 (50) | 3 (30) | 0.297 | 0.430 | 1.67 (0.59, 4.73) |
| M3 n = 13 | 2 (28.6) | 3 (50) | 0.529 | | 0.67 (0.17, 2.67) |
| Length of menstrual pain (mean (SD)) | | | | | |
| M entry n = 56 | 1.7 (1.6) | 1.2 (1.0) | 0.669 | | |
| M1 n = 40 | 1.46 (1.7) | 0.63 (1.4) | 0.108 | 0.238 | 0.83 (−0.2, 1.86) |
| M2 n = 36 | 0.9 (1.2) | 0.47 (1.1) | 0.271 | 0.258 | 0.43 (−0.36, 1.22) |
| M3 n = 15 | 0.57 (0.5) | 0.63 (1.1) | 0.906 | 0.587 | −0.06 (−1.02, 0.9) |
| Intensity of menstrual pain (mean (SD)) | | | | | |
| M entry n = 56 | 3 (1.3) | 2 (1.4) | 0.261 | | |
| M1 n = 23 | 3 (1.3) | 2 (1.4) | 0.146 | 0.285 | 1 (−0.37, 2.37) |
| M2 n = 14 | 1.91 (1.4) | 2.67 (1.5) | 0.423 | 0.141 | −0.76 (−2.76, 1.24) |
| M3 n = 7 | 1.5 (1.0) | 2.67 (1.5) | 0.272 | 0.840 | −1.17 (−3.6, 1.26) |

* indicates possible statistical significance, for example, $p < 0.05$.

protocol with a nonacupuncture control concluded that although "acupuncture did not increase the cumulative pregnancy rate, it decreased the time to achieve pregnancy" in subsequent IVF cycles. Although indications are that diet and exercise regimes may have positive effects on female fertility, studies where acupuncture and such lifestyle changes are used as comparators were not located by the authors.

The strengths of the study were that it addressed an underexplored research area using acupuncture to influence women's reproductive cycles outside ART; it used an intervention that approximated usual clinical practice of acupuncture; the participants welcomed the intervention and reported few adverse events. The limitations were that the study was underpowered and a sample size of 189 would be required to use pregnancy as an outcome measure. The adequacy of lifestyle modification as the comparator has not been established in other studies and this study indicated that measures to retain participants in the control group and ensure their commitment to fully complete assessments were inadequate. Because of the nature of an acupuncture pragmatic trial, participants were not blind to allocation.

## 7. Conclusion

The multiphasic fertility acupuncture protocol tested in this trial did positively influence the women who received it

TABLE 5: Secondary study endpoints by treatment group.

| | Acupuncture intervention $N = 28$ | Lifestyle only intervention $N = 28$ | $p$ value | Adjusted analysis |
|---|---|---|---|---|
| Pregnancy (%) | | | | |
| Incidence $n = 43$ | 4 (16) | $3^1$ (15) | 0.927 | 0.992 |
| Time from study entry to conception (weeks) $n = 43$ | 5.5 | 10.67 | 0.422 | 0.452 |
| Quality of life changes (MYMOP) $n = 43$ (mean (SD)) | | | | |
| Changes in symptom 1 | 1.27 (2.1) | 1.55 (1.5) | 0.628 | 0.775 |
| Changes in symptom 2 | 1.81 (1.4) | 1.40 (1.1) | 0.305 | 0.291 |
| Changes in activity | 1.80 (1.2) | 0.94 (1.2) | 0.033* | 0.047* |
| Changes in wellbeing | 0.95 (1.4) | 0.05 (1.4) | 0.043* | 0.042* |
| Change in MYMOP profile score | 1.47 (1.1) | 1.03 (0.8) | 0.156 | 0.165 |
| Lifestyle change (BMI) | | | | |
| Change in BMI (mean (SD)) | 0.0318 (1.1) | −0.75 (1.3) | 0.475 | 0.585 |
| Sustained lifestyle change at 12 months $n = 31$ (%) | 10 (53) | 6 (50) | 0.886 | |
| Acceptability of intervention $n$ (%) | | | | |
| Completion of exit interview | 22 (78.57) | 20 (71.43) | 0.314 | |
| Record of menstrual changes | 26 (92.86) | 16 (57.14) | 0.677 | |

[1] One of these pregnancies was achieved through IVF due to male factor problems for the couple. The participant advised the researcher after her pregnancy that she had used acupuncture prior to this conception, her first ever after years of IVF cycles.
* indicates possible statistical significance, for example, $p < 0.05$.

compared to the women who used lifestyle modification alone. It increased their fertility awareness and improved their wellbeing. Those who conceived did so in half the time of their lifestyle only peers. As a pilot study it offers a framework for greater exploration of acupuncture's capacity to influence women's reproduction but would require modification to include a more credible and acceptable control for this study population.

## Competing Interests

The authors declare that they have no competing interests.

## Acknowledgments

A postgraduate scholarship for women's health from the Centre for Complementary Medicine Research (now National Institute for Complementary Medicine) was received by the first author to complete her doctorate. Acupuncture supplies used in this research were donated by Helio Supply Company, Sydney.

## References

[1] M. C. Inhorn and P. Patrizio, "Infertility around the globe: new thinking on gender, reproductive technologies and global movements in the 21st century," *Human Reproduction Update*, 2015.

[2] A. R. White, "A review of controlled trials of acupuncture for women's reproductive health care," *Journal of Family Planning and Reproductive Health Care*, vol. 29, no. 4, pp. 233–236, 2003.

[3] E. W. S. So and E. H. Y. Ng, "Acupuncture in reproductive medicine," *Women's Health*, vol. 6, no. 4, pp. 551–563, 2010.

[4] A. Nandi, A. Shah, A. Gudi, and R. Homburg, "Acupuncture in IVF: a review of current literature," *Journal of Obstetrics & Gynaecology*, vol. 34, no. 7, pp. 555–561, 2014.

[5] C. A. Smith, M. Armour, and D. Betts, "Treatment of women's reproductive health conditions by Australian and New Zealand acupuncturists," *Complementary Therapies in Medicine*, vol. 22, no. 4, pp. 710–718, 2014.

[6] M. Bovey, A. Lorenc, and N. Robinson, "Extent of acupuncture practice for infertility in the United Kingdom: experiences and perceptions of the practitioners," *Fertility & Sterility*, vol. 94, no. 7, pp. 2569–2573, 2010.

[7] J. Lyttleton, *The Treatment of Infertility in Chinese Medicine*, Churchill Livingstone, New York, NY, USA, 2nd edition, 2013.

[8] L. Liang, *Contemporary Gynecology: An Integrated Chinese-Western Approach*, Blue Poppy Press, Boulder, Colo, USA, 2010.

[9] S. H. Chui, F. C. Chow, Y. T. Szeto, K. Chan, and C. W. K. Lam, "A case series of acupuncture treatment for female infertility with some cases supplemented with Chinese medicines," *European Journal of Integrative Medicine*, vol. 6, no. 3, pp. 337–341, 2014.

[10] A. Sahin, Y. Cayir, and F. Akcay, "Positive effects of acupuncture on menstrual irregularity and infertility in a patient with polycystic ovary syndrome," *Family Medicine & Medical Science Research*, vol. 3, no. 2, 2014.

[11] Y. Chen, Y. Fang, J. Yang, F. Wang, Y. Wang, and L. Yang, "Effect of acupuncture on premature ovarian failure: a pilot study," *Evidence-Based Complementary and Alternative Medicine*, vol. 2014, Article ID 718675, 6 pages, 2014.

[12] B. Chen and J. Yu, "Relationship between blood radioimmunoreactive β-endorphin and hand skin temperature during

the electro-acupuncture induction of ovulation," *Acupuncture & Electro-Therapeutics Research*, vol. 16, no. 1-2, pp. 1–5, 1991.

[13] I. Gerhard and F. Postneek, "Auricular acupuncture in the treatment of female infertility," *Gynecological Endocrinology*, vol. 6, no. 3, pp. 171–181, 1992.

[14] J. Lyttleton, *Treatment of Infertility with Chinese Medicine*, Churchill Livingstone, Edinburgh, UK, 2004.

[15] G. F. Homan, M. Davies, and R. Norman, "The impact of lifestyle factors on reproductive performance in the general population and those undergoing infertility treatment: a review," *Human Reproduction Update*, vol. 13, no. 3, pp. 209–223, 2007.

[16] K. Tremellan and K. Pearce, Eds., *Nutrition, Fertility, and Human Reproductive Function*, CRC Press, New York, NY, USA, 2015.

[17] M. Evans, C. Paterson, L. Wye et al., "Lifestyle and self-care advice within traditional acupuncture consultations: a qualitative observational study nested in a co-operative inquiry," *The Journal of Alternative and Complementary Medicine*, vol. 17, no. 6, pp. 519–529, 2011.

[18] M. Noakes and P. M. Clifton, *The CSIRO Total Wellbeing Diet*, CSIRO, 2005.

[19] E. Derbyshire and F. Bokhari, "Body weight—the importance of getting it right 'before' becoming pregnant," *Current Nutrition & Food Science*, vol. 7, no. 2, pp. 74–77, 2011.

[20] S. Cochrane, C. A. Smith, and A. Possamai-Inesedy, "Development of a fertility acupuncture protocol: defining an acupuncture treatment protocol to support and treat women experiencing conception delays," *Journal of Alternative & Complementary Medicine*, vol. 17, no. 4, pp. 329–337, 2011.

[21] P. Deadman, M. Al-Khafaji, and K. Baker, *A Manual of Acupuncture*, Journal of Chinese Medicine Publications, Hove, UK, 1998.

[22] K. K. S. Hui, E. E. Nixon, M. G. Vangel et al., "Characterization of the 'deqi' response in acupuncture," *BMC Complementary and Alternative Medicine*, vol. 7, article 33, 2007.

[23] C. Paterson, "Measuring outcomes in primary care: a patient generated measure, MYMOP, compared with the SF-36 health survey," *British Medical Journal*, vol. 312, no. 7037, pp. 1016–1020, 1996.

[24] S. Cochrane, C. A. Smith, A. Possamai-Inesedy, and A. Bensoussan, "Acupuncture and women's health: an overview of the role of acupuncture and its clinical management in women's reproductive health," *International Journal of Women's Health*, vol. 6, no. 1, pp. 313–325, 2014.

[25] L. Cai, R. Hai, B. Zhang, Y. Wen, M. Zeng, and M. Jiang, "Treatment of unexplained infertility by acupuncture in natural and control ovarian hyperstimulation cycles: a prospective analysis," *Advances in Reproductive Sciences*, vol. 2, no. 4, pp. 88–92, 2014.

# 2

# A Systematic Review on the Effects of Botanicals on Skeletal Muscle Health in Order to Prevent Sarcopenia

M. Rondanelli,[1] A. Miccono,[2] G. Peroni,[1] F. Guerriero,[3] P. Morazzoni,[4] A. Riva,[4] D. Guido,[1,5,6] and S. Perna[1]

[1]Department of Public Health, Experimental and Forensic Medicine, Section of Human Nutrition, Endocrinology and Nutrition Unit, Azienda di Servizi alla Persona, University of Pavia, 27100 Pavia, Italy
[2]Department of Clinical Sciences, Faculty of Medicine and Surgery, University of Milan, Milan, Italy
[3]Azienda di Servizi alla Persona, Pavia, Italy
[4]Research and Development Unit, Indena, 20139 Milan, Italy
[5]Department of Brain and Behavioral Sciences, Medical and Genomic Statistics Unit, University of Pavia, 27100 Pavia, Italy
[6]Department of Public Health, Experimental and Forensic Medicine, Biostatistics and Clinical Epidemiology Unit, University of Pavia, 27100 Pavia, Italy

Correspondence should be addressed to S. Perna; simoneperna@hotmail.it

Academic Editor: Hyunsu Bae

We performed a systematic review to evaluate the evidence-based medicine regarding the main botanical extracts and their nutraceutical compounds correlated to skeletal muscle health in order to identify novel strategies that effectively attenuate skeletal muscle loss and enhance muscle function and to improve the quality of life of older subjects. This review contains all eligible studies from 2010 to 2015 and included 57 publications. We focused our attention on effects of botanical extracts on growth and health of muscle and divided these effects into five categories: anti-inflammation, muscle damage prevention, antifatigue, muscle atrophy prevention, and muscle regeneration and differentiation.

## 1. Introduction

Sarcopenia is the loss of muscle protein mass and of muscle function and it occurs with increasing age, being a major component in the development of frailty [1]. It is a syndrome characterized by the progressive and generalized loss of skeletal muscle mass and strength with a risk of adverse outcomes such as physical disability, poor quality of life, and death [2]. Preventative diet, exercise, or treatment interventions particularly in middle-aged adults at the low end of the spectrum of muscle function may help to preserve mobility in later years and improve health span [3]. The therapeutic options for sarcopenia are unclear and constantly evolving. The most rational approach to delay the progression of sarcopenia is based on the combination of proper nutrition, possibly associated with the use of dietary supplements, and a regular exercise program [4]. Despite the major advantages offered by natural therapies with their long traditional use and poor physiological and psychological addiction as is commonly seen with conventional medicine [5], few studies have been performed on the topic of age-correlated pathologies of skeletal muscle. The aim of this review was to investigate the effectiveness of botanicals on skeletal muscle health focusing on possible therapeutics approaches to prevent sarcopenia.

## 2. Materials and Methods

The present systematic review was performed according to the steps by Egger et al. [6] (Table 1), as follows: (i) configuration of a working group: three operators skilled in clinical nutrition in the geriatric age, of whom one was acting as a methodological operator and two were participating as clinical operators; (ii) formulation of the revision question on the basis of considerations made in

TABLE 1: Summary of methodology.

| Step | General activities | Specific activities |
| --- | --- | --- |
| Step 1 | Configuration of a working group | Selection of three operators skilled in clinical nutrition: (i) One as methodological operator (ii) Two as clinical operators |
| Step 2 | Formulation of the revision question | Evaluation of the state of the art in metabolic and nutritional disorders of sarcopenia and their treatment with botanicals |
| Step 3 | Identification of relevant studies on PubMed | (a) Identification of the key words (sarcopenia, nutrients, and dietary supplement), allowing the definition of the interest field of the documents to be searched, grouped in inverted commas ("..."), and used separately or in combination (b) Use of the Boolean (a data type with only two possible values: true and false) AND operator, which allows the establishment of logical relations among concepts (c) Research modalities: advanced search (d) Limits: papers published in the last 20 years; in vitro, animal, and humans studies; languages: English (e) Manual search performed by the senior researchers experienced in clinical nutrition through the revision of reviews and individual articles on sarcopenia in the elderly, published in journals qualified in the Index Medicus |
| Step 4 | Analysis and presentation of the outcomes | The data extrapolated from the revised studies was investigated in the form of a narrative review of the reports and was collocated in tables |

the abstract: "sarcopenia and muscle mass, use of botanic extracts during aging"; (iii) identification of relevant studies: a research strategy was planned, on PubMed and Scopus, as follows: (a) definition of the key words (sarcopenia, muscle mass, inflammation, antioxidants, botanical extracts, phytotherapy, muscle atrophy, muscle fatigue, *Camellia sinensis*, *Vitis vinifera*, *Zingiber officinale*, *Citrus aurantium*, and *Panax quinquefolius*), allowing the definition of the interest field of the documents to be searched, grouped in inverted commas ("..."), and used separately or in combination; (b) use of the Boolean AND operator, which allows the establishment of logical relationships among concepts; (c) research modalities: advanced search; (d) limits: papers published until June 2015; humans, animals, in vivo, and in vitro studies; languages: English; (e) manual search performed by the senior researchers, experienced in clinical nutrition, through the revision of reviews and research articles on sarcopenia in the elderly, published in qualified journals of the Index Medicus.

Analysis and presentation of the outcomes had been done as follows: the data extrapolated from the revised studies were summarized in Tables 2–6; in particular, for each study, we specified the author and year of publication, the plant and the active principles, the models used, the posology, and the main results obtained. The analyses were carried out in the form of a narrative review of the reports. The flow diagram of narrative review of the literature has been reported in Figure 1. As shown in Figure 1, we consider several effects of botanical extracts on growth and health of muscle; we divided these effects into five categories: anti-inflammatory activity, muscle damage prevention, antifatigue, muscle atrophy prevention, and muscle regeneration and differentiation. After this, we examined the typology of the studies, that is, in vitro, animals (mice, rats), or human, and we classified the human data according to the different condition such as postmenopausal women, athletes or others. Another key

point was to identify the dosage of the extracts for each trial and the botanical compounds responsible for the activity. The use of the databases as PubMed or Scopus was determinant to enrich our review. At the end, we reported an analysis of all plants and their extracts that have a beneficial role in preventing sarcopenia or improve muscle health condition.

## 3. Results

*3.1. Screening and Selection Process of Study.* Of 120 articles identified, 57 studies met inclusion criteria (Figure 1), including 17 focused on anti-inflammation, 8 focused on muscle damage, 11 based on antifatigue effects, 7 based on muscle athorpy, and 15 based on muscle differentiation and regeneration (Figure 1).

As reported in Table 2, there are different effects on skeletal muscle for each botanical. At present, we evaluated in the literature over 70 different mechanisms of action.

*3.2. Anti-Inflammatory Activity.* This research has been carried out based on the keywords "skeletal muscle mass" and "inflammation" and "botanicals" or "plants" or "extracts"; 21 articles were sourced and 17 studies are taken into account. Among these papers, 3 studies are in in vitro setting, 4 in animals, 8 in humans, and two both in animals and in in vitro setting (Table 3).

Inflammation and oxidative stress induce muscle damage and muscle pain [18] and several botanicals (*Phlebodium decamanum*, *Citrus aurantium*, *Coffea arabica*, *Zingiber officinale*, *Eugenia punicifolia*, *Panax ginseng*, *Go-sha-jinki-Gan*, *Vitis vinifera*, and *Curcuma longa* L.) have a significant role in the prevention of this phenomenon.

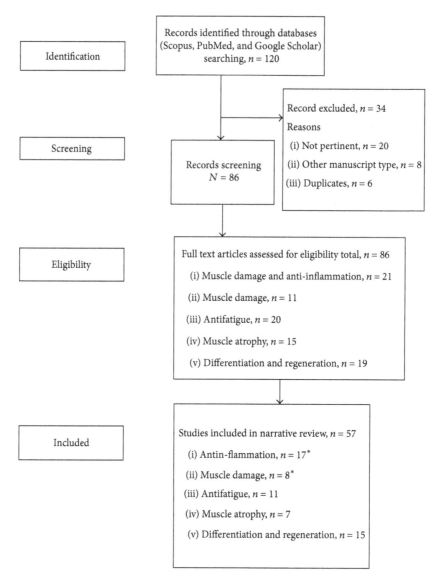

**Identification**

Records identified through databases (Scopus, PubMed, and Google Scholar) searching, $n = 120$

**Screening**

Records screening $N = 86$

Record excluded, $n = 34$

Reasons

(i) Not pertinent, $n = 20$

(ii) Other manuscript type, $n = 8$

(iii) Duplicates, $n = 6$

**Eligibility**

Full text articles assessed for eligibility total, $n = 86$

(i) Muscle damage and anti-inflammation, $n = 21$

(ii) Muscle damage, $n = 11$

(iii) Antifatigue, $n = 20$

(iv) Muscle atrophy, $n = 15$

(v) Differentiation and regeneration, $n = 19$

**Included**

Studies included in narrative review, $n = 57$

(i) Antin-flammation, $n = 17^{*}$

(ii) Muscle damage, $n = 8^{*}$

(iii) Antifatigue, $n = 11$

(iv) Muscle atrophy, $n = 7$

(v) Differentiation and regeneration, $n = 15$

$^{*}$One article is in both categories.

FIGURE 1: Flow diagram of narrative review of the literature.

Supplementation with *Phlebodium decamanum* (5 capsules of 400 mg) reduces inflammatory response and also the degree of oxidative stress in human during high-intensity exercise, through the decrease of 8-hydroxy-2′-deoxyguanosine and isoprostanes generation, the increase of antioxidant enzyme activities in erythrocyte and total antioxidant status in plasma, the decrease of tumor necrosis factor (TNF-$\alpha$), and the increase of soluble receptor II of TNF-$\alpha$ (sTNF-RII), but kept the levels of interleukin-6 (IL-6) and interleukin-1 antagonist receptor (IL-1ra) [18]. Other studies examine the anti-inflammatory effect of flavonoids isolated from *Citrus aurantium*, *Coffea arabica*, and *Zingiber officinale* on interleukins such as IL-1$\alpha$ and IL-6 and TNF-$\alpha$ on skeletal muscle cells. Specifically, the flavonoids (hesperidin, nobiletin, and naringin of *Citrus aurantium*, also known as sour orange) inhibit the inflammatory response

in lipopolysaccharide- (LPS-) induced L6 skeletal muscle cells. In addition, the flavonoids isolated from Korean *Citrus aurantium* L. inhibit significantly inducible nitric oxide synthase (iNOS), cyclooxygenase-2 (COX-2), IL-6, and TNF-$\alpha$ by blocking the nuclear factor-kappa B (NF-$\kappa$b) and by blocking mitogen-activated protein kinases (MAPKs) signal pathways. Another study in the same muscle cells demonstrates the anti-inflammatory role of flavonoids isolated from *Citrus aurantium* through the modulation in protein related to the immune response. Furthermore, the pretreatment with flavonoids resulted in a decreased level of cleaved caspase-3, which is induced by muscle inflammation and is involved in muscle proteolysis and atrophy. Also, *Zingiber officinale*, commonly known as ginger, showed interesting anti-inflammatory and analgesic effects in humans who ingested 2 grams of ginger or placebo after exercise; however, this extract

TABLE 2: Effects on skeletal muscle for each botanical.

| Effect | Botanicals | Physiology | Study | Authors |
| --- | --- | --- | --- | --- |
| Downregulation of LPS-induced COX-2 and iNOS expression | Korean *Citrus aurantium* L. | 10, 50, 75, and 100 μg/mL | Rat skeletal muscle cells | Kim et al., 2012 [7] |
| Suppression or inhibition of NF-κB | Korean *Citrus aurantium* L.<br>*Eugenia punicifolia*<br>*Camellia sinensis* | 10, 50, 75, and 100 μg/mL<br>2 mg/mL<br>0.25% or 0.5% green tea extract, at the age of 42 days | Rat skeletal muscle cells<br>Male mdx dystrophic mice<br>C57BL/6J and mdx mice | Kim et al., 2012 [7]<br>Leite et al., 2010 [8]<br>Evans et al., 2010 [9] |
| Increase of NF-κB | *Panax ginseng* | DS 20, 60, and 120 mg/kg | Rats | Yu et al., 2014 [10] |
| Induction of the phosporylation of AMPK | *Glycine max* | 100 μM | C2C12 myotubes | Hirasaka et al., 2013 [11] |
| Decrease of MURF-1 promoter activity | *Glycine max* | 100 μM | C2C12 myotubes | Hirasaka et al., 2013 [11] |
| Suppression of LPS-induced phosphorylation of the MAPKs (JNK, ERK, and p38 MAPK pERK) | Korean *Citrus aurantium* L.<br>*Eugenia punicifolia* | 10, 50, 75, and 100 μg/mL<br>100 μg/mL | Rat skeletal muscle cells<br>Mouse myoblastoma cells (C2C12) | Kim et al., 2012 [7]<br>Leite et al., 2014 [12] |
| Increase of ERK1/2 activity | Hachimijiogan (HJG) | HJG treatment (1–200 μg/mL) | Murine skeletal cells | Takeda et al., 2015 [13] |
| Activation of p38 MAPK signaling | *Broussonetia kazinoki* (pp38)<br>*Corydalis turtschaninovii* (p-p38) | KP in 2% HS for 48 h, 10–1000 nM<br>Various concentrations of THP | C2C12 and 10T1/2 cells<br>C2C12 myoblasts and fibroblast 10T1/2 | Hwang et al., 2015 [14]<br>Lee et al., 2014 [15] |
| Increase of myogenin | *Eugenia punicifolia* (17.5-kDa) | 2 mg/mL | Male mdx dystrophic mice | Leite et al., 2010 [8] |
| Increased expression of MHC, myogenin, and Troponin-T | *Broussonetia kazinoki*<br>*Corydalis turtschaninovii* | KP in 2% HS for 48 h, 10–1000 nM<br>Various concentrations of THP | C2C12 and 10T1/2 cells<br>C2C12 myoblasts and fibroblast 10T1/2 | Hwang et al., 2015 [14]<br>Lee et al., 2014 [15] |
| Decrease of the expression of TNF-α | Korean *Citrus aurantium* L.<br>*Vitis vinifera*<br>*Panax notoginseng*<br>*Phlebodium decumanum*<br>*Eugenia punicifolia*<br>Coffee<br>*Camellia sinensis*<br>*Rubus parvifolius* L. (RPL)<br>*Glycine max* | 10, 50, 75, and 100 μg/mL<br>100 μM<br>5 mg of Rg1<br>5 capsules of 400 mg (250 mg of leaf extract and 150 mg of rhizome extract)<br>2 mg/mL<br>The same amount of drink in control and coffee group for 4 weeks<br>0.5% w/w in diet for 3 weeks after downhill running<br>40 mg/kg and 20 mg/kg<br>100 μM | Rat skeletal muscle cells<br>Mouse C2C12 cells<br>Healthy young men ($N = 26$)<br>Amateur athletes ($N = 40$)<br>Male mdx dystrophic mice<br>C57BL/6 mice<br>Mice<br>Five-week-old male<br>C2C12 myotubes | Kim et al., 2012 [7]<br>Wang et al., 2014 [16]<br>Hou et al., 2015 [17]<br>Díaz-Castro et al., 2012 [18]<br>Leite et al., 2010 [8]<br>Guo et al., 2014 [19]<br>Haramizu et al., 2013 [20]<br>Chen et al., 2013 [21]<br>Hirasaka et al., 2013 [11] |

TABLE 2: Continued.

| Effect | Botanicals | Physiology | Study | Authors |
| --- | --- | --- | --- | --- |
| Increase in sTNF-RII | Phlebodium decumanum | 5 capsules of 400 mg (250 mg of leaf extract and 150 mg of rhizome extract) | Amateur athletes ($N = 40$) | Díaz-Castro et al., 2012 [18] |
| Decrease of IL-1α | Coffee | The same amount of drink in control and coffee group for 4 weeks | C57BL/6 mice | Guo et al., 2014 [19] |
| Decrease of IL-6 | Korean Citrus aurantium L. | 10, 50, 75, and 100 μg/mL | Rat skeletal muscle cells | Kim et al., 2012 [7] |
| | Curcumin (at 24 h) | 2.5 g twice daily | Men ($N = 17$) | Nicol et al., 2015 [22] |
| | Coffee | The same amount of drink in control and coffee group for 4 weeks | C57BL/6 mice | Guo et al., 2014 [19] |
| | Rubus parvifolius L. (RPL) | 40 mg/kg and 20 mg/kg | Five-week-old male | Chen et al., 2013 [21] |
| Increase of interleukin-6 (IL-6) | Curcumin (at 0 h and 48 h) | 2.5 g twice daily | Men ($N = 17$) | Nicol et al., 2015 [22] |
| Decrease of IL-8 | Curcumin | 1 g twice daily (corresponding to 200 mg curcumin twice a day) | Healthy, moderately active male ($N = 20$) | Drobnic et al., 2014 [23] |
| Decrease of IL-1β | Eugenia punicifolia (17.5-kDa) | 2 mg/mL | Male mdx dystrophic mice | Leite et al., 2010 [8] |
| | Panax ginseng | DS | Rats | Yu et al., 2014 [10] |
| | Camellia sinensis | 0.5% w/w in diet for 3 weeks after downhill running | Mice | Haramizu et al., 2013 [20] |
| Increase of IL-10 | Panax notoginseng | 5 mg of Rg1 | Healthy young men ($N = 26$) | Hou et al., 2015 [17] |
| | Panax ginseng | DS 20, 60, and 120 mg/kg | Rats | Yu et al., 2014 [10] |
| Decrease of MCP-1 | Camellia sinensis | 0.5% w/w in diet for 3 weeks after downhill running | Mice | Haramizu et al., 2013 [20] |
| Decreased MnSOD (only at high dose) | Panax ginseng | DS 20, 60, and 120 mg/kg | Rats | Yu et al., 2014 [10] |
| Decrease of the expression of cleaved caspase-3 | Korean Citrus aurantium L. | 100 μg | Rat skeletal muscle cells | Kim et al., 2013 [24] |
| | Eugenia punicifolia | 2 mg/mL | Male mdx dystrophic mice | Leite et al., 2010 [8] |
| Increased expression of antioxidant enzymes, such as GPx (not at high dose) and GCS | Panax ginseng | DS 20, 60, and 120 mg/kg | Rats | Yu et al., 2014 [10] |
| | Phlebodium decumanum (only GPx) | 5 capsules of 400 mg (250 mg of leaf extract and 150 mg of rhizome extract) | Amateur athletes ($N = 40$) | Díaz-Castro et al., 2012 [18] |
| Increase of MMP-9 and MMP-2 | Eugenia punicifolia | 100 μg/mL | Mouse myoblastoma cells (C2C12) | Leite et al., 2014 [12] |
| Reduced MMP-9 | Eugenia punicifolia | 2 mg/mL | C57BL/10 mice | Leite et al., 2014 [12] |
| Reduced MMP-9 and MMP-2 | Eugenia punicifolia | 2 mg/mL | Male mdx dystrophic mice | Leite et al., 2010 [8] |
| Increase of citrate synthase (CS) activity | Panax notoginseng | 5 mg of Rg1 | Healthy young men ($N = 26$) | Hou et al., 2015 [17] |

TABLE 2: Continued.

| Effect | Botanicals | Physiology | Study | Authors |
|---|---|---|---|---|
| Attenuation of the increases in mRNAs encoding Ly6G and CD68 observed at 24 h after downhill running | Camellia sinensis | 0.5% w/w in diet for 3 weeks after downhill running | Mice | Haramizu et al., 2013 [20] |
| Increase of p27 and pAkt | Eugenia punicifolia | 100 µg/mL | Mouse myoblastoma cells (C2C12) | Leite et al., 2014 [12] |
| | Corydalis turtschaninovii (only pAkt) | Various concentrations of THP | C2C12 myoblasts and fibroblast 10T1/2 | Lee et al., 2014 [15] |
| Reduction of Cyclin D1 | Eugenia punicifolia | 100 µg/mL | Mouse myoblastoma cells (C2C12) | Leite et al., 2014 [12] |
| Increased expression of pAkt and pFoxO3a | Camellia sinensis | 10–150 µM | C2C12 myotubes | Mirza et al., 2014 [25] |
| Decrease in MPO activity | Camellia sinensis | 0.5% w/w in diet for 3 weeks after downhill running | Mice | Haramizu et al., 2013 [20] |
| Decreased caspase-3 expression | Vitis vinifera | 0.4 mg per gram body mass per day | Mice (male C57BL/6J mice) | Ballak et al., 2015 [26] |
| Upregulation of phosphorylation of Akt, p70S6K, mTOR, and 4E-BP1 | Vitis vinifera | 100 µM | Mouse C2C12 cells | Wang et al., 2014 [16] |
| | Coffee | Coffee solution 10, 30, 50, and 100 µg/mL | Mouse myosatellite cells | Guo et al., 2014 [19] |
| Prevention of HSPB1 phosphorylation | Pinus pinaster | 0.05 mg/mL | Human muscle satellite cells | Poussard et al., 2013 [27] |
| Decrease in FoxO1 protein and promotion of FoxO1 phosphorylation | Vitis vinifera | 100 µM | Mouse C2C12 cells | Wang et al., 2014 [16] |
| Decreased MURF-1 and MAFbx | Camellia sinensis | 10–150 µM | C2C12 myotubes | Mirza et al., 2014 [25] |
| Increased MURF-1 | Go-sha-jinki-Gan (GJG) (only PGC-1$\alpha$) | 4% (w/w) | Male SAMP8, SAMR1 mice | Kishida et al., 2015 [28] |
| Increase of the expression of MAFbx/atrogin1 | Chestnuts flour | Polyphenols (100 nM) or tocopherols (100 nM) | C2C12 myotube cells | Frati et al., 2014 [29] |
| Decreased expression of proteasomes 20S and 19S | Camellia sinensis | 10–150 µM | C2C12 myotubes | Mirza et al., 2014 [25] |
| Decreased peak CK serum or activity | Curcumin | 150 mg before and 12 h after each eccentric exercise | Untrained young men | Tanabe et al., 2015 [30] |
| | Curcumin | 2.5 g twice daily | Men (N = 17) | Nicol et al., 2015 [22] |
| | Curcumin | 200 mg/kg/day | Male Wistar rats | Boz et al., 2014 [31] |
| Decrease plasma-serum ammonia levels | Pumpkin (Cucurbita moschata) fruit | 0, 50, 100, and 250 mg/kg/day for 14 days | Male ICR mice | Wang et al., 2012 [32] |
| | Angelica sinensis | 0.41 g/kg/day (Ex-AS1) and 2.05 g/kg/day (Ex-AS5), 6 weeks | Male ICR strain mice | Yeh et al., 2014 [33] |
| | Rubus parvifolius L. (RPL) | 40 mg/kg and 20 mg/kg | Five-week-old male | Chen et al., 2013 [21] |
| Increase in blood creatine kinase | Zingiber officinale Roscoe | 4 g of ginger once a day for 5 days | 20 non-weight trained participants | Matsumura et al., 2015 [34] |
| | Eriobotrya japonica | 50 mg/kg/day | Young (5-month-old) and aged (18-19-month-old) rats | Sung et al., 2015 [35] |

TABLE 2: Continued.

| Effect | Botanicals | Physiology | Study | Authors |
|---|---|---|---|---|
| Increase in serum creatinine | Ashwagandha (Withania somnifera) (WS) | 750 mg/day × 10 days; 1000 mg/day × 10 days; 1250 mg/day × 10 days | Eighteen apparently healthy volunteers | Raut et al., 2012 [36] |
| Decrease of serum creatine kinase activity | Pumpkin (Cucurbita moschata) fruit | 0, 50, 100, and 250 mg/kg/day for 14 days | Male ICR mice | Wang et al., 2012 [32] |
| | Salvia officinalis | 100, 200, and 300 mg/kg BW | 50 rats | JiPing, 2011 [37] |
| | Angelica sinensis | 0.41 g/kg/day (Ex-AS1) and 2.05 g/kg/day (Ex-AS5), 6 weeks | Male ICR strain mice | Yeh et al., 2014 [33] |
| | Camellia sinensis | 0.25% or 0.5% green tea extract at the age of 42 days | C57BL/6J and mdx mice | Evans et al., 2010 [9] |
| | Withania somnifera | 500 mg of the whole root extract twice daily; 750 mg twice daily | 35 individuals | Mishra and Trikamji, 2013 [5] |
| | Korean mistletoe (Viscum album subsp. coloratum) | KME at 400 or 1000 mg/(kg·d) for 1 week and 25, 40, 200, and 400 mg/kg | ICR mice | Jung et al., 2012 [38] |
| Decrease in plasma lactate or lactic acid | Aegle marmelos (L.) Corr. | 100, 200, and 400 mg/kg BW for 21 d | BALB/c mice | Nallamuthu et al., 2014 [39] |
| | Pumpkin (Cucurbita moschata) fruit | 0, 50, 100, and 250 mg/kg/day for 14 days | Male ICR mice | Wang et al., 2012 [32] |
| | Tao-Hong-Si-Wu-Tang (THSWT) | 5, 10, and 20 mL/ kg body weight for 28 days | 32 male mice | Li et al., 2013 [40] |
| | Rubus parvifolius L. (RPL) | 40 mg/kg and 20 mg/kg | Five-week-old male | Chen et al., 2013 [21] |
| | Angelica sinensis | 0.41 g/kg/day (Ex-AS1) and 2.05 g/kg/day (Ex-AS5), 6 weeks | Male ICR strain mice | Yeh et al., 2014 [33] |
| Increase in LDH and lactic acid | Panax ginseng | 10 mg/kg | Rat | Tan et al., 2013 [41] |
| | Acanthopanax senticosus (LDH) | 500 mg/kg and 200 mg/kg; 280 mg/kg or 70 mg/kg; 70 mg/kg or 280 mg/kg | Five-week-old male ICR mice | Huang et al., 2011 [42] |
| | Rubus parvifolius L. (RPL) | 40 mg/kg and 20 mg/kg | Five-week-old male | Chen et al., 2013 [21] |
| Decreased myoglobin levels | Curcumin | 200 mg/kg/day | Male Wistar rats | Boz et al., 2014 [31] |
| Decreased MDA levels in liver tissue | Curcumin | 200 mg/kg/day | Male Wistar rats | Boz et al., 2014 [31] |
| | Aegle marmelos (L.) Corr. | 100, 200, and 400 mg/kg BW for 21 days | BALB/c mice | Nallamuthu et al., 2014 [39] |
| | Curcuma longa | 20–40 μg kg$^{-1}$ of curcumin | Wistar rats ($n = 130$) | Vitadello et al., 2014 [43] |
| Increased MDA | Panax ginseng | 10 mg/kg | Rat | Tan et al., 2013 [41] |
| Increased availability of serum free fatty acid | Aegle marmelos (L.) Corr. | 400 mg/kg BW for 21 days | BALB/c mice | Nallamuthu et al., 2014 [39] |

TABLE 2: Continued.

| Effect | Botanicals | Physiology | Study | Authors |
|---|---|---|---|---|
| Decreased level of TG | Acanthopanax senticosus | 500 mg/kg and 200 mg/kg; 280 mg/kg or 70 mg/kg; 70 mg/kg or 280 mg/kg | Five-week-old male ICR mice | Huang et al., 2011 [42] |
| | Rubus parvifolius L. (RPL) | 40 mg/kg and 20 mg/kg | Five-week-old male | Chen et al., 2013 [21] |
| | Ashwagandha (Withania somnifera) (WS) | 750 mg/day × 10 days; 1000 mg/day × 10 days; 1250 mg/day × 10 days | Eighteen apparently healthy volunteers | Raut et al., 2012 [36] |
| Decrease in glucose and insulin | Panax notoginseng | 5 mg of Rg1 | Healthy young men ($N = 26$) | Hou et al., 2015 [17] |
| Increase in blood glucose | Pumpkin (Cucurbita moschata) fruit | 0, 50, 100, and 250 mg/kg/day for 14 days | Male ICR mice | Wang et al., 2012 [32] |
| | Angelica sinensis | 0.41 g/kg/day (Ex-AS1) and 2.05 g/kg/day (Ex-AS5), 6 weeks | Male ICR strain mice | Yeh et al., 2014 [33] |
| Increase in citrate synthase (CS) activity | Panax notoginseng | 5 mg of Rg1 | Healthy young men ($N = 26$) | Hou et al., 2015 [17] |
| Rate of glycogen accumulation | Panax notoginseng | 5 mg of Rg1 | Healthy young men ($N = 26$) | Hou et al., 2015 [17] |
| Increase in glycogen content of liver and muscle | Aegle marmelos (L.) Corr. | 100, 200, and 400 mg/kg BW for 21 d | BALB/c mice | Nallamuthu et al., 2014 [39] |
| | Pumpkin (Cucurbita moschata) fruit | 0, 50, 100, and 250 mg/kg/day for 14 days | Male ICR mice | Wang et al., 2012 [32] |
| | Panax ginseng | 10 mg/kg | Rat | Tan et al., 2013 [41] |
| | Tao-Hong-Si-Wu-Tang (THSWT) | 5, 10, and 20 mL/kg body weight for 28 days | 32 male mice | Li et al., 2013 [40] |
| | Angelica sinensis | 0.41 g/kg/day (Ex-AS1) and 2.05 g/kg/day (Ex-AS5), 6 weeks | Male ICR strain mice | Yeh et al., 2014 [33] |
| | Rubus parvifolius L. (RPL) | 40 mg/kg and 20 mg/kg | Five-week-old male | Chen et al., 2013 [21] |
| Increase in cholinesterase (ChE) | Salvia officinalis | 100, 200, and 300 mg/kg BW | 50 rats | JiPing, 2011 [37] |
| Upregulation of HSP70 mRNA levels or induction of the expression of Hsp-70 | Rhodiola rosea | 10 μg/mL of Rhodiolife | Murine skeletal muscle cells | Hernández-Santana et al., 2014 [44] |
| | Cichorium intybus (Cii) | 5, 10, 25, and 50 μg/mL | C2C12 myoblast | Lee et al., 2013 [45] |
| Downregulation of Hsp-70 | Aegle marmelos (L.) Corr. | 100, 200, and 400 mg/kg BW for 21 days | BALB/c mice | Nallamuthu et al., 2014 [39] |
| Prevention of calpain upregulation | Pinus pinaster | Oligopin (0.05 mg/mL) | Cultured human skeletal muscle satellite cells | Dargelos et al., 2010 [46] |
| Inhibition of the level of ceramide | Cichorium intybus (Cii) | 5, 10, 25, and 50 μg/mL | C2C12 myoblast | Lee et al., 2013 [45] |
| Suppression or mitigation of the increases in plasma CPK, AST, ALT, and MDA levels after downhill running | Camellia sinensis | 0.5% w/w in diet for 3 weeks after downhill running | Mice | Haramizu et al., 2013 [20] |
| | Chlorella (only CPK) | 1% Chlorella-supplemented diet (CSD group) | Transgenic mice | Nakashima et al., 2014 [47] |
| Reduction of the levels of carbonylated protein | Camellia sinensis | 0.5% w/w in diet for 3 weeks after downhill running | Mice | Haramizu et al., 2013 [20] |
| | Curcuma longa | 20–40 μg kg$^{-1}$ of curcumin | Wistar rats ($n = 130$) | Vitadello et al., 2014 [43] |
| | Camellia sinensis | GTE (50 mg/kg body weight) | Sixty male rats | Alway et al., 2015 [48] |

TABLE 2: Continued.

| Effect | Botanicals | Physiology | Study | Authors |
| --- | --- | --- | --- | --- |
| Attenuation of hydrogen peroxide concentration | Curcuma longa | 3 mg | Male C57BL/6 mice | Kawanishi et al., 2013 [49] |
| Attenuation of NADPH-oxidase mRNA expression | Curcuma longa | 3 mg | Male C57BL/6 mice | Kawanishi et al., 2013 [49] |
| Attenuation of F4/80 mRNA expression | Curcuma longa | 3 mg | Male C57BL/6 mice | Kawanishi et al., 2013 [49] |
| Counteraction of the increase of BiP, ATF4, XBP1u, and XBP1s mRNA | Camellia sinensis | Green tea extract (0.5% w/vol) | Twelve-week-old female C57BL/6J mice | Rodriguez et al., 2014 [50] |
| Increase in the mitochondrial oxygen consumption rate | Korean mistletoe (Viscum album subsp. coloratum) | 6 $\mu$g/mL | L6 cells and C2C12 cells, mice | Jung et al., 2012 [38] |
| Increase of the expression of peroxisome proliferator-activated receptor coactivator- (PGC-) 1$\alpha$ and SIRT-1 | Korean mistletoe (Viscum album subsp. coloratum) | 6 $\mu$g/mL | L6 cells and C2C12 cells, mice | Jung et al., 2012 [38] |
| | Vitis vinifera | 0.05% trans-resveratrol for 10 months | Middle-aged (18 months) C57/BL6 mice | Jackson et al., 2011 [51] |
| | Glycine max | 100 $\mu$M | C2C12 myotubes | Hirasaka et al., 2013 [11] |
| | Vitis vinifera | 125 mg/kg/day | Thirty-six male rats | Bennett et al., 2013 [52] |
| Decrease of PGC-1$\alpha$ expression | Go-sha-jinki-Gan (GJG) (only PGC-1$\alpha$) | 4% (w/w) | Male SAMP8, SAMR1 mice | Kishida et al., 2015 [28] |
| Decrease of BUN | Aegle marmelos (L.) Corr. | 400 mg/kg BW for 21 days | BALB/c mice | Nallamuthu et al., 2014 [39] |
| | Pumpkin (Cucurbita moschata) fruit | 0, 50, 100, and 250 mg/kg/day for 14 days | Male ICR mice | Wang et al., 2012 [32] |
| | Tao-Hong-Si-Wu-Tang (THSWT) | 5, 10, and 20 mL/kg body weight for 28 days | 32 male mice | Li et al., 2013 [40] |
| | Acanthopanax senticosus | 500 mg/kg and 200 mg/kg; 280 mg/kg or 70 mg/kg; 70 mg/kg or 280 mg/kg | Five-week-old male ICR mice | Huang et al., 2011 [42] |
| | Ashwagandha (Withania somnifera) (WS) | 750 mg/day × 10 days; 1000 mg/day × 10 days; 1250 mg/day × 10 days | Eighteen apparently healthy volunteers | Raut et al., 2012 [36] |
| Increase of SOD and catalase | Aegle marmelos (L.) Corr. | 100, 200, and 400 mg/kg BW for 21 d | BALB/c mice | Nallamuthu et al., 2014 [39] |
| | Panax ginseng (only SOD) | 10 mg/kg | Rat | Tan et al., 2013 [41] |
| | Salvia officinalis (SOD and GSHPx) | 100, 200, and 300 mg/kg BW | 50 rats | JiPing, 2011 [37] |
| Upregulation of GLUT-4 and AMPK-1$\alpha$ | Aegle marmelos (L.) Corr. | 100, 200, and 400 mg/kg BW for 21 d | BALB/c mice | Nallamuthu et al., 2014 [39] |
| Decrease in SUN levels | Rubus parvifolius L. (RPL) | 40 mg/kg and 20 mg/kg | Five-week-old male | Chen et al., 2013 [21] |
| Increase of Grp94 protein | Curcuma longa | 20–40 $\mu$g kg$^{-1}$ of curcumin | Wistar rats ($n = 130$) | Vitadello et al., 2014 [43] |
| Decrease in myostatin and $\beta$-galactosidase | Camellia sinensis | 1 mg/kg b.i.d. | Young and old C57BL/6 male mice | Gutierrez-Salmean et al., 2014 [53] |
| Increase in the ratio of plasma follistatin/myostatin | Camellia sinensis | 25 mg of pure Epi (~1 mg/kg/day) | Human subjects ($n = 6$) | Gutierrez-Salmean et al., 2014 [53] |
| Decrease in cross-sectional area (CSA) | Eriobotrya japonica | 50 mg/kg/day | Young (5-month-old) and aged (18-19-month-old) rats | Sung et al., 2015 [35] |

TABLE 3: Botanicals with anti-inflammatory effects on skeletal muscle.

| Paper | Botanical | Compound | Model | Physiology | Main results |
|---|---|---|---|---|---|
| | | | In vitro | | |
| Kim et al., 2012 [7] | Korean *Citrus aurantium* L. | Flavonoids (hesperidin, nobiletin, and naringin) | Rat skeletal muscle cells | Flavonoids 10, 50, 75, and 100 $\mu$g/mL | Decrease in the production of inducible nitric oxide synthase, cyclooxygenase-2, TNF-$\alpha$, and IL-6. |
| Kim et al., 2013 [24] | Korean *Citrus aurantium* L. | Flavonoids (naringin, hesperidin, poncirin, isosinnesetin, and hexamethoxyflavone) | Rat skeletal muscle cells | 100 $\mu$g | Protection of cell-structure related proteins and decrease in level of cleaved caspase-3. |
| Leite et al., 2014 [12] | *Eugenia punicifolia* | Pentacyclic triterpenes (barbinervic acid) | Mouse myoblastoma cells (C2C12) | Ep-CM 100 $\mu$g/mL | Reduction of C2C12 cell density and proliferation. Increase of metalloproteases activity: MMP-9 (128 $\pm$ 14%, $p < 0.005$) and MMP-2 (110 $\pm$ 18%, $p < 0.005$). |
| Wang et al., 2014 [16] | *Vitis vinifera* | Resveratrol (3,5,40-trihydroxystilbene) | Mouse C2C12 cells | Resveratrol 100 $\mu$M | Counteraction of TNF-$\alpha$ induced muscle protein loss and reversion of declining expression of Akt, mTOR, p70S6K, 4E-BP1, and FoXO1. |
| Guo et al., 2014 [19] | Coffee | Chlorogenic acid, anhydrous caffeine, and polyphenols | Mouse myosatellite cells | Coffee solution 10, 30, 50, and 100 $\mu$g/mL | Increase in cell proliferation rate, enhancement of the DNA synthesis of the proliferating satellite cells, and increase of the activation level of Akt. |
| | | | Animals | | |
| Yu et al., 2014 [10] | *Panax ginseng* | Dammarane steroids (DS) | Rats | DS 20, 60, and 120 mg/kg | Anti-inflammatory effects on skeletal muscle following muscle-damaging exercise. |
| Kishida et al., 2015 [28] | Go-sha-jinki-Gan (GJG) | Paeoniflorin, loganin, and total alkaloids | Male SAMP8, SAMR1 mice | GJG 4% (w/w) | Reduction of the loss of skeletal muscle mass and amelioration of the increase in slow skeletal muscle fibers. |
| Guo et al., 2014 [19] | Coffee | Coffee bean, chlorogenic acid, anhydrous caffeine, and polyphenols | C57BL/6 mice | The same amount of drink in control and coffee group for 4 weeks | Improvement in grip strength; faster regeneration of injured skeletal muscles. Decrease in the levels of interleukins. |
| Leite et al., 2010 [8] | *Eugenia punicifolia* | Dichloromethane fraction | Male mdx dystrophic mice | Ep-CM 2 mg/mL | Reduction of MMP-9 (62 $\pm$ 12%, $p < 0.005$) and MMP-2 (58 $\pm$ 10%, $p < 0.005$) activities. Reduction of TNF-$\alpha$ production (42 $\pm$ 9%, $p < 0.01$) and NF-$\kappa$B expression (48 $\pm$ 7%, $p < 0.005$). |
| Leite et al., 2014 [12] | *Eugenia punicifolia* | Pentacyclic triterpenes (barbinervic acid) | C57BL/10 mice | Ep-CM 2 mg/mL | Reduction of MMP-9 activity (35 $\pm$ 7%, $p < 0.05$) but difference concerning MMP-2 activity in the muscular lesion; reduction of the inflammatory lesion area. |
| Boz et al., 2014 [31] | Curcumin | Curcumin | Male Wistar rats | 200 mg/kg/day | Decrease of CK activity ($p > 0.05$) and significant decrease of myoglobin levels ($p < 0.05$). |

TABLE 3: Continued.

| Paper | Botanical | Compound | Model | Physiology | Main results |
|---|---|---|---|---|---|
| | | | Humans | | |
| Diaz-Castro et al., 2012 [18] | *Phlebodium decumanum* | Polyphenols, terpenoids, and flavonoids | Amateur athletes (N = 40) | 5 capsules of 400 mg (250 mg of leaf extract and 150 mg of rhizome extract) | Reduction of oxidative stress ($p < 0.0001$). Reduction in the inflammatory response. Decrease of TNF-$\alpha$ before and after the high-intensity exercise. Increase in sTNF-RII. |
| Hou et al., 2015 [17] | *Panax notoginseng* | Ginsenosides Rg1 | Healthy young men (N = 26) | 5 mg of Rg1 | Increase in exercise time to exhaustion (Rg1 $38.3 \pm 6.7$ min versus placebo $31.8 \pm 5.0$ min). Improvement in meal tolerance during recovery ($p < 0.05$). |
| Black et al., 2010 [54] | *Zingiber officinale* Roscoe | Gingerols and shogaols | Individuals (N = 28) | 2 g of ginger after exercise | Postexercise reduction in arm pain the following day (13%; $-5.9 \pm 8$ mm). |
| Black et al., 2010 [54] | *Zingiber officinale* Roscoe | Gingerols and shogaols | 34 participants in study 1; 40 participants in study 2 | 2 g for 11 consecutive days after exercise | Decrease in pain-intensity ratings 24 hours after eccentric exercise in both studies ($p < 0.05$). |
| Pumpa et al., 2013 [55] | *Panax notoginseng* | Saponins (ginsenosides) | Well-trained male volunteers (N = 20) | 4 g of *P. notoginseng* | Decrease in IL-6 24 h after the downhill run (placebo). Decrease in TNF-$\alpha$ 24 h after the downhill run (placebo). |
| Drobnic et al., 2014 [23] | Curcumin | Phytosome delivery system (Meriva) | Healthy, moderately active male (N = 20) | 1 g twice daily (corresponding to 200 mg curcumin twice a day) | Significant decrease in pain intensity for the right and left anterior thigh ($4.4 \pm 2.5$ and $4.4 \pm 2.4$, $p < 0.05$). Lower increase in hsPCR levels at 24 hours (116.2%). Lower increase of IL-8 levels at 2 hours ($196.8 \pm 66.1$ pg/mL, $p < 0.05$). |
| Nicol et al., 2015 [22] | Curcumin | Curcuminoids | Men (N = 17) | 2.5 g twice daily | Moderate-to-large reduction in pain during single-leg squat (VAS scale $-1.4$ to $-1.7$; 90% CI: $\pm1.0$), gluteal stretch ($-1.0$ to $-1.9$; $\pm0.9$), and squat jump ($-1.5$ to $-1.1$; $\pm1.2$) and reduction in creatine kinase activity ($-22$–29%; $\pm21$-22%). Increase in IL-6 concentrations at 0 h (31%; $\pm29$%) and 48 h (32%; $\pm29$%), but decrease in IL-6 at 24 h relative to postexercise period ($-20$%; $\pm18$%). |
| Tanabe et al., 2015 [30] | Curcumin | Curcuminoids (Theracurmin) | Untrained young men (N = 14) | 150 mg before and 12 h after each eccentric exercise | Faster recovery of maximum voluntary contraction torque (e.g., 4 days after exercise: $-31 \pm 13$% versus $-15 \pm 15$%), lower peak serum CK activity (peak: $7684 \pm 8959$ IU/L versus $3398 \pm 3562$ IU/L, $p < 0.05$). No significant changes in IL-6 and TNF-$\alpha$ after exercise. |

TABLE 4: Botanicals with counterbalancing muscle damage effects.

| Paper | Botanical | Compound | Model | Physiology | Main results |
|---|---|---|---|---|---|
| | | | | In vitro | |
| Hernández-Santana et al., 2014 [44] | Rhodiola rosea | RR extracts: rosavins and salidroside | Murine skeletal muscle cells | 1–100 $\mu$g/mL and others | Upregulation of HSP70 mRNA levels and enhancement of the expression by exposure to $H_2O_2$ ($p < 0.05$). Maintenance of HSP70 protein levels in pretreated cell cultures compared to controls ($\sim$50%). |
| Dargelos et al., 2010 [46] | Pinus pinaster | Polyphenols | Cultured human skeletal muscle satellite cells | Oligopin (0.05 mg/mL) | Restoration of cell viability ($55.2 \pm 3.2$% versus $42.3 \pm 4.8$% in $H_2O_2$ treated cells). Abolishment of $H_2O_2$ induced apoptotic cell death. |
| | | | | Animals | |
| Haramizu et al., 2013 [20] | Camellia sinensis | Catechins: epigallocatechin gallate, epigallocatechin, epicatechin gallate, epicatechin, gallocatechin, and gallocatechin gallate | Mice | 0.5% w/w in diet for 3 weeks after downhill running | Mitigation of the running-induced decrease in voluntary wheel-running activity by 35%. Maintenance of endurance running capacity ($214 \pm 9$ versus $189 \pm 10$ min, $p < 0.05$). |
| Kawanishi et al., 2013 [49] | Curcuma longa | Curcumin | Male C57BL/6 mice | 3 mg | Decrease of hydrogen peroxide concentration and NADPH-oxidase mRNA expression ($p < 0.05$). |
| Rodriguez et al., 2014 [50] | Camellia sinensis | Green tea extracts | Twelve-week-old female C57BL/6J mice | Green tea extract (0.5% w/vol) | Decrease of BiP, ATF4, XBP1u, and XBP1s mRNA. No activity on CHOP mRNA. |
| | | | | Humans | |
| Shanely et al., 2014 [56] | Rhodiola rosea | Rosavin, salidroside, syringin, triandrin, and tyrosol | 55 subjects (48 completing all aspects of the study) | 600 mg/day for 30 days prior to, on the day of, and after 7 days of the marathon | No effects on DOMS increased ($p = 0.700$). |
| Pumpa et al., 2013 [55] | Panax notoginseng | Saponins (ginsenosides) | Twenty well-trained male volunteers | 4000 mg of P. notoginseng capsules | Lower IL-6 concentrations 24 h after the downhill run in the placebo group. |
| Matsumura et al., 2015 [34] | Zingiber officinale Roscoe | Gingerols and shogaols | 20 non-weight trained participants | 4 g of ginger once a day for 5 days | Acceleration in the recovery of muscle strength following intense exercise. |

TABLE 5: Botanicals with antifatigue activity on skeletal muscle.

| Paper | Botanical | Compound | Model | Physiology | Main results |
|---|---|---|---|---|---|
| | | | | In vitro | |
| Jung et al., 2012 [38] | Korean mistletoe (*Viscum album* subsp. *coloratum*) | KME (Korean mistletoe extract) | L6 cells and C2C12 cells, mice | $6\,\mu g/mL$ | Acceleration of OCR (37%). Significant increase in PGC-1$\alpha$ mRNA expression. 9.3-fold increase in SIRT1 expression. |
| | | | | Animals | |
| Nallamuthu et al., 2014 [39] | *Aegle marmelos* (L.) Corr. | Polyphenols | BALB/c mice | 100, 200, and 400 mg/kg BW for 21 d | Increase in the duration of swimming time to exhaustion by 23.4 and 47.5% for medium and higher doses, respectively. |
| Wang et al., 2012 [32] | Pumpkin (*Cucurbita moschata*) fruit | *C. moschata* fruit extract (CME) | Male ICR mice | 0, 50, 100, and 250 mg/kg/day for 14 days | Dose-dependent increase in swimming time ($p = 0.0006$). |
| Tan et al., 2013 [41] | *Panax ginseng* | Ginsenoside Rb1 (GRb1) | Rat | 10 mg/kg | Significant decrease of maximum grip strength of the MG group and the GG group ($p < 0.05$). |
| Li et al., 2013 [40] | Tao-Hong-Si-Wu-Tang (THSWT) | | 32 male mice | 5, 10, and 20 mL/kg body weight for 28 days | Significant increase of exhaustive swimming times ($p < 0.05$). |
| JiPing, 2011 [37] | *Salvia officinalis* | | 50 rats | 100, 200, and 300 mg/kg BW | Reduction of lipid peroxidation, LDH, and CK. |
| Yeh et al., 2014 [33] | *Angelica sinensis* | Ferulic acid | Male ICR strain mice | 0.41 g/kg/day (Ex-AS1) and 2.05 g/kg/day (Ex-AS5), 6 weeks | Slight increase of grip strength ($p = 0.0616$), at the higher AS doses, longer exercise performance (1.49, $p = 0.0116$). |
| Huang et al., 2011 [42] | *Acanthopanax senticosus* | Eleutheroside E, eleutheroside E$_2$ | Five-week-old male ICR mice | 500 mg/kg and 200 mg/kg; 280 mg/kg or 70 mg/kg; 70 mg/kg or 280 mg/kg | Increase of swimming time to exhaustion at high dose ($p < 0.01$). |
| Chen et al., 2013 [21] | *Rubus parvifolius* L. (RPL) | Three saponins (nigaichigoside, suavissimoside, and coreanoside) | Five-week-old male | 40 mg/kg and 20 mg/kg | Delays of SUN and LA accumulation, decrease in TG level, and increase in HG and LDH. Suppression of inflammatory cytokine production. |
| Jung et al., 2012 [38] | Korean mistletoe (*Viscum album* subsp. *coloratum*) | | ICR mice | KME at 400 or 1000 mg/(kg·d) for 1 week and 25, 40, 200, and 400 mg/kg | Induction of mitochondrial activity and improvement in endurance. |
| Jackson et al., 2011 [51] | *Vitis vinifera* | Resveratrol | Middle-aged (18 months old) C57/BL6 mice | 0.05% trans-resveratrol for 10 months | Protection against oxidative stress through the upregulation of MnSOD. Increase in the muscles activity in animals that were 28 months of age by an additional ~40% ($p \leq 0.05$). |
| | | | | Humans | |
| Raut et al., 2012 [36] | Ashwagandha (*Withania somnifera*) (WS) | | Eighteen apparently healthy volunteers | 750 mg/day × 10 days; 1000 mg/day × 10 days; 1250 mg/day × 10 days | Increase in serum creatinine and blood urea nitrogen. Significant decrease in total cholesterol. |

TABLE 6: Botanicals with effects on muscle atrophy.

| Paper | Botanical | Compound | Model | Physiology | Main results |
|---|---|---|---|---|---|
| | | | In vitro | | |
| Lee et al., 2013 [45] | *Cichorium intybus* (Cii) | | C2C12 myoblast | 5, 10, 25, and 50 $\mu$g/mL | Prevention of cell viability loss. |
| Hirasaka et al., 2013 [11] | *Glycine max* | Isoflavone (genistein and daidzein) | C2C12 myotubes | 100 $\mu$M | Approximately 2-fold increase of SIRT1 mRNA expression. |
| Mirza et al., 2014 [25] | *Camellia sinensis* | Epigallocatechin-3-gallate | C2C12 myotubes | 10–150 $\mu$M | Reduction of the expression of proteasome 19S and 20S subunits. Reduction of the expression of MuRF-1 and MAFbx. |
| Frati et al., 2014 [29] | Chestnuts flour | Chestnuts flour extract polyphenols or tocopherols or SL-s | C2C12 myotube cells | Polyphenols (100 nM) or tocopherols (100 nM) | Counterbalance of cell atrophy. Γ-Tocopherol and sphingolipids positively affect skeletal muscle cell atrophy. |
| | | | Animals | | |
| Vitadello et al., 2014 [43] | *Curcuma longa* | Curcumins | Wistar rats ($n = 130$) | 20–40 $\mu$g kg$^{-1}$ of curcumin | About twofold increase of Grp 94 in muscles of ambulatory rats ($p < 0.05$). Counteracted loss of soleus mass and myofiber cross-sectional area by 30% ($p \leq 0.02$). |
| Nakashima et al., 2014 [47] | *Chlorella* | | Transgenic mice | 1% *Chlorella*-supplemented diet (CSD group) | Improvement of skeletal muscle atrophy and cytochrome C oxidase activity. Recovery of body weight, enhancement of oxidative stress, and increase of CPK. |
| | | | Humans | | |
| Choquette et al., 2013 [57] | *Glycine max* | Isoflavones (daidzein, glycitein, and genistein) | 70 women | Isoflavones (70 mg/day) and exercise | No effects. |

has no remarkable effect after single administration. In fact, only a moderate reduction in the progression of muscle pain from 24 h to 48 h following eccentric exercise was observed in participants who consumed ginger 24 h after exercise, and this effect was not enhanced by heat-treated ginger. In mice, *Coffea* decreases the levels of interleukins IL-1$\alpha$ and IL-6 and TNF-$\alpha$, which are correlated with muscle weight and grip strength. Using mice cells in vitro, coffee increases the number of proliferating cells and augmented DNA synthesis through the Akt signaling pathway. As a result, there is a combination of augmented satellite cell activation and decreased inflammatory levels by coffee treatment; it has anti-inflammatory effects both because it has antioxidant properties and because it has compounds, such as kahweol, with immunomodulatory properties [7, 19, 24, 54, 61]. Also, *Eugenia punicifolia* showed anti-inflammatory properties in the gastrocnemius muscle of mdx dystrophic mice; in particular, the activity of dichloromethane fraction of *Eugenia punicifolia* (Ep-CM), in mice, decreases metalloprotease-9 and metalloprotease-2 activities (indicators of local inflammation and tissue remodeling, resp.) and levels of tumor necrosis factor-$\alpha$ and NF-$\kappa$B transcription factor [8]; isolated pentacyclic triterpene from *Eugenia punicifolia* reduces myoblast cells proliferation, has no effects on apoptosis, and increases matrix metalloproteases and muscular area (MMP-9 and MMP-2) [12]. As shown in the study by Yu et al. [10], Dammarane steroids (DS) of *Panax ginseng* produce anti-inflammatory effects in rats, following muscle damage exercise, because they potentiate inflammation at baseline but exerted anti-inflammatory effects on skeletal muscle following muscle-damaging exercise. Another study has also highlighted the effect of steroid Rg1 (capsule with 5 mg of Rg1), an ergogenic component of ginseng, in healthy human against exercise challenge: the extract can minimize unwanted lipid peroxidation and attenuate proinflammatory shift under exercise challenge and so it ameliorates the postexercise recovery and mitochondria enzyme adaptation probably because the incorporation of the bulky steroid moiety of Rg1 into cellular membrane lipid may enhance molecular complexity and mechanical stability of the cell and mitochondrial membranes [17]. *Panax notoginseng*, as shown by Pumpa et al., seems to have no particular effects on interleukins, indicators of inflammation and muscle damage, in well-trained males after a bout of eccentric exercise designed to induce delayed-onset muscle soreness (DOMS) (in the experiment, 400 mg of *Panax notoginseng* was used) [55]. Even *Go-sha-jinki-Gan* (GJG) maintains the area of muscle fibers in the soleus via normalizing signal transduction through the insulin-growth factor (IGF-1) Akt axis, the suppression of inflammation, and the maintenance of mitochondrial-related transcription factors in mice [28]. A positive effect on cell atrophy caused by TNF-$\alpha$ was shown with resveratrol (in *Vitis vinifera*) supplementation in a muscle cell line (regulating the Akt/mTOR/FoxO1 signaling pathways together with inhibition of the atrophy-related ubiquitin ligase) [16].

Finally, several studies have investigated the mechanisms by which curcumin, a constituent of turmeric (*Curcuma longa* L.), exerts its beneficial effect on muscle [62]. Early experimental study demonstrated that curcumin suppresses the activation of NF-$\kappa$B, an effect of critical relevance in DOMS relief, since NF-$\kappa$B appears to be involved in the regulation of proteolysis and inflammation in muscle [62]. Therefore, inhibition of NF-$\kappa$B by curcumin may result in a muscle-protective effect. Consistently, it has been suggested that curcumin may prevent loss of muscle mass during sepsis and endotoxaemia and may stimulate muscle regeneration after traumatic injury [62]. Other mechanisms potentially responsible for the anti-inflammatory and antioxidant properties of curcumin include induction of heat-shock response [62], reduction in the expression of the proinflammatory enzyme cyclooxygenase-2 (COX-2), and promotion of the antioxidant response by activation of the transcription factor Nrf2 [63]. More recent studies confirm that curcumin can reduce inflammation and decrease some of the negative effects associated with eccentric exercise-induced muscle damage, including the release of proinflammatory cytokines and markers of muscle injury like creatine kinase (CK), as shown in animal models [31] and in in vitro settings [64].

The three studies that have been conducted until now in humans [22, 23, 30] have shown that curcumin, at the dosages of 1 g twice daily (as the Phytosome® delivery system, Meriva®) and 2.5 g twice daily, and 150 mg of solid-lipid nanoparticle curcumin (Theracurmin®), respectively, can prevent DOMS with some evidence of enhanced recovery of muscle performance, maximal voluntary contraction loss, and serum creatine kinase activity increase.

In conclusion, the muscle that makes activities undergoes an increase in inflammation that can damage the muscle itself. It is important to counteract the inflammatory activity in order to preserve the muscle from numerous types of damage. Several animal and in vitro studies have investigated the efficacy of botanicals with recognized anti-inflammatory activity (such as *Phlebodium decamanum*, *Citrus aurantium*, *Coffea arabica*, *Zingiber officinale*, *Eugenia punicifolia*, *Panax ginseng*, *Go-sha-jinki-Gan*, *Vitis vinifera*, and *Curcuma longa* L.) on inflammation secondary to muscle activity (Table 2). These botanical extracts exerted their effects through different biochemical pathways, specifically decreasing interleukins or aging on transcriptional factors. Human studies were performed using four botanicals (*Panax ginseng*, *Zingiber officinale*, *Phlebodium decumanum*, and *Curcuma longa* L.) showing that (1) the daily consumption of raw and heat-treated *Zingiber* resulted in moderate-to-large reductions in muscle pain after exercise-induced muscle injury; (2) *Phlebodium* supplementation for both professional and amateur athletes performing strenuous exercise resulted in reducing the undesirable effects of the oxidative stress and inflammation signaling elicited during high-intensity exercise; (3) *Panax notoginseng* did not convincingly have an effect on performance, muscular pain, or assessed blood markers in well-trained males after an intense bout of eccentric exercise that induced delayed-onset muscle soreness (DOMS); (4) curcumin could prevent DOMS enhancing the recovery of muscle performance and the maximal voluntary contraction loss and modulating the serum creatine kinase activity increase.

All these clinical studies considered the reduction of inflammation and consequently muscle pain after a strenuous exercise and not in sarcopenic subjects, but this is a good starting point for the future utilization of these plants in the elderly.

*3.3. Muscle Damage Prevention.* This research has been carried out based on the keywords "skeletal muscle mass" and "damage" and "botanicals" or "plants" or "extracts"; 11 articles were sourced and 8 studies have been taken into consideration. Among these, 2 studies are in in vitro setting, 3 in animals, and 3 in humans (Table 4).

A recent study by Kawanishi et al. has clarified properties of *curcumin* after downhill running-induced muscle damage in mice. This study underlines how curcumin has an antioxidant effect in mice following downhill running-induced muscle damage; however, no differences in plasma creatine kinase (CK) and plasma lactate dehydrogenase (LDH), as markers of muscle damage, were observed. Curcumin administration immediately after downhill running did not prevent muscle damage but significantly attenuates the concentration of hydrogen peroxide and NADPH-oxidase gene expression; therefore, curcumin may be beneficial for the prevention of oxidative stress in downhill running-induced skeletal muscle damage [49]. Two recent studies in humans by Pumpa et al. [34] and Matsumura et al. [55] investigated the effects of *Panax notoginseng* (4000 mg) and *Zingiber officinale* (4 g for 5 days) on delayed-onset muscle soreness (DOMS); *Zingiber officinale* supplementation could have accelerated the recovery of maximal strength following muscle damage but did not prevent delayed muscle damage. The authors concluded that there is no evidence to support the use of *Panax* as a preventive option for DOMS and its related inflammation. *Rhodiola rosea* (600 mg/d) did not attenuate the postmarathon decrease in muscle function, the increases in muscle damage, the extracellular heatshock protein (eHSP72), or the plasma cytokines in human experienced runners [56]; however, the same plant modulates in vitro the expression of molecular factors (chaperone HSP70) such as heatshock proteins (HSP) in order to protect C2 C12 myotubes cells against peroxide-induced oxidative stress, suggesting a potential antioxidant role [44]. Finally, Haramizu et al. demonstrated that catechins of *Camellia sinensis* attenuate downhill running-induced muscle damage in mice, perhaps through their antioxidant properties, hastening recovery of physical performance [20]. A typical example of muscle damage is the cellular dysfunction caused by lipid excess. Lipid excess activates endoplasmatic reticulum (ER) stress in skeletal muscle and, as a consequence, accumulation of unfolded or misfolded proteins in ER lumen. Rodriguez et al. demonstrated that epigallocatechin-3-gallate (EGCG) from *Camellia sinensis* could protect mice muscle against ER stress, especially thanks to its antioxidant properties [50]. Dargelos et al. investigate the role of a natural antioxidant extracted from pine bark (*Pinus pinaster*) in cultured human skeletal muscle satellite cells. Results showed that this polyphenolic extract is able to protect cells from oxidative stress ($H_2O_2$) damage and prevent the apoptosis and the activation of calpains mediated by $H_2O_2$ [46].

In conclusion (Table 3), until today, important studies were made on humans and animals for the prevention of muscle damage. Most of the plants used (*Curcuma longa, Panax notoginseng, Zingiber officinale, Rhodiola rosea, Camellia sinensis*, and *Pinus pinaster*) act on DOMS, thanks to their antioxidant properties. In human, *Panax notoginseng* seems to have no effect as a preventive option for DOMS, and *Rhodiola rosea* does not attenuate muscle damage. Further studies are needed but we can say that botanical supplementation, thanks to its antioxidant properties, could be useful to prevent sarcopenia due to the fact that the loss of muscle mass in aging is driven also by oxidative stress, as it happens after strenuous exercise.

*3.4. Antifatigue.* This research has been carried out based on the keywords "skeletal muscle mass" and "fatigue" and "botanicals" or "plants" or "extracts"; 20 articles were sourced and 11 studies are taken into account. Among these, only one study is made in humans, one in in vitro settings, and one both in in vitro settings and in animals and the others are made in animals (Table 5).

Tan et al. in 2013 investigated for the first time the role of ginsenoside Rb1 (Grb1) in *Panax quinquefolius*, as antifatigue agent, on postoperative fatigue syndrome (POFS) in a rat model induced by major small intestinal resection, through its antioxidant properties and the improvement of energy metabolism. Grb1 enhances maximum grip strength and increases the activity of lactate dehydrogenase and other biochemical parameters. The results suggested that GRb1 improves the maintenance of normal pH range in muscle tissue by reducing the accumulation of lactic acid (LA) and attenuates LA induced side effects of various biochemical and physiological processes, which impair bodily performance [41]. In accordance, the study by Nallamuthu et al. demonstrated the antifatigue properties in mice of *A. marmelos* fruit, most probably manifested by delaying the accumulation of serum lactic acid, increasing the fat utilization, and upregulating the skeletal muscle metabolic regulators [39]. Likewise, *Salvia sativa, Angelica sinensis, Cucurbita moschata, Withania somnifera*, and *Acanthopanax senticosus* extracts exhibit different antifatigue effects. All of these studies, with the exception of *Withania somnifera*, are performed in animals (rats or mice). These studies demonstrate that the antioxidant properties of plants play an important role in reducing fatigue. *Salvia* reduces lipid peroxidation, lactate dehydrogenase, creatine kinase activities, enhanced antioxidant enzymes, and cholinesterase (ChE) activities in the skeletal muscle of endurance exercise rats; similar effects have been observed for other extracts, with some differences between each other, in which, additionally, antifatigue is measured also by forelimb grip strength and exhaustive swimming time as well as serum levels of lactate, ammonia, glucose, and creatine kinase after a 15 min swimming exercise. Specifically, the mechanisms of *Acanthopanax* (also called *Eleutherococcus senticosus* or Siberian ginseng) are the reduction of the level of triglycerides by increasing fat utilization, the delay of the accumulation of blood urea nitrogen (BUN), and the increase of the lactate dehydrogenase (LDH) to reduce the accumulation of lactic acid in muscle and then protect the muscle tissue [32, 33, 36, 37, 42]. Strange but active is Tao-Hong-Si-Wu-Tang that shows antifatigue activity in mice due to extended exhaustive swimming time, the increase of liver and muscle glycogen contents, and the decrease of the lactic acid (BLA) and urea nitrogen (BUN) plasmatic contents [40]. Also, Chen et al. define the antifatigue property of *Rubus parvifolius* L. (RPL) in experiment with mice, finding that total saponins from RPL possess potent capabilities to alleviate fatigue induced by forced swimming and that nigaichigoside F1 was responsible for the pharmacological effect. The underlying mechanisms include delays in the accumulation of serum urea nitrogen (SUN) and lactic acid (LA), a decrease in TG level by increasing fat consumption, increases in hepatic glycogen (HG) and LDH so that lactic acid accumulation was decreased, the reduction of ammonia in the muscle, and the suppression of increased immune activation and inflammatory cytokine production [21]. *Viscum album* subsp. *coloratum* increase mitochondrial oxygen consumption rate (OCR) in L6 cells and increase the expression of peroxisome proliferator-activated receptor c coactivator- (PGC-) 1a and silent mating type information regulation 2 homolog 1 (SIRT1), two major regulators of mitochondria function, in C2C12 cells, suggesting that this extract has great potential as a novel mitochondria-activating agent and could exert the antifatigue effect [38]. Jackson et al. try to understand how *Vitis vinifera* and its compound resveratrol could prevent muscle fatigue. Resveratrol has a protective effect against aging-induced oxidative stress in skeletal muscle, likely through the upregulation of manganese superoxide dismutase (MnSOD) activity, reducing hydrogen peroxide, and lipid peroxidation levels in muscle samples, but sarcopenia was not attenuated by resveratrol [51].

*Withania somnifera* (gradual escalating doses from 750 to 1250 mg/day) in humans has demonstrated muscle strengthening and lipid lowering [36].

In conclusion, there are several preclinical lines of evidence that botanical extracts, such as *Panax quinquefolius*, *A. marmelos* fruit, *Salvia sativa*, *Angelica sinensis*, *Phalaenopsis cornu-cervi*, *Cucurbita moschata*, *Withania somnifera*, *Acanthopanax senticosus*, deer antler extract, Tao-Hong-Si-Wu-Tang, *Rubus parvifolius* L., velvet antler extract, *Viscum album* subsp. *coloratum*, and *Vitis vinifera*, can reduce the muscle's fatigue, after intense exercise or simply in a condition of loss of muscle mass, as in sarcopenia (Table 4). Commonly, these properties are due to their antioxidant effects: in general, these plants reduce lipid peroxidation, lactic acid, and serum levels of ammonia and creatine kinase and increase liver and muscle glycogen. The only study found in human was that of Raut et al., in which supplementation with *Withania somnifera* (with gradual escalating doses from 750 to 1250 mg/day) seems to have good effects on antifatigue, but this is a preliminary study. Until today, the role of plants in antifatigue in clinical studies has been not deeply documented and so it is difficult to recommend particular supplementation.

*3.5. Muscle Atrophy Prevention.* This research has been carried out based on the keywords "skeletal muscle mass" and "atrophy" and "botanicals" or "plants" or "extracts"; 15 articles were sourced and 7 studies are taken into account. Among these, 4 are in in vitro settings and 2 are in animals and only one is in human (Table 6).

*Curcuma longa* can prevent muscle atrophy. It stimulates glucose-regulated protein 94 kDa (Grp94) expression in myogenic cells, whose levels decrease significantly in unloaded muscle, and it is involved in attenuation of myofiber atrophy in rats [43]. Also, *Camellia sinensis* extracts in rats appear to counteract the increased protein degradation (linked with its ability to downregulate key components of the ubiquitin proteasome proteolytic pathway) [25]. Instead, *Cichorium intybus* extract prevents skeletal muscle atrophy in vitro, probably increasing heat-shock protein-70 (Hsp-70) production and inhibiting the level of ceramide: Hsp-70, in fact, has a positive effect on reducing oxidative stress of cells and ceramide is involved in the regulation of cell death [45]. Also, chestnut sweet flour (rich in γ-tocopherol) protects from skeletal muscle cell atrophy, but this protection appears not to be due to a general antioxidant action, but maintaining cellular redox homeostasis through the regulation of NADPH oxidase, mitochondrial integrity [29]. Isoflavones are the most important phytochemicals in *Glycine max* for preventing muscle atrophy. These products could induce in vitro the expression of SIRT-1, a sirtuin that normally deacetylates p65, in order to reduce the activity of MuRF-1 related to muscle atrophy. Overall, they suppress MuRF-1 promoter activity and myotube atrophy induced by TNF-$\alpha$ in C2C12 myotubes [11]. However, a study performed by Choquette et al. demonstrated that, in postmenopausal women, only exercise, but not soy isoflavones (70 mg/day), could improve muscle strength and reduce risks of mobility impairments [57]. In addition, consumption of *Chlorella*, a unicellular green alga, could prevent age-related muscle atrophy in mice, because it contains various antioxidant substances, including carotenoids and vitamins and plastoquinone that has been shown to hold greater antioxidant properties. *Chlorella* contains also amino acids such as the brain chain amino acids (BCAA) valine, leucine, and isoleucine, which are important components of actin and myosin, the fundamental muscle proteins, and may be important in prevention of sarcopenia. Finally, *Chlorella* also prevents mitochondrial dysfunction [47].

In conclusion, it is clear that botanical extracts can prevent the atrophy of muscle, after intense exercise or simply in a condition of loss of muscle mass, as in sarcopenia. We considered several botanicals (*Curcuma longa*, *Camellia sinensis*, *Cichorium intybus*, chestnut sweet flour, *Glycine max*, and *Chlorella*): most of them have important antioxidant properties, which prevent muscle's atrophy. However, the only study made on human, using *Glycine max*, did not show positive results and so other researches are needed to substantiate the use of botanicals supplementation to prevent muscle atrophy.

*3.6. Muscle Regeneration and Differentiation.* This research has been carried out based on the keywords "skeletal muscle mass" and "regeneration" and "botanicals" or "plants" or "extracts"; 19 articles were sourced and 15 studies are taken into account. Among these, 4 are in in vitro settings, 7 in animals, and 3 in human and one is both in animals and in humans (Table 7). Nutraceutical compounds by *C. sinensis* in mice decrease myostatin and $\beta$-galactosidase and increase levels of markers of muscle; instead, in humans, they (7-day treatment with epicatechin at 1 mg/kg/day) increase hand grip strength and the ratio of plasma follistatin/myostatin [53] and regulate NF-$\kappa$B activity in regenerating muscle fibers [9]. *Camellia* also induces changes in satellite cell number and it improves muscle recovery following a period of atrophy in old rats and decreases oxidative stress, but this is insufficient to improve muscle recovery following a period of atrophy [48]. Also, an increase in myogenin (due to a supplement of *Vitis vinifera* resveratrol extracts) served to stimulate differentiation to compensate for an impaired function of satellite cells (SCs) in the old muscles [26]. An article by Ballak et al., about resveratrol, says that this compound does not rescue the hypertrophic response and even reduces the number of satellite cells in hypertrophied muscle of mice [26]. Also, *Ferula hermonis* Boiss. and *Vitis vinifera* significantly increase muscle weight and enhance the growth of skeletal muscle fibers or fiber size (increase the fiber cross-sectional area of type IIA and IIB fibers) and nuclear number in order to enhance the growth of skeletal muscle [52, 58]. It is noteworthy that proanthocyanidins of *Vitis* have been used in a clinical trial. An increase of muscle mass and the improvement of several physical conditions have been observed in middle-aged women (with at least one menopausal symptom) treated with doses from 100 to 200 mg/d [60]. *Broussonetia kazinoki* (*B. kazinoki*), *Corydalis turtschaninovii*, and Hachimijiogan, in vitro, promote myogenic differentiation through activation of key promyogenic kinase (p38 MAPK) or ERK1/2 and MyoD transcription activities (MyoD family transcription factors play a key role in promoting myoblast differentiation) without affecting the Akt signaling pathway [13–15]. Another in vitro study, performed by Poussard et al., indicated Oligopin, a *pine bark* extract, as natural antioxidant; in fact, with aging, oxidative stress produces disruption of cytoskeleton and phosphorylated heat-shock protein beta-1 (HSPB1) may help to repair injured structures. Furthermore, Oligopin prevents the stress-induced phosphorylation of HSPB-1 in human cells [27]. Curcumin (*Curcuma longa*) may modulate the entry into apoptosis during immobilization and stimulate initial steps of muscle regeneration, aging on proteins and enzyme such as proteasome chymotrypsin-like activity and proapoptotic smac/DIABLO protein levels, and apoptosome-linked caspase-9 activities [59]. Another study was performed in humans with *Withania somnifera*: it seems to improve muscle strength and endurance for the aged subjects and so it could be used in preventing sarcopenia (500–750 mg twice daily for three months) [5]. Finally, Kim et al. demonstrate that physical exercise combined with tea catechin supplementation (350 mL of a tea beverage fortified with 540 mg of catechins) had a beneficial effect on physical function measured by walking ability and muscle mass in women with sarcopenia [65].

Lastly, a very recent study [35] demonstrated in animal models that loquat (*Eriobotrya japonica*) leaf extract (LE) diminished the age-associated loss of grip strength and enhanced muscle mass and muscle creatine kinase

(CK) activity. Histochemical analysis revealed that loquat (*Eriobotrya japonica*) leaf extract (LE) abrogated the age-associated decrease in cross-sectional area (CSA) and decreased the amount of connective tissue in the muscle of aged rats. Moreover, in order to investigate the mode of action, C2C12 murine myoblasts were used to evaluate the myogenic potential of LE. The expression levels of myogenic proteins (MyoD and myogenin) and functional myosin heavy chain (MyHC) were measured by western blot analysis. LE enhanced MyoD, myogenin, and MyHC expression. The changes in the expression of myogenic genes corresponded to an increase in the activity of CK, a myogenic differentiation marker. Finally, loquat (*Eriobotrya japonica*) leaf extract (LE) activated the Akt/mammalian target of rapamycin (mTOR) signaling pathway, which is involved in muscle protein synthesis during myogenesis. These findings suggest that loquat (*Eriobotrya japonica*) leaf extract (LE) attenuates sarcopenia by promoting myogenic differentiation and subsequently promoting muscle protein synthesis.

In conclusion, there are several preclinical lines of evidence for a variety of plants (*Camellia sinensis*, *Vitis vinifera*, *Ferula hermonis* Boiss., grape seed, *Broussonetia kazinoki*, *Corydalis turtschaninovii*, Hachimijiogan, *pine bark*, *Curcuma longa*, *Withania somnifera*, and *Eriobotrya japonica*), but only four studies are available in humans: two of these were conducted with supplementation of *Camellia sinensis* products, one with *Withania somnifera* and one with *grape seed*. In particular, the use of *Withania somnifera* (50–750 mg twice a day) resulted in improving muscle strength in human and also the supplementation with 540 mg of catechin from *Camellia sinensis* induced positive physical improvement. The second study demonstrated an improvement in grip strength, but it was only an experimental study with 25 mg of pure EGCG. Finally, the clinical trial with *grape seed* (100–200 mg/d) seemed to increase muscle mass and improve other physical conditions during menopause. For muscle regeneration, the main studies to take into account were those performed by Kim et al. and by Mishra et al., in which sarcopenic subjects have been enrolled. However, it is clear that the supplementation with EGCG should be complementary to appropriate physical exercise in order to reach the beneficial effects on muscle mass and that further studies are needed also for *Withania* supplementation.

## 4. Discussion

Currently, only diet and exercise are recognized as an effective means to counteract loss of muscle [53]. Regarding exercise, it is important to note that exercise-induced muscle damage (EIMD) can be caused by eccentric type or unaccustomed (novel) exercise and results in decrements in muscle force production, development of delayed-onset muscle soreness (DOMS) and swelling, rise in passive tension, and an increase in blood intramuscular proteins [66].

Delayed-onset muscle soreness is generally considered a hallmark sign of EIMD [67], and it is thought that DOMS is partially related to direct muscle fiber damage, and its magnitude appears to vary with the type, duration, and intensity of exercise [68].

TABLE 7: Botanicals with effects on muscle regeneration.

| Paper | Botanical | Compound | Model | Physiology | Results |
|---|---|---|---|---|---|
| | | | In vitro | | |
| Hwang et al., 2015 [14] | *Broussonetia kazinoki* | Kazinol-P (KP) | C2C12 and 10T1/2 cells | KP in 2% HS for 48 h, 10–1000 nM | Increase of expression of MHC, myogenin, and Troponin-T. Increase in the level of an actively phosphorylated form of p38 MAPK (pp38) in a dose-dependent manner. |
| Lee et al., 2014 [15] | *Corydalis turtschaninovii* | Tetrahydropalmatine (THP) | C2C12 myoblasts and fibroblast 10T1/2 | Various concentrations of THP | Enhancement of the expression of muscle-specific proteins, including MHC, MyoD, and myogenin. Increase in the levels of phosphorylated p38 MAPK. |
| Takeda et al., 2015 [13] | Hachimijiogan (HJG) | | Murine skeletal cells | HJG treatment (1–200 μg/mL) | 1.23-fold increase in the cell number. |
| Poussard et al., 2013 [27] | *Pinus pinaster* | Natural antioxidant: short oligomers of catechin and epicatechin | Human muscle satellite cells | 0.05 mg/mL | Block of the apoptosis and the protein oxidation. Recovery of HSPB1. |
| | | | Animals | | |
| Allouh, 2011 [58] | *Ferula hermonis* | Ferutinin, teferdin, teferin, and epoxy-benz | Adult male rats | 60 mg/kg/rat | Significant increase in muscle weight, fiber size, and nuclear number. |
| Bennett et al., 2013 [52] | *Vitis vinifera* | Resveratrol (3,5,4′-trihydroxystilbene) | Thirty-six male rats | 125 mg/kg/day | Favorable changes to type IIA and type IIB muscle fiber CSA and reduction of apoptotic signaling in muscles of old animal. |
| Alway et al., 2015 [48] | *Camellia sinensis* | Epicatechin, gallocatechin, epigallocatechin, epicatechin-3-gallate, and epigallocatechin-3-gallate | Sixty male rats | GTE (50 mg/kg body weight) | Counterbalance of the loss of hind limb plantaris muscle mass ($p < 0.05$) and tetanic force ($p < 0.05$) during HLS. Improvement of muscle fiber cross-sectional area in both plantaris ($p < 0.05$) and soleus after HLS. |
| Evans et al., 2010 [9] | *Camellia sinensis* | Gallocatechin, epigallocatechin, epicatechin, and epigallocatechin gallate | C57BL/6J and mdx mice | 0.25% or 0.5% green tea extract | Increase in the area of normal fiber morphology ($p \le 0.05$). Decrease in the area of regenerating fibers ($p \le 0.05$). |
| Ballak et al., 2015 [26] | *Vitis vinifera* | Resveratrol | Mice (male C57BL/6J mice) | 0.4 mg per gram body mass per day | No modification of the age-related decrease in muscle force, specific tension, or mass. |
| Gutierrez-Salmean et al., 2014 [53] | *Camellia sinensis* | Epicatechin | Young and old C57BL/6 male mice | 1 mg/kg b.i.d. | Significant decrease of myostatin levels in young and old mice (15% and 21%, resp.). Significant decrease of SA-β-Gal in old SkM (22%). |
| Vazeille et al., 2012 [59] | *Curcuma longa* | Curcumin | Male Wistar rats | 1 mg/kg body weight | Improvement of recovery during reloading. |
| Sung et al., 2015 [35] | *Eriobotrya japonica* | Leaf extract | Young (5-month-old) and aged (18-19-month-old) rats | 50 mg/kg/day | Enhancement in MyoD, myogenin, and MyHC expression. Activation of mTOR signaling pathway, which is involved in muscle protein synthesis during myogenesis. |

TABLE 7: Continued.

| Paper | Botanical | Compound | Model | Physiology | Results |
|-------|-----------|----------|-------|------------|---------|
| | | | | Humans | |
| Terauchi et al., 2014 [60] | Grape seeds | Proanthocyanidin of grape seeds | 91 women | 100 or 200 mg/d proanthocyanidin | Changes in lean mass and muscle mass from baseline to 8 weeks significantly higher in treated groups. |
| Gutierrez-Salmean et al., 2014 [53] | Camellia sinensis | Epicatechin | Human subjects ($n = 6$) | 25 mg of pure Epi (~1 mg/kg/day) | Increase in bilateral hand strength of ~7%. Significant increase ($49.2 \pm 16.6\%$) in the ratio of plasma follistatin/myostatin levels. |
| Kim et al., 2013 [24] | Camellia sinensis | Catechins | 128 women | 540 mg of catechins daily | Significant group × time interactions in TUG ($p = 0.005$), usual walking speed ($p = 0.007$), and maximum walking speed ($p < 0.001$). |
| Mishra and Trikamji, 2013 [5] | Withania somnifera | Alkaloids and steroidal lactones | 35 individuals | 500 mg of the whole root extract twice daily; 750 mg twice daily | Improvement of the strength and functioning of the muscle. |

The inflammatory response to EIMD results in the release into blood of reactive species from both neutrophils and macrophages and an array of cytokines from the injured muscle including tumor necrosis factor- (TNF-) $\alpha$, interleukin- (IL-) $1\beta$, and IL-6, which contribute to low-grade systemic inflammation and oxidative stress [69]. The proinflammatory and prooxidant response can provoke secondary tissue damage [70], thus prolonging the regenerative process, which is generally characterized by restoration of muscle strength and resolution of inflammation [70]. All these phenomena must be avoided in elderly sarcopenic subjects and so it is critical in this population to better preserve skeletal muscle and muscle function.

In this review, we focused our attention on effects of several botanicals on growth and health of muscle and we divided these effects into five categories: anti-inflammation, muscle damage prevention, antifatigue, muscle atrophy prevention, and muscle regeneration and differentiation.

To date, although the animal studies and in vitro studies are numerous and promising, studies in humans evaluating the effectiveness of anti-inflammatory and antioxidant activities of botanicals on welfare of skeletal muscle are still very few.

Although only relatively few human studies have been published on the potential use of botanicals for the prevention and treatment of muscle function, the present review is important because it highlights the need of continued efforts to find effective treatment of this debilitating condition. The available results, in particular considering human studies, suggest that the botanicals that may be potentially useful dietary supplements to prevent loss of muscle mass and function are curcumin from *Curcuma longa*, alkaloids and steroidal lactones from *Withania somnifera* (Solanaceae), catechins from *Camellia sinensis*, proanthocyanidin of *grape seeds*, and gingerols and shogaols from *Zingiber officinale*.

It should be noted that this review is not claiming that the use of these botanicals has been proven to prevent and treat loss of muscle mass and muscle function, but we believe that early and preliminary observations are promising. Further researches will support the use of these botanicals in the management of age-related muscle dysfunction and this may open the possibility of treating age-related loss of muscle mass and function with supplements.

## Conflict of Interests

The authors declare no conflict of interests regarding the publication of this paper.

## References

[1] Y. Rolland, S. Czerwinski, G. Abellan Van Kan et al., "Sarcopenia: its assessment, etiology, pathogenesis, consequences and future perspectives," *The Journal of Nutrition Health and Aging*, vol. 12, no. 7, pp. 433–450, 2008.

[2] A. J. Cruz-Jentoft, J. P. Baeyens, J. M. Bauer et al., "European working group on sarcopenia in older people. Sarcopenia: European consensus on definition and diagnosis: report of the European working group on sarcopenia in older people," *Age and Ageing*, vol. 39, no. 4, pp. 412–423, 2010.

[3] R. A. McGregor, D. Cameron-Smith, and S. D. Poppitt, "It is not just muscle mass: a review of muscle quality, composition and metabolism during ageing as determinants of muscle function and mobility in later life," *Longevity & Healthspan*, vol. 3, no. 1, article 9, 2014.

[4] M. Rondanelli, M. Faliva, F. Monteferrario et al., "Novel insights on nutrient management of sarcopenia in elderly," *BioMed Research International*, vol. 2015, Article ID 524948, 14 pages, 2015.

[5] S. K. Mishra and B. Trikamji, "A clinical trial with *Withania somnifera* (Solanaceae) extract in the management of sarcopenia," *Signpost Open Access Journal of Organic and Biomolecular Chemistry*, vol. 1, pp. 187–194, 2013.

[6] M. Egger, K. Dickersin, and G. D. Smith, "Problems and limitations in conducting systematic reviews," in *Systematic Reviews in Health Care: Meta-Analysis in Context*, M. Egger, G. D. Smith and, and D. G. altman, Eds., chapter 3, BMJ Books, London, UK, 2nd edition, 2001.

[7] J.-A. Kim, H.-S. Park, S.-R. Kang et al., "Suppressive effect of flavonoids from Korean citrus *aurantium* L. on the expression of inflammatory mediators in L6 skeletal muscle cells," *Phytotherapy Research*, vol. 26, no. 12, pp. 1904–1912, 2012.

[8] P. E. C. Leite, K. B. de Almeida, J. Lagrota-Candido et al., "Anti-inflammatory activity of *Eugenia punicifolia* extract on muscular lesion of mdx dystrophic mice," *Journal of Cellular Biochemistry*, vol. 111, no. 6, pp. 1652–1660, 2010.

[9] N. P. Evans, J. A. Call, J. Bassaganya-Riera, J. L. Robertson, and R. W. Grange, "Green tea extract decreases muscle pathology and NF-$\kappa$B immunostaining in regenerating muscle fibers of mdx mice," *Clinical Nutrition*, vol. 29, no. 3, pp. 391–398, 2010.

[10] S.-H. Yu, C.-Y. Huang, S.-D. Lee et al., "Decreased eccentric exercise-induced macrophage infiltration in skeletal muscle after supplementation with a class of ginseng-derived steroids," *PLoS ONE*, vol. 9, no. 12, Article ID e114649, 2014.

[11] K. Hirasaka, T. Maeda, C. Ikeda et al., "Isoflavones derived from soy beans prevent MuRF1-mediated muscle atrophy in C2C12 myotubes through SIRT1 activation," *Journal of Nutritional Science and Vitaminology*, vol. 59, no. 4, pp. 317–324, 2013.

[12] P. E. Leite, K. G. Lima-Araújo, G. R. França, J. Lagrota-Candido, W. C. Santos, and T. Quirico-Santos, "Implant of polymer containing pentacyclic triterpenes from *Eugenia punicifolia* inhibits inflammation and activates skeletal muscle remodeling," *Archivum Immunologiae et Therapiae Experimentalis*, vol. 62, no. 6, pp. 483–491, 2014.

[13] T. Takeda, K. Tsuji, B. Li, M. Tadakawa, and N. Yaegashi, "Proliferative effect of Hachimijiogan, a Japanese herbal medicine, in C2C12 skeletal muscle cells," *Clinical Interventions in Aging*, vol. 10, pp. 445–451, 2015.

[14] J. Hwang, S.-J. Lee, M. Yoo et al., "Kazinol-P from *Broussonetia kazinoki* enhances skeletal muscle differentiation via p38MAPK and MyoD," *Biochemical and Biophysical Research Communications*, vol. 456, no. 1, pp. 471–475, 2015.

[15] S.-J. Lee, M. Yoo, G.-Y. Go et al., "Tetrahydropalmatine promotes myoblast differentiation through activation of p38MAPK and MyoD," *Biochemical and Biophysical Research Communications*, vol. 455, no. 3-4, pp. 147–152, 2014.

[16] D.-T. Wang, Y. Yin, Y.-J. Yang et al., "Resveratrol prevents TNF-$\alpha$-induced muscle atrophy via regulation of Akt/mTOR/FoxO1 signaling in C2C12 myotubes," *International Immunopharmacology*, vol. 19, no. 2, pp. 206–213, 2014.

[17] C.-W. Hou, S.-D. Lee, C.-L. Kao et al., "Improved inflammatory balance of human skeletal muscle during exercise after supplementations of the ginseng-based steroid rg1," *PLoS ONE*, vol. 10, no. 1, Article ID e0116387, 2015.

[18] J. Díaz-Castro, R. Guisado, N. Kajarabille et al., "*Phlebodium decumanum* is a natural supplement that ameliorates the oxidative stress and inflammatory signalling induced by strenuous exercise in adult humans," *European Journal of Applied Physiology*, vol. 112, no. 8, pp. 3119–3128, 2012.

[19] Y. Guo, K. Niu, T. Okazaki et al., "Coffee treatment prevents the progression of sarcopenia in aged mice in vivo and in vitro," *Experimental Gerontology*, vol. 50, no. 1, pp. 1–8, 2014.

[20] S. Haramizu, N. Ota, T. Hase, and T. Murase, "Catechins suppress muscle inflammation and hasten performance recovery after exercise," *Medicine and Science in Sports and Exercise*, vol. 45, no. 9, pp. 1694–1702, 2013.

[21] J. Chen, X. Wang, Y. Cai et al., "Bioactivity-guided fractionation of physical fatigue-attenuating components from *Rubus parvifolius* L.," *Molecules*, vol. 18, no. 9, pp. 11624–11638, 2013.

[22] L. M. Nicol, D. S. Rowlands, R. Fazakerly, and J. Kellett, "Curcumin supplementation likely attenuates delayed onset muscle soreness (DOMS)," *European Journal of Applied Physiology*, vol. 115, no. 8, pp. 1769–1777, 2015.

[23] F. Drobnic, J. Riera, G. Appendino et al., "Reduction of delayed onset muscle soreness by a novel curcumin delivery system (Meriva⁵): a randomised, placebo-controlled trial," *Journal of the International Society of Sports Nutrition*, vol. 11, article 31, 2014.

[24] J. A. Kim, H. S. Park, K. I. Park et al., "Proteome analysis of the anti-inflammatory response of flavonoids isolated from Korean *Citrus aurantium* L. in lipopolysaccharide-induced L6rat skeletal muscle cells," *The American Journal of Chinese Medicine*, vol. 41, no. 4, pp. 901–912, 2013.

[25] K. A. Mirza, S. L. Pereira, N. K. Edens, and M. J. Tisdale, "Attenuation of muscle wasting in murine $C_2C_{12}$ myotubes by epigallocatechin-3-gallate," *Journal of Cachexia, Sarcopenia and Muscle*, vol. 5, no. 4, pp. 339–345, 2014.

[26] S. B. Ballak, R. T. Jaspers, L. Deldicque et al., "Blunted hypertrophic response in old mouse muscle is associated with a lower satellite cell density and is not alleviated by resveratrol," *Experimental Gerontology*, vol. 62, pp. 23–31, 2015.

[27] S. Poussard, A. Pires-Alves, R. Diallo, J.-W. Dupuy, and E. Dargelos, "A natural antioxidant pine bark extract, oligopin⁵, regulates the stress chaperone HSPB1 in human skeletal muscle cells: a proteomics approach," *Phytotherapy Research*, vol. 27, no. 10, pp. 1529–1535, 2013.

[28] Y. Kishida, S. Kagawa, J. Arimitsua et al., "Go-sha-jinki-Gan (GJG), a traditional Japanese herbal medicine, protects against sarcopenia in senescence-accelerated mice," *Phytomedicine*, vol. 22, no. 1, pp. 16–22, 2015.

[29] A. Frati, D. Landi, C. Marinelli et al., "Nutraceutical properties of chestnut flours: beneficial effects on skeletal muscle atrophy," *Food and Function*, vol. 5, no. 11, pp. 2870–2882, 2014.

[30] Y. Tanabe, S. Maeda, N. Akazawa et al., "Attenuation of indirect markers of eccentric exercise-induced muscle damage by curcumin," *European Journal of Applied Physiology*, vol. 115, no. 9, pp. 1949–1957, 2015.

[31] I. Boz, M. Belviranli, and N. Okudan, "Curcumin modulates muscle damage but not oxidative stress and antioxidant defense following eccentric exercise in rats," *International Journal for Vitamin and Nutrition Research*, vol. 84, no. 3-4, pp. 163–172, 2014.

[32] S.-Y. Wang, W.-C. Huang, C.-C. Liu et al., "Pumpkin (*Cucurbita moschata*) fruit extract improves physical fatigue and exercise performance in mice," *Molecules*, vol. 17, no. 10, pp. 11864–11876, 2012.

[33] T.-S. Yeh, C.-C. Huang, H.-L. Chuang, and M.-C. Hsu, "Angelica sinensis improves exercise performance and protects against physical fatigue in trained mice," *Molecules*, vol. 19, no. 4, pp. 3926–3939, 2014.

[34] M. D. Matsumura, G. S. Zavorsky, and J. M. Smoliga, "The effects of pre-exercise ginger supplementation on muscle damage and delayed onset muscle soreness," *Phytotherapy Research*, vol. 29, no. 6, pp. 887–893, 2015.

[35] B. Sung, S. Y. Hwang, M. J. Kim et al., "Loquat leaf extract enhances myogenic differentiation, improves muscle function and attenuates muscle loss in aged rats," *International Journal of Molecular Medicine*, vol. 36, no. 3, pp. 792–800, 2015.

[36] A. A. Raut, N. N. Rege, F. M. Tadvi et al., "Exploratory study to evaluate tolerability, safety, and activity of Ashwagandha (*Withania somnifera*) in healthy volunteers," *Journal of Ayurveda and Integrative Medicine*, vol. 3, no. 3, pp. 111–114, 2012.

[37] S. JiPing, "Antifatigue effect of aqueous extract of salvia in endurance training rats' skeletal muscle," *International Journal of Physical Sciences*, vol. 6, no. 11, pp. 2697–2700, 2011.

[38] H.-Y. Jung, A.-N. Lee, T.-J. Song et al., "Korean mistletoe (*Viscum album coloratum*) extract improves endurance capacity in mice by stimulating mitochondrial activity," *Journal of Medicinal Food*, vol. 15, no. 7, pp. 621–628, 2012.

[39] I. Nallamuthu, A. Tamatam, and F. Khanum, "Effect of hydroalcoholic extract of *Aegle marmelos* fruit on radical scavenging activity and exercise-endurance capacity in mice," *Pharmaceutical Biology*, vol. 52, no. 5, pp. 551–559, 2014.

[40] S. S. Li, Z. C. Chen, and C. H. Zhang, "Effect of Tao-Hong-Si-Wu-Tang, a traditional Chinese herbal medicine formula, on physical fatigue in mice," *African Journal of Traditional, Complementary and Alternative Medicines*, vol. 10, no. 1, pp. 60–65, 2013.

[41] S. Tan, F. Zhou, N. Li et al., "Anti-fatigue effect of ginsenoside Rb1 on postoperative fatigue syndrome induced by major small intestinal resection in rat," *Biological & Pharmaceutical Bulletin*, vol. 36, no. 10, pp. 1634–1639, 2013.

[42] L.-Z. Huang, B.-K. Huang, Q. Ye, and L.-P. Qin, "Bioactivity-guided fractionation for anti-fatigue property of *Acanthopanax senticosus*," *Journal of Ethnopharmacology*, vol. 133, no. 1, pp. 213–219, 2011.

[43] M. Vitadello, E. Germinario, B. Ravara, L. D. Libera, D. Danieli-Betto, and L. Gorza, "Curcumin counteracts loss of force and atrophy of hindlimb unloaded rat soleus by hampering neuronal nitric oxide synthase untethering from sarcolemma," *The Journal of Physiology*, vol. 592, no. 12, pp. 2637–2652, 2014.

[44] A. Hernández-Santana, V. Pérez-López, J. M. Zubeldia, and M. Jiménez-Del-Rio, "A rhodiola rosea root extract protects skeletal muscle cells against chemically induced oxidative stress by modulating heat shock protein 70 (HSP70) expression," *Phytotherapy Research*, vol. 28, no. 4, pp. 623–628, 2014.

[45] Y.-H. Lee, D.-H. Kim, Y. S. Kim, and T.-J. Kim, "Prevention of oxidative stress-induced apoptosis of C2C12 myoblasts by a *Cichorium intybus* root extract," *Bioscience, Biotechnology and Biochemistry*, vol. 77, no. 2, pp. 375–377, 2013.

[46] E. Dargelos, C. Brulé, P. Stuelsatz et al., "Up-regulation of calcium-dependent proteolysis in human myoblasts under acute oxidative stress," *Experimental Cell Research*, vol. 316, no. 1, pp. 115–125, 2010.

[47] Y. Nakashima, I. Ohsawa, K. Nishimaki et al., "Preventive effects of *Chlorella* on skeletal muscle atrophy in muscle-specific mitochondrial aldehyde dehydrogenase 2 activity-deficient mice," *BMC complementary and alternative medicine*, vol. 14, article 390, 2014.

[48] S. E. Alway, B. T. Bennett, J. C. Wilson et al., "Green tea extract attenuates muscle loss and improves muscle function during disuse, but fails to improve muscle recovery following unloading in aged rats," *Journal of Applied Physiology*, vol. 118, no. 3, pp. 319–330, 2015.

[49] N. Kawanishi, K. Kato, M. Takahashi et al., "Curcumin attenuates oxidative stress following downhill running-induced muscle damage," *Biochemical and Biophysical Research Communications*, vol. 441, no. 3, pp. 573–578, 2013.

[50] J. Rodriguez, H. Gilson, C. Jamart et al., "Pomegranate and green tea extracts protect against ER stress induced by a high-fat diet in skeletal muscle of mice," *European Journal of Nutrition*, vol. 54, pp. 377–389, 2014.

[51] J. R. Jackson, M. J. Ryan, and S. E. Alway, "Long-term supplementation with resveratrol alleviates oxidative stress but does not attenuate sarcopenia in aged mice," *Journals of Gerontology. Series A Biological Sciences and Medical Sciences*, vol. 66, no. 7, pp. 751–764, 2011.

[52] B. T. Bennett, J. S. Mohamed, and S. E. Alway, "Effects of resveratrol on the recovery of muscle mass following disuse in the plantaris muscle of aged rats," *PLoS ONE*, vol. 8, no. 12, Article ID e83518, 2013.

[53] G. Gutierrez-Salmean, T. P. Ciaraldi, L. Nogueira et al., "Effects of (-)-epicatechin on molecular modulators of skeletal muscle growth and differentiation," *The Journal of Nutritional Biochemistry*, vol. 25, no. 1, pp. 91–94, 2014.

[54] C. D. Black, M. P. Herring, D. J. Hurley, and P. J. O'Connor, "Ginger (*Zingiber officinale*) reduces muscle pain caused by eccentric exercise," *The Journal of Pain*, vol. 11, no. 9, pp. 894–903, 2010.

[55] K. L. Pumpa, K. E. Fallon, A. Bensoussan, and S. Papalia, "The effects of *Panax notoginseng* on delayed onset muscle soreness and muscle damage in well-trained males: a double blind randomised controlled trial," *Complementary Therapies in Medicine*, vol. 21, no. 3, pp. 131–140, 2013.

[56] R. A. Shanely, D. C. Nieman, K. A. Zwetsloot et al., "Evaluation of *Rhodiola rosea* supplementation on skeletal muscle damage and inflammation in runners following a competitive marathon," *Brain, Behavior, and Immunity*, vol. 39, pp. 204–210, 2014.

[57] S. Choquette, T. Dion, M. Brochu, and I. J. Dionne, "Soy isoflavones and exercise to improve physical capacity in post-menopausal women," *Climacteric*, vol. 16, no. 1, pp. 70–77, 2013.

[58] M. Z. Allouh, "Effect of *Ferula hermonis* root extract on rat skeletal muscle adaptation to exercise," *Experimental Biology and Medicine*, vol. 236, no. 12, pp. 1373–1378, 2011.

[59] E. Vazeille, L. Slimani, A. Claustre et al., "Curcumin treatment prevents increased proteasome and apoptosome activities in rat skeletal muscle during reloading and improves subsequent recovery," *The Journal of Nutritional Biochemistry*, vol. 23, no. 3, pp. 245–251, 2012.

[60] M. Terauchi, N. Horiguchi, A. Kajiyama et al., "Effects of grape seed proanthocyanidin extract on menopausal symptoms, body composition, and cardiovascular parameters in middle-aged women: a randomized, double-blind, placebo-controlled pilot study," *Menopause*, vol. 21, no. 9, pp. 990–996, 2014.

[61] C. D. Black and P. J. O'Connor, "Acute effects of dietary ginger on muscle pain induced by eccentric exercise," *Phytotherapy Research*, vol. 24, no. 11, pp. 1620–1626, 2010.

[62] N. Alamdari, P. O'Neal, and P.-O. Hasselgren, "Curcumin and muscle wasting—a new role for an old drug?" *Nutrition*, vol. 25, no. 2, pp. 125–129, 2009.

[63] A. Shehzad and Y. S. Lee, "Molecular mechanisms of curcumin action: signal transduction," *BioFactors*, vol. 39, no. 1, pp. 27–36, 2013.

[64] M. Peleli, I.-K. Aggeli, A. N. Matralis, A. P. Kourounakis, I. Beis, and C. Gaitanaki, "Evaluation of two novel antioxidants with differential effects on curcumin-induced apoptosis in C2 skeletal myoblasts; involvement of JNKs," *Bioorganic and Medicinal Chemistry*, vol. 23, no. 3, pp. 390–400, 2015.

[65] H. Kim, T. Suzuki, K. Saito et al., "Effects of exercise and tea catechins on muscle mass, strength and walking ability in community-dwelling elderly Japanese sarcopenic women: a randomized controlled trial," *Geriatrics & Gerontology International*, vol. 13, no. 2, pp. 458–465, 2013.

[66] G. Howatson and K. A. van Someren, "The prevention and treatment of exercise-induced muscle damage," *Sports Medicine*, vol. 38, no. 6, pp. 483–503, 2008.

[67] G. L. Warren, D. A. Lowe, and R. B. Armstrong, "Measurement tools used in the study of eccentric contraction-induced injury," *Sports Medicine*, vol. 27, no. 1, pp. 43–59, 1999.

[68] K. Cheung, P. A. Hume, and L. Maxwell, "Delayed onset muscle soreness: treatment strategies and performance factors," *Sports Medicine*, vol. 33, no. 2, pp. 145–164, 2003.

[69] L. Hirose, K. Nosaka, M. Newton et al., "Changes in inflammatory mediators following eccentric exercise of the elbow flexors," *Exercise Immunology Review*, vol. 10, pp. 75–90, 2004.

[70] P. M. Clarkson and M. J. Hubal, "Exercise-induced muscle damage in humans," *American Journal of Physical Medicine & Rehabilitation*, vol. 81, no. 11, pp. S52–S69, 2002.

# 3

# Guizhi Fuling Wan, a Traditional Chinese Herbal Formula, Sensitizes Cisplatin-Resistant Human Ovarian Cancer Cells through Inactivation of the PI3K/AKT/mTOR Pathway

**Li Han,**[1] **Xiaojuan Guo,**[1] **Hua Bian,**[1] **Lei Yang,**[1]
**Zhong Chen,**[2] **Wenhua Zang,**[1] **and Jingke Yang**[3]

[1]*Zhang Zhongjing College of Chinese Medicine, Nanyang Institute of Technology, 80 Changjiang Road, Nanyang 473004, China*
[2]*College of Pharmaceutical Science, Soochow University, 199 Ren-ai Road, Suzhou 215123, China*
[3]*Affiliated Cancer Hospital, Zhengzhou University, Dongming Road 127, Zhengzhou 450008, China*

Correspondence should be addressed to Li Han; hanlxv@live.com

Academic Editor: Youn C. Kim

The aim of the study was to explore the possible mechanisms that Guizhi Fuling Wan (GFW) enhances the sensitivity of the SKOV3/DDP ovarian cancer cells and the resistant xenograft tumours to cisplatin. Rat medicated sera containing GFW were prepared by administering GFW to rats, and the primary bioactive constituents of the sera were gallic acid, paeonol, and paeoniflorin analysed by HPLC/QqQ MS. Cell counting kit-8 analysis was shown that coincubation of the sera with cisplatin/paclitaxel enhanced significantly the cytotoxic effect of cisplatin or paclitaxel in SKOV3/DDP cells. The presence of the rat medicated sera containing GFW resulted in an increase in rhodamine 123 accumulation by flow cytometric assays and a decrease in the protein levels of P-gp, phosphorylation of AKT at Ser473, and mTOR in a dose-dependent manner in SKOV3/DDP cells by western blot analysis, but the sera had no effect on the protein levels of PI3K p110α and total AKT. The low dose of GFW enhanced the anticancer efficacy of cisplatin and paclitaxel treatment in resistant SKOV3/DDP xenograft tumours. GFW could sensitize cisplatin-resistant SKOV3/DDP cells by inhibiting the protein level and function of P-gp, which may be medicated through inactivation of the PI3K/AKT/mTOR pathway.

## 1. Introduction

Ovarian cancer (OC) is the most lethal of the gynaecological malignancies, largely due to the concealed pathogenesis of OC and advanced stage (FIGO stages III and IV) at diagnosis in most patients [1]. The standard of care in the initial chemotherapeutic management of advanced OC is the combination of a platinum agent (carboplatin or cisplatin) and a taxane agent (paclitaxel or docetaxel) given intravenously [2]. Most ovarian cancer patients will respond to initial chemotherapy, but the long-term survival remains poor as a result of recurrence and drug resistance, leading to a 5-year survival rate of 46% [3]. Stordal et al. demonstrated that the recurrence/drug resistance in OC patients treated with first-line platinum/taxane

chemotherapy was related to the overexpression of P-glycoprotein (P-gp) [4]. Other studies have shown that the main mechanism of drug resistance was also due to P-gp expression in doxorubicin-, vincristine-, and paclitaxel-resistant OC cell lines [5] and in OC patients [6]. Because P-gp overexpression plays an important role in the recurrence or drug resistance in OC chemotherapy, it is a problem that should be solved quickly to identify P-gp inhibitors and then improve the chemotherapy sensitivity for OC patients.

Unfortunately, there are no agents currently available to "block" P-gp-mediated resistance in the clinic, although four generations of P-gp inhibitors have been developed, and most of them have shown considerable *in vitro* success. The failure may be attributed to nonspecific toxicity, adverse drug interaction, and numerous pharmacokinetic issues associated with the use of P-gp inhibitors in the conducted clinical trials [7]. Thus, novel P-gp inhibitors with proven efficacy and minimal toxicity and/or adverse effects are urgently required to overcome P-gp-mediated resistance in cancer chemotherapy.

Guizhi Fuling Wan (GFW; Gyejibokryeong-hwan in Korean and Keishi-bukuryo-gan in Japan) is a well-known traditional Chinese herbal formula, comprising the five herbs *Ramulus Cinnamomi cassiae, Scierotium Poriae cocos, Radix Albus paeoniae Lactiflorae, Cortex Radicis moutan,* and *Semen Pruni persicae.* GFW originally appeared in *Essential Pre-scriptions from the Golden Cabinet* (Jinkui Yaolue), a classic clinical book of traditional Chinese medicine (TCM), written by Zhang Zhongjing (150–219 AD) at the end of the Eastern Han Dynasty. GFW has been used extensively throughout Asia in the treatment of blood stasis, and it has been proven to be very safe and effective with fewer harmful side effects. Modern medical research has shown that GFW has various therapeutic effects on conditions such as inflammatory skin disorders [8], endometriosis [9], diabetes-mellitus-induced neuropathology [10], and atherosclerosis [11]. GFW capsules are currently being assessed for the efficacy, safety, and dose-response in the treatment of primary dysmenorrhea by the USA Food and Drug Administration (FDA) [12, 13]. In the recent years, it was reported that catechin, one of the chemical constituents of GFW, is a potent P-gp inhibitor [14]. Moreover, it was demonstrated that the main bioactive constituents of GFW in rat plasma include gallic acid, amygdalin, albiflorin, paeoniflorin, paeonol, cinnamic acid, dehydrotumulosic acid, tumulosic acid, and polyporic acid C [15, 16], while gallic acid, paeonol, and dehydrotumulosic acid were found to have a potent P-gp inhibition effect on mul-tidrug resistance (MDR) cell lines [17–19], and paeoniflorin was found to modulate MDR of the human gastric cancer cell line SGC7901/vincristine (VCR) effectively at nontoxic concentrations via inhibiting the activation of NF-kappaB and subsequently downregulating its target genes *MDR1,* which encodes P-gp [20]. Therefore, accumulating studies have shown that GFW may be a formula demonstrating a P-gp inhibition effect, a finding that has not yet been reported elsewhere.

Recently, more and more researchers have come to realize that drug resistance is a complex phenomenon involving multiple mechanisms, including the activation of multiple signalling pathways. Growing evidence has suggested that the phosphatidylinositol 3-kinase (PI3K)/AKT/mammalian target of rapamycin (mTOR) pathway, wherein *MDR1* and NF-kappaB are downstream factors of this pathway, is closely related to the occurrence of drug resistance in cancer [21–23]. It was also found that cisplatin resistance to OC was related to the PI3K/AKT/mTOR pathway [22]. However, the effect of GFW on the pathway has never been explored.

The aims of the present experiments were to investi-gate whether GFW has inhibitory effects on P-gp and to identify the underlying molecular mechanisms involving the PI3K/AKT/mTOR pathway in human MDR OC cell lines, SKOV3/DDP, and mouse xenograft model generated from SKOV3/DDP cells.

## 2. Materials and Methods

*2.1. Plant Materials and Preparation of the GFW Extract.* The five herbals forming GFW—that is, *Ramulus Cinnamomi cas-siae* (Batch number 201409), *Scierotium Poriae cocos* (Batch number 201410), *Radix Albus paeoniae Lactiflorae* (Batch number 201410), *Cortex Radicis moutan* (Batch number 201409), and *Semen Pruni persicae* (Batch number 201408)—were purchased from the Zhang Zhongjing Pharmacy Chain-Like Limited Company (Nanyang, China). The origin of these herbals was taxonomically double confirmed by Professor Xianzhang Huang, a plant taxonomist from the Zhang Zhongjing College of Chinese Medicine, Nanyang Institute of Technology, where the voucher specimens were deposited.

GFW was prepared in accordance with the process as stated in the Chinese Pharmacopeia (2010 Edition) [24]. Briefly, *Cortex Radicis moutan* was submerged in water and submitted to water distillation (WD) for 1 h with a standard apparatus for extracting volatile oil. The dregs of *Cortex Radicis moutan* were put together with *Ramulus Cinnamomi cassiae, Scierotium Poriae cocos, Radix Albus paeoniae Lac-tiflorae,* and *Semen Pruni persicae* and then were extracted twice (60 min per time) by refluxing with 90% ethanol (EtOH). The EtOH extracts were combined, filtered, and evaporated under reduced pressure to the appropriate vol-ume. The dregs of the five herbs were extracted subsequently twice (60 min per time) with water. The water extracts were combined, filtered, and evaporated under reduced pressure to the appropriate volume. The concentrated EtOH extract was next combined with the water extract and volatile oil uniformly, and the concentration was adjusted to 1.5 g/mL corresponding to the crude herbs. The mixed solution was used for animal studies and preparing the rat medicated sera.

*2.2. Cell Culture.* The human OC SKOV3 cell line and its cisplatin-resistant SKOV3/DDP cell line were obtained from the Chinese Academy of Medical Sciences and Peking Union Medical College. The cells were cultured in RPMI 1640 (Gibco BRL, Grand Island, NY, USA) supplemented with 10% (v/v) foetal bovine sera (FBS; Hyclone, Logan, UT, USA) at 37°C in a humidified atmosphere containing 5% $CO_2$. To maintain resistance, SKOV3/DDP cells were cultured in medium containing $1 \mu g$/mL cisplatin (Qilu Pharmaceutical Co., Ltd., Shandong, China).

*2.3. Preparation of Rat Medicated Sera.* The rat medicated sera were prepared according to the published protocols [25]. Briefly, 60 Wistar female rats, aged between 6 and 8 weeks old and weighing 220~250 g, were randomly divided into four groups (15 rats per group): the control group was given normal saline by gavage, and low-dose (LD) GFW group, middle-dose (MD) GFW group, and high-dose (HD) GFW group were given the mixed GFW solution by gavage at dosages of $4 \text{ g·kg}^{-1}\text{·d}^{-1}$, $8 \text{ g·kg}^{-1}\text{·d}^{-1}$, and $16 \text{ g·kg}^{-1}\text{·d}^{-1}$, respectively. The animals were supplied by the Henan Exper-imental Animal Center (Zhengzhou, China) and maintained in an air-conditioned room with a controlled temperature of $22 \pm 2°C$, a humidity level of 45% to 65%, and a 12-/12-hour light/dark cycle. After 5 days of administration, the rats were anaesthetized, and the blood was collected from the abdominal aorta and centrifuged. The collected sera were aliquoted into 1 mL Eppendorf tubes and preserved at $-80°C$ for future use. This study was carried out in strict accordance with the recommendations in the Guide for the Care and Use of Laboratory Animals of the National Institutes of Health. The protocol was approved by the Committee on the Ethics of Animal Experiments of the Nanyang Institute of Technology (Permit number: 2014-L38). The whole surgery was performed under sodium pentobarbital anaesthesia, and all efforts were made to minimize suffering.

### 2.4. Bioactive Constituents of GFW Analysis by HPLC/QqQ MS.
An aliquot of $100 \mu L$ of LD sera was pipetted into a 1.5 mL capped polypropylene tube, $400 \mu L$ of methanol was added, and the contents were mixed by vortexing for 30 s. After centrifuging at $12,000 \times g$ for 5 min, $400 \mu L$ of the supernatant was transferred to a 10 mL glass tube and evaporated to dryness under a steam of nitrogen at $+50°C$. The residue was redissolved with $100 \mu L$ of the mobile phase and briefly vortexed. After centrifuging at $13,000 \times g$ for 5 min at room temperature again, the supernatant was transferred into a glass autosampler vial and $20 \mu L$ aliquot of supernatant was injected into the HPLC/Q-TOF MS system. Gallic acid (catalogue #91215, Sigma-Aldrich, St. Louis, MO, USA), paeoniflorin (catalogue #P0038, Sigma-Aldrich), and paeonol (catalogue #H35803, Sigma-Aldrich) were separately prepared in $100 \mu L$ of blank sera to obtain concentrations of 20.0, 10.0, and 40.0 ng/mL, respectively. The spiked sera were prepared as mentioned above for the LD sera and were analysed by the same system.

The HPLC was a ThermoFisher ACCELA LC system. The mobile phase consists of a mixed aqueous solution of methanol-ammonium acetate (5 mM). The flow rate was set at 0.3 mL/min. The column temperature was maintained at $30°C$. Detection was achieved using a ThermoFisher TSQ Quantum Ultra Triple-Quadrupole Mass Spectrometer with an electrospray ionization (ESI) interface in the negative-ion mode. The parameter settings were as follows: spray voltage, 2,000 V; capillary temperature, $400°C$; sheath gas (nitrogen), 40 arbitrary units; auxiliary gas (nitrogen), 10 arbitrary units; vaporizer temperature, room temperature. Detection of the compounds was performed in the selected-ion monitoring (SIM) mode with $m/z$ 169.0 $[M - H]^-$ for gallic acid, $m/z$ 479.4 $[M - H]^-$ for paeoniflorin, and $m/z$ 167.0 $[M - H]^-$ for paeonol. ThermoFisher LCQUAN software was used to analyse the chromatograms.

### 2.5. Cytotoxicity Assay.
The ability of the rat medicated sera containing GFW to potentiate cisplatin or paclitaxel (Hisun Pharmaceutical Co., Ltd., Zhejiang, China) cytotoxicity was evaluated in SKOV3/DDP and SKOV3 cells using cell counting kit-8 (CCK-8) (Sigma-Aldrich, St. Louis, MO, USA) assay [26]. Briefly, the cells were harvested in the exponential growth phase and were seeded into 96-well plates at a density of $1.0 \times 10^4$ cells per well. The supernatant was

removed after the cells adhered to the wall, and then FBS-free RPMI 1640 medium was added followed by incubation for another 24 hours at $37°C$. Additionally, the cells were treated with the rat medicated control sera, the LD, MD, and HD sera, the LD sera, or verapamil (VER, Harvest Pharmaceutical Co., Ltd., Shanghai, China; $5 \mu mol/L$) plus cisplatin or paclitaxel. The sera volume ratio for incubation is 10%. After incubation at $37°C$ for 72 hours, WST-8 [2-(2-methoxy-4-nitrophenyl)-3-(4-nitrophenyl)-5-(2, 4-disulfophenyl)-2H tetrazolium, monosodium salt], which can be bioreduced by cellular dehydrogenases to an orange formazan product, which is then dissolved in cell culture medium, was added to the cells at a volume ratio of 1 : 10 to incubate for 2.5 hours. The optical density (OD) was measured at 450 nm using an enzyme immunoassay analyser (Dynatech MR4100, USA). Cell viability (% of control) was calculated as follows: $(OD_{test} - OD_{blank})/(OD_{control} - OD_{blank})$ and growth inhibition rate was calculated as follows: 1 − cell viability%. The concentrations required to inhibit growth by 50% ($IC_{50}$ values) were calculated from the cytotoxicity curves using Bliss's method. The resistance fold values, used as the parameter for resistance, were calculated by dividing the $IC_{50}$ of SKOV3/DDP cells by the $IC_{50}$ of SKOV3 cells to cisplatin or paclitaxel or other combinations as above. The reversal fold values, used as the potency parameter for reversal, were calculated by dividing the $IC_{50}$ of cisplatin or paclitaxel alone by the $IC_{50}$ of cisplatin or paclitaxel in combination with the LD sera or VER.

### 2.6. Flow Cytometric Assay of Rhodamine 123 Cellular Accumulation.
The assay to analyse the function of P-gp in SKOV3/DDP cells was carried out using a modified method as previously described [27]. Briefly, the cells were adjusted to a density of $2 \times 10^6$/mL, resuspended in serum-free medium, and distributed as 0.5 mL aliquots into 1 mL Eppendorf tubes. The LD, MD, and HD sera, VER ($5 \mu mol/L$), and vehicle were added to the aliquoted samples, and the samples were incubated at $37°C$ for 24 h before rhodamine 123 (Rho123; Sigma-Aldrich, St. Louis, MO, USA) was added at a final concentration of 0.5 $\mu g$/mL. The tubes were incubated further at $37°C$ for 1 h, and then the samples were transferred to 4 mL flow cytometry tubes and washed twice with ice-cold phosphate-buffered saline (PBS) before being resuspended in 0.5 mL of PBS. Flow cytometry analysis was carried out to evaluate the mean fluorescence intensity (MFI) of Rho123 in SKOV3/DDP cell using the EPICS XL-MCL flow cytometer (Beckman Coulter, Fullerton, CA, USA). All analyses were performed in duplicate in at least three separate experiments. The data were analysed using Expo32 ADC software (Beckman Coulter, Fullerton, CA, USA).

### 2.7. Western Blotting Assay.
Western blotting analyses of P-gp, PI3K, AKT, phospho-AKT (p-AKT), and mTOR proteins were performed using a slight modification of the method described previously [28]. Briefly, SKOV3/DDP cells were seeded into 6-well plates at a density of $2.0 \times 10^6$ cells per well and were treated with the rat medicated control sera, the LD, MD, and HD sera for 72 h, and then the

cells were lysed using RIPA lysis buffer (Beyotime Institute of Biotechnology, China). The protein concentrations were determined using the bicinchoninic acid assay (BCA; Santa Cruz Biotechnology, USA). A total of $40\,\mu g$ of proteins was electrophoresed via sodium dodecyl sulphate polyacrylamide gel electrophoresis (SDS-PAGE) and transferred onto nitro-cellulose membranes (Millipore, USA), which were then blocked with 5% skimmed milk powder for 1 hour at room temperature. The membranes were next incubated with rabbit polyclonal antibody to PI3K p110$\alpha$ (clone H-201, catalogue #sc-7174, 1:500 dilution; Santa Cruz Biotechnology), AKT (clone H-136, catalogue #sc-8312, 1:1000 dilution; Santa Cruz Biotechnology), p-AKT (Ser473, catalogue #sc-33437, 1:1000 dilution; Santa Cruz Biotechnology), mTOR (clone H-266, catalogue #sc-8319, 1:1000 dilution; Santa Cruz Biotechnology), or mouse monoclonal antibody to human P-gp (catalogue #sc-55510, 1:500 dilution; Santa Cruz Biotechnology) and $\beta$-actin (catalogue #sc-47778, 1:500 dilution; Santa Cruz Biotechnology) at 4°C overnight. Following primary antibody incubation, the membranes were washed with TBST, and goat anti-rabbit IRDye 800CW (926-32211, 1:5000 dilution) or goat anti-mouse IRDye 680LT secondary antibody (926-68020, 1:10000 dilution; Li-COR Biosciences, NE, USA) was added, respectively. After incubation at room temperature for 2 hours, the bands were detected using the Odyssey Infrared Fluorescent Western Blots Imaging System from Li-COR Bioscience (Lincoln, NE, USA). The optical density of each band was measured with a computer-assisted imaging analysis system (Quantity One, Bio-Rad, Hemel Hempstead, UK) and the relative protein levels were normalized to optical density of $\beta$-actin.

*2.8. In Vivo Tumour Xenografts and Reversing Efficacy Test.* The ability of GFW to potentiate the antitumour activity of cisplatin/paclitaxel was evaluated using the SKOV3/DDP xenografts as described previously [29]. Briefly, female BALB/c nude mice, aged between 3 and 4 weeks and weighing 20~22 g, were housed in standard microisolator conditions free of pathogens and used in accordance with the Animal Care and Use protocol approved by Nanyang Institute of Technology. Next, $2 \times 10^7$ SKOV3/DDP cells were injected into the left flanks of each mouse selected for the experiment. When the tumours reached a diameter of circa 6 mm (approximately 116 mm$^3$), the mice were randomly divided into different treatment groups comprising 10 mice in each group: a control group (normal saline administered orally and consecutively for 21 days), a single LD GFW group at dosage of $4\,\text{g}\cdot\text{kg}^{-1}\cdot\text{d}^{-1}$ administered orally for 21 days, a cisplatin (10 mg/kg administered intraperitoneally (i.p.) per 4 days) plus paclitaxel (15 mg/kg administered intravenously (i.v.) per 3 days) group, a combination of cisplatin, paclitaxel, and LD GFW group, and a combination of cisplatin, paclitaxel, and VER ($5.0\,\text{mg}\cdot\text{kg}^{-1}$ administrated i.v. for 21 days) group. The animals were weighed, and the tumour length ($L$) and width ($W$) were measured every 4 days. The tumour volume ($TV$) was calculated according to published article [30] as follows: $TV = 1/2 \times L \times W^2$. After the last treatment, tumours were resected and weighted. The percent

of tumour growth inhibition was calculated by comparing the average tumour weights of the treated groups with those of the tumour-bearing control group. Tumour growth in saline treated control animals was taken to be at 100%.

*2.9. Statistical Analysis.* For all of the experiments, the data are presented as the mean ± SD. Tests for significant differences between the groups were performed using one-way ANOVA with multiple comparisons (Fisher's pairwise comparisons) using SPSS 20.0. A minimum $P$ value of 0.05 was estimated as the significance level for all tests. Graphic representations were performed using GraphPad Prism version 6.01 for Windows.

## 3. Results

*3.1. Bioactive Constituents in Rat Medicated Sera after the Administration of GFW.* We investigated whether the 3 potent MDR inhibitors, gallic acid, paeonol, and paeoniflorin in GFW, would be present in rat medicated sera after the administration of GFW. The chromatograms of the blank sera, spiked sera samples, and rat medicated sera samples after the oral administration of GFW are shown in Figure 1. Blank sera samples were screened and found to be free of interference from endogenous components or other sources at the same mass transitions (Figure 1(a)); the retention times (RTs) for gallic acid, paeonol, and paeoniflorin standards (Figure 1(b)) in the spiked sera samples were the same as those detected for three bioactive constituents in the rat medicated sera (Figure 1(c)), indicating that the 3 potent MDR inhibitors were present in the rat medicated sera.

*3.2. In Vitro Reversing Effects.* The ability of the rat medicated sera containing GFW to reverse the resistance against SKOV3/DDP cells was investigated, and the LD sera were used to study the reversing effect because they have the lowest growth inhibition effect on SKOV3 and SKOV3/DDP cells (less than 5%, Figure 2). The resistance fold of SKOV3/DDP cells to cisplatin and paclitaxel was approximately 4.13 and 3.85 compared with that of the SKOV3 cells. In the drug-resistant SKOV3/DDP cells, coincubation of the LD sera or VER with cisplatin or paclitaxel enhanced significantly the cytotoxic effect of cisplatin or paclitaxel ($P < 0.01$, Table 1). However, there is no significant difference between the LD sera in combination with cisplatin or paclitaxel and VER in combination with cisplatin or paclitaxel, although the reversal fold of the former was lower than those of the latter. These results indicate that the LD sera have similar reversing effect with VER *in vitro*.

*3.3. Flow Cytometric Assay of Rho123 Accumulation in SKOV3/DDP Cells.* The rat medicated sera containing GFW corresponding to different oral dosages were examined in a short-term Rho123 accumulation assay for their P-gp inhibitory effect on SKOV3/DDP cells. The results are displayed in Figure 3. The presence of the rat medicated sera containing GFW resulted in an increase in Rho123 accumulation in a dose-dependent manner in SKOV3/DDP

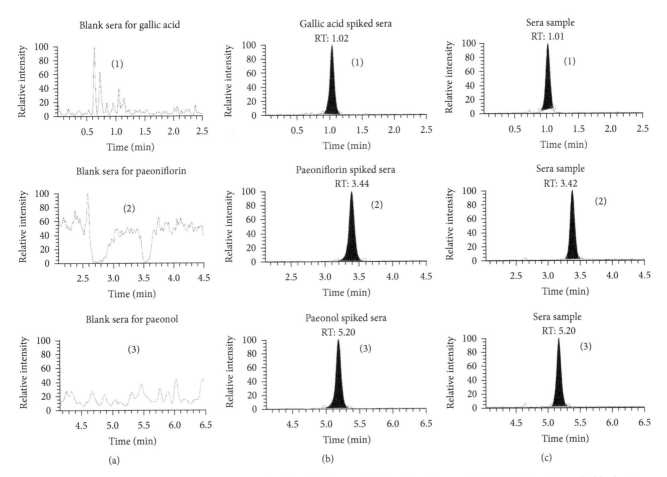

FIGURE 1: Typical chromatograms of HPLC/QqQ MS of gallic acid (1), paeoniflorin, (2) and paeonol (3). (a) Blank rat sera; (b) blank rat sera spiked with gallic acid, paeoniflorin, and paeonol; (c) rat sera sample obtained 30 min after the last oral administration of low-dose GFW.

TABLE 1: Cytotoxicity of the LD sera or VER in combination with cisplatin or paclitaxel in SKOV3 and SKOV3/DDP cells *in vitro*.

| Drug and concentration | $IC_{50}$ (mg·L$^{-1}$) | | Resistance fold | Reversal fold |
|---|---|---|---|---|
| | SKOV3 | SKOV3/DDP | | |
| Cisplatin | $3.58 \pm 0.12$ | $14.79 \pm 0.41^{**}$ | 4.13 | |
| Paclitaxel | $1.78 \pm 0.31$ | $6.86 \pm 0.22^{**}$ | 3.85 | |
| LD sera + cisplatin | $3.22 \pm 0.08$ | $4.39 \pm 0.17^{**}$ | 1.36 | 3.04 |
| LD sera + paclitaxel | $1.59 \pm 0.27$ | $2.33 \pm 0.42^{**}$ | 1.47 | 2.62 |
| VER + cisplatin | $3.34 \pm 0.13$ | $4.09 \pm 0.29^{#}$ | 1.22 | 3.39 |
| VER + paclitaxel | $1.69 \pm 0.24$ | $1.95 \pm 0.30^{#}$ | 1.18 | 3.26 |

LD, low-dose. VER, verapamil. $^{**}P < 0.01$ compared with each other, $^{#}P < 0.01$ compared with each other.

cells, manifesting as peaks moving far away from the vertical-axis, and the MFI increased with the dose of the rat medicated sera. The effect of increasing Rho123 accumulation by the LD sera was similar to that of VER, manifesting the MFIs between them have no significant difference ($P > 0.05$). These results suggest that P-gp function was inhibited by the rat medicated sera containing GFW. In these short-term experiments, no signs of toxicity or cell damage were observed directly in microscope after stained with trypan blue.

3.4. *GFW Disrupts the PI3K/AKT/mTOR Signalling Pathway.* We employed Western blotting to test whether the PI3K/AKT/mTOR signalling pathway was involved in the reversing effect of the rat medicated sera containing GFW. As shown in Figure 4, the levels of P-gp and p-AKT at Ser473 as well as the expression of mTOR, a known downstream target of AKT, in SKOV3/DDP cells, were increased significantly compared with those in SKOV3 cells ($P < 0.05$). After treated with the rat medicated sera containing GFW in SKOV3/DDP cells, the levels of P-gp, p-AKT, and mTOR were decreased

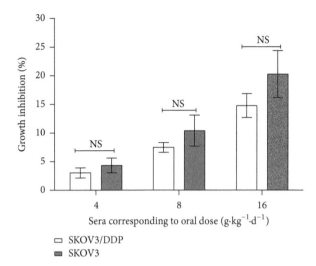

FIGURE 2: Effect of the rat medicated sera containing GFW corresponding to different oral dosages on the proliferation of SKOV3 and SKOV3/DDP cells. After treatment, the cells were washed and cultured for 72 h at 37°C in 96-well plates. The values correspond to the mean ± SD of three independent experiments. Significant differences between the means are specified by capped lines; NS indicates no significant.

in a dose-dependent manner ($P < 0.01$, $P < 0.05$). Whereas the levels of PI3K p110$\alpha$ and total AKT in SKOV3/DDP cells were not different compared with those in SKOV3 cells ($P > 0.05$), no changes were observed after SKOV3/DDP cells were treated with the rat medicated sera ($P > 0.05$). These results indicated that the sera inhibited MDR in SKOV3/DDP cells possibly through the downregulation of P-gp expression and the involvement of the PI3K/AKT/mTOR signalling pathway.

*3.5. In Vivo Efficacy Evaluation.* The ability of GFW to reverse MDR *in vivo* was tested in BALB/c xenograft nude mice generated with SKOV3/DDP cells. Compared with mice treated with saline, mice treated with a single LD of GFW showed no reduction in tumour growth and no death was observed with 21 days of administration. A similar outcome was obtained by measuring the weight of the mice and excised tumours at the end of the administration ($P > 0.05$). However, 2/10 mice died in the saline treatment group at the end of the administration; this may result from progression of disease. These results suggest that LD GFW has no apparent antitumour effect and may own the property of low toxicity on tested animals.

The combination of cisplatin and paclitaxel showed tumour growth inhibition of 40.66% at the end of the administration in the resistant SKOV3/DDP xenograft tumours, and the average tumour volume was decreased significantly along with 21 days of administration, while 3/10 mice died, and the average weight of the mice was reduced significantly at the end of the administration compared with that in the mice treated with saline ($P < 0.01$); this may result from chemotherapeutic toxicities of cisplatin and paclitaxel. By contrast, no mice died, and the average weight of the mice showed no significant decrease at the end of the

administration in the combination cisplatin, paclitaxel, and LD GFW group ($P > 0.05$); however, the tumour growth inhibition increased to 66.2% at the end of the administration compared with that in the mice treated with saline. In the meanwhile, a similar tumour growth inhibition effect was observed in the combinative treatment of cisplatin, paclitaxel, and VER group; however, also 4/10 mice died at the end of administration in this group (Figures 5(a), 5(b), and 5(c)). These *in vivo* findings demonstrated that LD GFW enhances the anticancer efficacy of cisplatin and paclitaxel treatment in resistant SKOV3/DDP xenograft tumours with mice body weights being maintained.

## 4. Discussion

In recent years, interest in the potential of plants and herbal medicine as a source of novel medicinal agents has grown significantly. Substantive research, aimed at utilizing this vast natural resource, is being carried out worldwide. In the development of anticancer agents, a wide range of plant-derived cytotoxic agents and/or MDR inhibitors were discovered from plant extracts. However, a large amount of time and effort is required before these agents can reach the market for clinical use due to insufficient evidence supporting their safety. For example, the development of camptothecins and taxanes as drugs for clinical use took over twenty years [31].

TCM has more than 2,000-year history of dealing with diseases and has evolved over time to become the second largest health care system in the world, after modern Western medicine. In general, treatment with Western medicine is not satisfactory for chronic diseases such as cardiovascular disease, type 2 diabetes mellitus, chronic pain, and cancer; TCM may offer an effective option [32, 33]. In addition, the long history of TCM use may dramatically reduce the time to its clinical use, if a TCM formula is found that has new therapeutic effects apart from its traditional usage. GFW is a TCM formula used in China, Japan, and other Asian countries that has been proven to be very safe and effective with fewer harmful side effects according to its long history of use. Recently, GFW was reported to improve the curative effect of chemotherapy with lower side effects when combined with cisplatin in OC patients during a 3-month treatment cycle, but the exact mechanism is unknown [34]. We suspect that enhancement of the effect may be involved in certain mechanisms delaying and/or overcoming MDR in chemotherapy. To address the possible mechanisms, a novel seropharmacology method arising recently for pharmacological study was adopted to study TCM *in vitro* using animal-medicated sera [35]. TCM formulas typically comprise more than 3 herbs, making their extracts contain hundreds or thousands of components; for example, GFW was found to contain 27 main components, including monoterpene glycosides, acetophenones, galloyl glucose, and even some isomers in its extract [36]. The essence of seropharmacology is to administer TCM to experimental animals (generally rabbits or rats), followed by harvesting the animal sera after a period of time. The sera are then applied to different cell lines

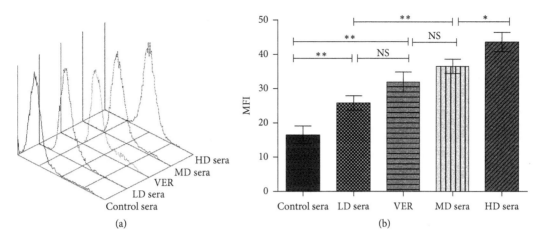

(a)                                    (b)

FIGURE 3: P-gp function changes in SKOV3/DDP cells after treatment for 24 h with verapamil or the rat medicated sera containing GFW corresponding to oral doses by flow cytometric analyses. (a) Representative flow cytometry overlay plot is shown. The P-gp inhibition effect increased along with the peaks moving far away from the vertical-axis. (b) Bar graph of mean fluorescence intensities (MFIs) of Rho123 in SKOV3/DDP cells with different treated groups. The results are the mean ± SD of 3 independent experiments. $^{**}P < 0.01$, $^{*}P < 0.05$; NS, no difference. LD sera represent the rat medicated sera corresponding to the GFW dosage of $4 \, \text{g·kg}^{-1} \cdot \text{d}^{-1}$. MD sera represent the rat medicated sera corresponding to the GFW dosage of $8 \, \text{g·kg}^{-1} \cdot \text{d}^{-1}$. HD sera represent the rat medicated sera corresponding to the GFW dosage of $16 \, \text{g·kg}^{-1} \cdot \text{d}^{-1}$.

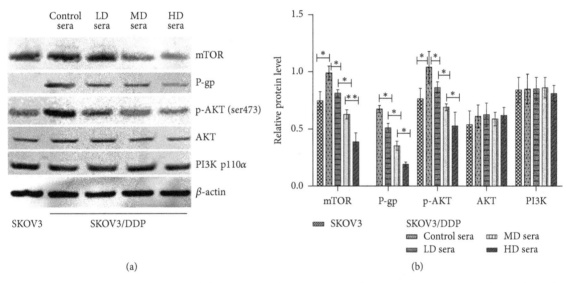

(a)                                    (b)

FIGURE 4: Rat medicated sera containing GFW inhibit MDR involved in P-gp and the PI3K/AKT/mTOR signalling pathway by Western blotting analysis in SKOV3/DDP cells after treated for 72 h. (a) Representative Western blotting gel results. (b) Bar graphs for relative protein levels. The results are the mean ± SD of at least 3 independent experiments. $\beta$-actin was used as an endogenous control and densitometric values were normalized by $\beta$-actin. $^{**}P < 0.01$, $^{*}P < 0.05$. LD sera represent the rat medicated sera corresponding to the GFW dosage of $4 \, \text{g·kg}^{-1} \cdot \text{d}^{-1}$. MD sera represent the rat medicated sera corresponding to the GFW dosage of $8 \, \text{g·kg}^{-1} \cdot \text{d}^{-1}$. HD sera represent the rat medicated sera corresponding to the GFW dosage of $16 \, \text{g·kg}^{-1} \cdot \text{d}^{-1}$.

for molecular mechanism studies. The advantage of seropharmacology for TCM study is the use of a TCM formula as a whole and the focus on the actual pharmaceutical ingredients or internal biological metabolic compounds of the formula, avoiding the isolation of individual components which may remove other potential key components that may not be detected using current technologies. We found that the 3 potent MDR inhibitors, gallic acid, paeonol, and paeoniflorin, in GFW extract were present in the rat medicated sera after

the administration of GFW (Figure 1) by HPLC/QqQ MS technology.

The *in vitro* reversal effects of the rat medicated sera containing GFW were studied with first-line chemotherapeutical drugs for OC, cisplatin and paclitaxel, in SKOV3/DDP cells and its parental cisplatin-sensitive counterpart. We found that the sera containing GFW significantly restored the sensitivity of SKOV3/DDP cells to cisplatin and paclitaxel. However, in SKOV3 cells, the rat medicated sera containing GFW

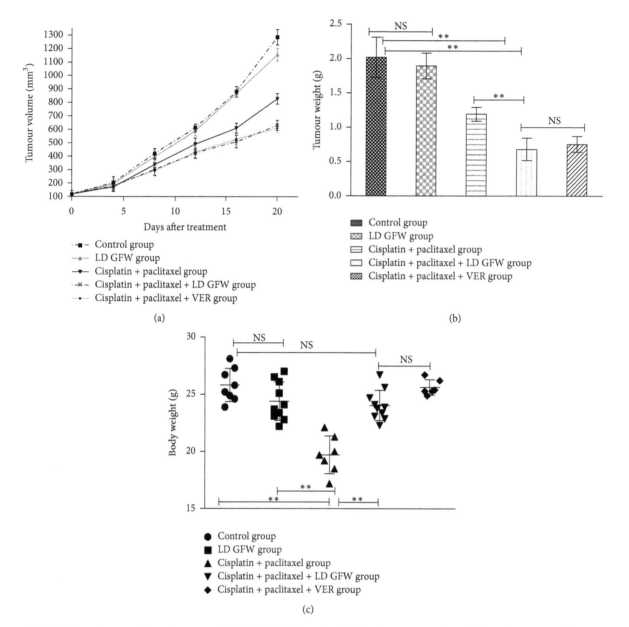

FIGURE 5: Inhibition of xenograft ovarian cancer by GFW. BALB/c nude mice bearing tumours formed by SKOV3/DDP cells were given saline as controls, a single GFW dosage of $4\,g\cdot kg^{-1}\cdot d^{-1}$(LD GFW), cisplatin (10 mg/kg administered intraperitoneally (i.p.) per 4 days) and paclitaxel (15 mg/kg administered i.v. per 3 days), combination of cisplatin, paclitaxel, and LD GFW, or combination of cisplatin, paclitaxel, and VER (5.0 mg·kg$^{-1}$ administrated i.v. for 21 days) ($n = 10$). The figures show the average tumour volumes along with the days after different treatments (a), average excised tumour weights (b), and body weights (c) of mice at the end of observation. $^{**}P < 0.01$; NS, no difference.

had no significant effect on drug cytotoxicity. Moreover, we showed that GFW could overcome the resistance of cisplatin and paclitaxel in xenograft tumour models generated with SKOV3/DDP cells (Figures 5(a) and 5(b)). The reversal effect of the rat medicated sera containing GFW was similar to those of the known MDR inhibitor, verapamil, which was popularly used as a positive control for research on inhibition of P-gp function [37, 38]. Since a median lethal dose of VER for the i.v. administration in mouse was reported to be 7.6 mg·kg$^{-1}$ [39], a single i.v. dose of 2.5 mg·kg$^{-1}$ VER still caused the death of 40% of animals in the *in vivo*

efficacy test, which may result from the cardiotoxicity of VER [40]; instead, no mice died in the combinative treatment of cisplatin, paclitaxel, and LD of GFW group. These data suggest, for the first time, that GFW may be an efficacious reversal TCM formula for ovarian cancer *in vitro* and *in vivo*.

P-gp modulation is thought to be an effective strategy to reverse MDR by inhibiting P-gp function and/or expression [41], reducing the clearance of anticancer drugs by cancer cells and then dramatically increasing their toxicity. Rho123 has been used as a marker for detecting the changes in P-gp function due to its low toxicity and specificity for P-gp [42, 43]. Some authors have reported that Rho123 is a substrate for both MRP and P-gp [44], but it was also reported that Rho123 is transported approximately 10 times higher by P-gp than by MRP1, and it is useless for the test of MRP1 activity [45]. In this study, we demonstrated that Rho123 accumulation was increased in a dose-dependent manner after adding the rat medicated sera containing GFW in SKOV3/DDP cells, suggesting that GFW reverses MDR through the inhibiting of P-gp function.

The PI3K/AKT/mTOR pathway is crucial for the regulation of chemoresistance in various cancers [46]. Activated receptor tyrosine kinase (RTK) associates with the p85 SH2-domain-containing subunit and recruits and activates the p110 catalytic domain of PI3K. Activated PI3K phosphorylates membrane phosphatidylinositol-4,5-bisphosphate (PIP2) in the 30 position, which acts as a docking site for phosphoinositide-dependent kinase 1 (PDK1) and AKT. AKT is activated by PDK and regulates downstream effectors, such as *MDR1*, which regulates drug resistance [21, 47]. mTOR participates in cell survival and proliferation, in part, through its ability to control AKT activity by the phosphorylation of AKT at Ser473 [48]. The inhibition of AKT phosphorylation could significantly downregulate the expression of P-gp and thus partially reverse MDR [49]. Due to its mechanistic activity involving these crucial pathways that directly or indirectly interplay with P-gp activities, we posed a potent functional effect for GFW to affect such interaction. Our results demonstrated that the rat medicated sera containing GFW could inhibit the protein levels of P-gp, p-AKT at Ser473 and mTOR, which were significantly different between SKOV3/DDP cells and their parental cisplatin-sensitive counterpart, in a dose-dependent manner in SKOV3/DDP cells, while no effect has been shown on the protein levels of PI3K p110α and total AKT, which were not significantly different between SKOV3/DDP and their parental cisplatin-sensitive counterpart, suggesting that the effect of MDR reversal by GFW may occur through inhibition of the activated PI3K/AKT/mTOR signalling pathway.

In summary, this study demonstrates, for the first time, the reversal MDR potential of GFW for ovarian cancer *in vitro* and *in vivo* by inhibiting the protein expression and function of P-gp, which may act through the inactivation of the PI3K/AKT/mTOR signalling pathway. The combination of cisplatin and/or paclitaxel and GFW may provide a therapeutic benefit against cisplatin-resistant ovarian cancers after further validation.

## Ethical Approval

The authors further confirm that any aspect of the work covered in this paper that has involved experimental animals has been conducted with the ethical approval of all relevant bodies and that such approvals are acknowledged within the paper.

## Disclosure

The authors further confirm that the order of authors listed in the paper has been approved by all of them.

## Competing Interests

The authors declare that they have no competing interests.

## Authors' Contributions

Li Han and Hua Bian conceived and designed the experiments. Li Han, Xiaojuan Guo, and Jingke Yang performed the experiments. Lei Yang analysed the data. Zhong Chen and Wenhua Zang contributed reagents, materials, and analysis tools. Li Han wrote the paper.

## Acknowledgments

This work was supported by the Henan Province Foundation and Advanced Technology Research Program (Grant no. 152300410179).

## References

[1] D. Jelovac and D. K. Armstrong, "Recent progress in the diagnosis and treatment of ovarian cancer," *CA: A Cancer Journal for Clinicians*, vol. 61, no. 3, pp. 183–203, 2011.

[2] B. T. Hennessy, R. L. Coleman, and M. Markman, "Ovarian cancer," *The Lancet*, vol. 374, no. 9698, pp. 1371–1382, 2009.

[3] R. C. Bast Jr., "Molecular approaches to personalizing management of ovarian cancer," *Annals of Oncology*, vol. 22, no. 8, pp. 5–15, 2011.

[4] B. Stordal, M. Hamon, V. McEneaney et al., "Resistance to paclitaxel in a cisplatin-resistant ovarian cancer cell line is mediated by P-glycoprotein," *PLoS ONE*, vol. 7, no. 7, Article ID e40717, 2012.

[5] R. Januchowski, K. Wojtowicz, P. Sujka-Kordowska, M. Andrzejewska, and M. Zabel, "MDR gene expression analysis of six drug-resistant ovarian cancer cell lines," *BioMed Research International*, vol. 2013, Article ID 241763, 2013.

[6] L. Xu, J. Cai, Q. Yang et al., "Prognostic significance of several biomarkers in epithelial ovarian cancer: a meta-analysis of published studies," *Journal of Cancer Research and Clinical Oncology*, vol. 139, no. 8, pp. 1257–1277, 2013.

[7] Z. Binkhathlan and A. Lavasanifar, "P-glycoprotein inhibition as a therapeutic approach for overcoming multidrug resistance in cancer: current status and future perspectives," *Current Cancer Drug Targets*, vol. 13, no. 3, pp. 326–346, 2013.

[8] S.-J. Jeong, H.-S. Lim, C.-S. Seo et al., "Anti-inflammatory actions of herbal formula Gyejibokryeong-hwan regulated by inhibiting chemokine production and STAT1 activation in HaCaT cells," *Biological & Pharmaceutical Bulletin*, vol. 38, no. 3, pp. 425–434, 2015.

[9] C. Hu, Z. Wang, Z. Pang et al., "Guizhi fuling capsule, an ancient Chinese formula, attenuates endometriosis in rats via induction of apoptosis," *Climacteric*, vol. 17, no. 4, pp. 410–416, 2014.

[10] K.-J. Wu, Y.-F. Chen, H.-Y. Tsai, C.-R. Wu, and W. G. Wood, "Guizhi-Fuling-Wan, a traditional Chinese herbal medicine, ameliorates memory deficits and neuronal apoptosis in the streptozotocin-induced hyperglycemic rodents via the decrease of bax/bcl2 ratio and caspase-3 expression," *Evidence-Based Complementary and Alternative Medicine*, vol. 2012, Article ID 656150, 2012.

[11] Y. Nagata, H. Goto, H. Hikiami et al., "Effect of keishibukuryo-gan on endothelial function in patients with at least one

component of the diagnostic criteria for metabolic syndrome: a controlled clinical trial with crossover design," *Evidence-Based Complementary and Alternative Medicine*, vol. 2012, Article ID 359282, 10 pages, 2012.

[12] ClinicalTrials, ClinicalTrials.gov. Effect of KYG0395 on primary dysmenorrhea, https://clinicaltrials.gov/ct2/show/study/NCT01588236?term=KYG0395&rank=1.

[13] X. Lei, J. Chen, C.-X. Liu, J. Lin, J. Lou, and H.-C. Shang, "Status and thoughts of Chinese patent medicines seeking approval in the US market," *Chinese Journal of Integrative Medicine*, vol. 20, no. 6, pp. 403–408, 2014.

[14] S. Y. Eid, M. Z. El-Readi, E. E. M. N. Eldin, S. H. Fatani, and M. Wink, "Influence of combinations of digitonin with selected phenolics, terpenoids, and alkaloids on the expression and activity of P-glycoprotein in leukaemia and colon cancer cells," *Phytomedicine*, vol. 21, no. 1, pp. 47–61, 2013.

[15] F. Xiao, Q. Li, K. Liang et al., "Comparative pharmacokinetics of three triterpene acids in rat plasma after oral administration of Poria extract and its formulated herbal preparation: GuiZhi-FuLing capsule," *Fitoterapia*, vol. 83, no. 1, pp. 117–124, 2012.

[16] L. Zhao, Z. Xiong, Y. Sui et al., "Simultaneous determination of six bioactive constituents of Guizhi Fuling Capsule in rat plasma by UHPLC-MS/MS: application to a pharmacokinetic study," *Journal of Chromatography B: Analytical Technologies in the Biomedical and Life Sciences*, vol. 1001, pp. 49–57, 2015.

[17] J. Cai, S. Chen, W. Zhang et al., "Paeonol reverses paclitaxel resistance in human breast cancer cells by regulating the expression of transgelin 2," *Phytomedicine*, vol. 21, no. 7, pp. 984–991, 2014.

[18] E. Chieli, N. Romiti, I. Rodeiro, and G. Garrido, "In vitro modulation of ABCB1/P-glycoprotein expression by polyphenols from *Mangifera indica*," *Chemico-Biological Interactions*, vol. 186, no. 3, pp. 287–294, 2010.

[19] H. E. Shan, Z. Qing-lin, L. U. Yu-xin, C. Xiao-chen, and H. Yuan, "Isolation and identification of ethanolic extract of Poria cocos and its reversal of multidrug resistance of KBV200 cells," *International Journal of Pharmaceutical Research*, vol. 39, no. 1, pp. 49–55, 2012.

[20] S. Fang, W. Zhu, Y. Zhang, Y. Shu, and P. Liu, "Paeoniflorin modulates multidrug resistance of a human gastric cancer cell line via the inhibition of NF-κB activation," *Molecular Medicine Reports*, vol. 5, no. 2, pp. 351–356, 2012.

[21] H. A. Burris III, "Overcoming acquired resistance to anticancer therapy: Focus on the PI3K/AKT/mTOR pathway," *Cancer Chemotherapy and Pharmacology*, vol. 71, no. 4, pp. 829–842, 2013.

[22] M. Liu, Z. Qi, B. Liu et al., "RY-2f, an isoflavone analog, overcomes cisplatin resistance to inhibit ovarian tumorigenesis via targeting the PI3K/AKT/mTOR signaling pathway," *Oncotarget*, vol. 6, no. 28, pp. 25281–25294, 2015.

[23] S. T. Wilks, "Potential of overcoming resistance to HER2-targeted therapies through the PI3K/Akt/mTOR pathway," *The Breast*, vol. 24, no. 5, pp. 548–555, 2015.

[24] National Commission of Chinese Pharmacopoeia, *Pharmacopoeia of Peoples Republic of China*, vol. 1, China Medical Science and Technology Press, Beijing, China, 2010.

[25] X. Hu, H. Lu, Y.-L. Deng, Q. Wan, and S.-M. Yie, "Effect of rat medicated serum containing Zuo Gui wan and/or you Gui Wan on the differentiation of stem cells derived from human first trimester umbilical cord into oocyte-like cells in vitro," *Evidence-Based Complementary and Alternative Medicine*, vol. 2015, Article ID 825805, 17 pages, 2015.

[26] G. Liu, P. Du, and Z. Zhang, "Myeloid differentiation factor 88 promotes cisplatin chemoresistance in ovarian cancer," *Cell Biochemistry and Biophysics*, vol. 71, no. 2, pp. 963–969, 2015.

[27] L. Han, Y. F. Wang, Y. Zhang et al., "Increased expression and function of P-glycoprotein in peripheral blood CD56+ cells is associated with the chemoresistance of non-small-cell lung cancer," *Cancer Chemotherapy and Pharmacology*, vol. 70, no. 3, pp. 365–372, 2012.

[28] L. Han, Y. Wang, X. Guo et al., "Downregulation of MDR1 gene by cepharanthine hydrochloride is related to the activation of c-Jun/JNK in K562/ADR cells," *BioMed Research International*, vol. 2014, Article ID 164391, 2014.

[29] N. Gyémánt, H. Engi, Z. Schelz et al., "In vitro and in vivo multidrug resistance reversal activity by a Betti-base derivative of tylosin," *British Journal of Cancer*, vol. 103, no. 2, pp. 178–185, 2010.

[30] H. Li, Z. Yan, W. Ning et al., "Using rhodamine 123 accumulation in CD8$^+$ cells as a surrogate indicator to study the P-glycoprotein modulating effect of cepharanthine hydrochloride in vivo," *Journal of Biomedicine and Biotechnology*, vol. 2011, Article ID 281651, 7 pages, 2011.

[31] G. M. Cragg and D. J. Newman, "Plants as a source of anti-cancer agents," *Journal of Ethnopharmacology*, vol. 100, no. 1-2, pp. 72–79, 2005.

[32] J.-J. Zhang, Q. Meng, W. Chang, and C.-H. Wan, "Clinical assessment of the efficacy of anti-cancer treatment: current status and perspectives," *Chinese Journal of Cancer*, vol. 29, no. 2, pp. 234–238, 2010.

[33] X. Mao, X. Q. Zhang, and N. Lin, "Application and perspectives of traditional Chinese medicine in the treatment of liver cancer," *Cancer Translational Medicine*, vol. 1, no. 3, pp. 101–107, 2015.

[34] T. Min, "Clinical observation on the treatment of 28 cases of oophoroma with Guizhifuling pills and adjuvant chemotherapy," *Anti-Tumor Pharmacy*, vol. 1, no. 6, pp. 520–523, 2011.

[35] H. Xu, Q. Wu, C. Peng, and L. Zhou, "Study on the antiviral activity of San Huang Yi Gan Capsule against hepatitis B virus with seropharmacological method," *BMC Complementary and Alternative Medicine*, vol. 13, article 239, 2013.

[36] L. Chen, D. Wang, J. Wu, B. Yu, and D. Zhu, "Identification of multiple constituents in the traditional Chinese medicine formula GuiZhiFuLing-Wan by HPLC-DAD-MS/MS," *Journal of Pharmaceutical and Biomedical Analysis*, vol. 49, no. 2, pp. 267–275, 2009.

[37] T. Tsuruo, H. Iida, S. Tsukagoshi, and Y. Sakurai, "Overcoming of vincristine resistance in P388 leukemia in vivo and in vitro through enhanced cytotoxicity of vincristine and vinblastine by verapamil," *Cancer Research*, vol. 41, no. 5, pp. 1967–1972, 1981.

[38] W. Kishimoto, N. Ishiguro, E. Ludwig-Schwellinger, T. Ebner, K. Maeda, and Y. Sugiyama, "Usefulness of a model-based approach for estimating in vitro P-glycoprotein inhibition potency in a transcellular transport assay," *Journal of Pharmaceutical Sciences*, vol. 105, no. 2, pp. 891–896, 2016.

[39] M. J. O'Neil, *The Merck Index: An Encyclopedia of Chemicals, Drugs, and Biologicals*, Merck and Co, Whitehouse Station, NJ, USA, 2006.

[40] P. P. Jadhav and S. Bohra, "Cardiotoxicity of verapamil in renal failure: a case report and review of the literature," *Cases Journal*, vol. 2, no. 9, article 6312, 2009.

[41] R. Callaghan, F. Luk, and M. Bebawy, "Inhibition of the multidrug resistance P-glycoprotein: time for a change of strategy?" *Drug Metabolism and Disposition*, vol. 42, no. 4, pp. 623–631, 2014.

[42] L. Han, X. Guo, H. Bian, Y. Zhou, T. Li, and J. Yang, "Changed expression and function of P-gp in peripheral blood CD56$^+$ cells predicting chemoresistance in non-Hodgkin lymphoma patients," *Cancer Biomarkers*, vol. 15, no. 3, pp. 289–297, 2015.

[43] J. Kasaian, F. Mosaffa, J. Behravan et al., "Reversal of P-glycoprotein-mediated multidrug resistance in MCF-7/Adr cancer cells by sesquiterpene coumarins," *Fitoterapia*, vol. 103, pp. 149–154, 2015.

[44] R. Daoud, C. Kast, P. Gros, and E. Georges, "Rhodamine 123 binds to multiple sites in the multidrug resistance protein (MRP1)," *Biochemistry*, vol. 39, no. 50, pp. 15344–15352, 2000.

[45] A. L. Dogan, O. Legrand, A.-M. Faussat, J.-Y. Perrot, and J.-P. Marie, "Evaluation and comparison of MRP1 activity with three fluorescent dyes and three modulators in leukemic cell lines," *Leukemia Research*, vol. 28, no. 6, pp. 619–622, 2004.

[46] S. T. Wilks, "Potential of overcoming resistance to HER2-targeted therapies through the PI3K/Akt/mTOR pathway," *The Breast*, vol. 24, no. 5, pp. 548–555, 2015.

[47] P. L. Tazzari, A. Cappellini, F. Ricci et al., "Multidrug resistance-associated protein 1 expression is under the control of the phosphoinositide 3 kinase/Akt signal transduction network in human acute myelogenous leukemia blasts," *Leukemia*, vol. 21, no. 3, pp. 427–438, 2007.

[48] A. Riaz, K. S. Zeller, and S. Johansson, "Receptor-specific mechanisms regulate phosphorylation of AKT at ser473: role of RICTOR in $\beta$1 integrin-mediated cell survival," *PLoS ONE*, vol. 7, no. 2, article e32081, 2012.

[49] M. B. Aldonza, J. Y. Hong, S. Y. Bae et al., "Suppression of MAPK signaling and reversal of mTOR-dependent MDR1-associated multidrug resistance by 21alpha-methylmelianodiol in lung cancer cells," *PloS ONE*, vol. 10, no. 6, Article ID e0127841, 2015.

# 4

# Effects of Jia-Wei-Xiao-Yao-San on the Peripheral and Lymphatic Pharmacokinetics of Paclitaxel in Rats

**Mei-Ling Hou,[1] Chia-Ming Lu,[1] and Tung-Hu Tsai[1,2,3,4]**

[1]Institute of Traditional Medicine, National Yang-Ming University, No. 155, Section 2, Li-Nong Street, Taipei 112, Taiwan
[2]Graduate Institute of Acupuncture Science, China Medical University, No. 91, Hsueh-Shih Road, Taichung 404, Taiwan
[3]School of Pharmacy, College of Pharmacy, Kaohsiung Medical University, No. 100, Shih-Chuan 1st Road, Kaohsiung 807, Taiwan
[4]Department of Education and Research, Taipei City Hospital, No. 145, Zhengzhou Road, Datong District, Taipei 103, Taiwan

Correspondence should be addressed to Tung-Hu Tsai; thtsai@ym.edu.tw

Academic Editor: José L. Ríos

Paclitaxel is effective against breast cancer. The herbal medicine, Jia-Wei-Xiao-Yao-San (JWXYS), is the most frequent prescription used to relieve the symptoms of breast cancer treatments. The aim of the study was to investigate the herb-drug interaction effects of a herbal medicine on the distribution of paclitaxel to lymph. A validated ultraperformance liquid chromatography with tandem mass spectrometry (UPLC-MS/MS) method was used to determine the paclitaxel levels in rat plasma and lymph after intravenous infusion of paclitaxel alone with or without 7 days of JWXYS pretreatment. The pharmacokinetic results indicate that paclitaxel concentrations in plasma exceeded those in lymph by approximately 3.6-fold. The biodistribution of paclitaxel from plasma to lymph was $39 \pm 5\%$; however, this increased to $45 \pm 4\%$ with JWXYS pretreatment. With JWXYS pretreatment, the AUC and $C_{max}$ of paclitaxel in plasma were significantly reduced by approximately 1.5-fold, compared to paclitaxel alone. Additionally, JWXYS decreased the AUC and $C_{max}$ of paclitaxel in lymph. However, the lymph absorption rate of paclitaxel with or without JWXYS pretreatment was not significantly changed ($27 \pm 3$ and $30 \pm 2\%$, resp.). Our findings demonstrate that when paclitaxel is prescribed concurrently with herbal medicine, monitoring of the blood pharmacokinetics of paclitaxel is recommended.

## 1. Introduction

Cancer is a global health problem. Surgery, chemotherapy, and radiotherapy are still the major conventional cancer therapies [1]. Paclitaxel is a natural product used as a chemotherapeutic agent against various malignant tumors including ovarian, breast, and non-small-cell lung cancers. The antitumor activity of paclitaxel is attributed to microtubule stabilization [2]. Although chemotherapy and radiotherapy are effective treatments against cancer, these treatments can cause serious side effects and complications, including fatigue, pain, diarrhea, nausea, vomiting, and hair loss, that cannot be ignored [1, 3, 4]. Thus, increasing evidence demonstrates that herbal medicines can be used as adjuvant therapies to ameliorate the chemotherapy-induced side effects [5–7].

According to a survey from the National Health Insurance (NHI) database in Taiwan, Traditional Chinese Medicine (TCM) is frequently prescribed to people with cancer as a remedy for alleviating symptoms or improving quality of life [8]. The results demonstrate that the Chinese herbal formula Jia-Wei-Xiao-Yao-San (JWXYS) is the most frequently prescribed formula for treating breast cancer [8, 9]. Generally, JWXYS relieves climacteric symptoms including panic, dysphoria, and hot flashes in postmenopausal women [6]. Recently, JWXYS has been prescribed as an alternative treatment for chronic diseases [6, 8, 9].

Paclitaxel is a P-glycoprotein (P-gp) substrate and is metabolized via cytochrome P450 (CYP) 2C8 and the 3A4 subfamily [10]. Coadministration of drugs that modulate the activity of CYP enzymes is likely to have undesirable clinical consequences [5, 11, 12]. The study suggested that oral administration of some phenolic substances might increase paclitaxel blood concentration during chemotherapy [13]. Various clinical factors including lymph node invasion and tumor size are essential in determining the best therapeutic option for breast cancer patients [3, 4]. Differences in pharmacokinetics, and drug distribution in particular, may cause poor efficacy of the chemotherapeutic drug at the targeted site [3, 4]. The pharmacokinetics of paclitaxel in rats and humans has been investigated [14–16]; however, information regarding the distribution of paclitaxel in lymph remains limited. In addition, JWXYS is the most frequent prescription used to relieve symptoms in women being treated for breast cancer [8]. It is possible that JWXYS and paclitaxel may interact to exhibit adverse effects in the clinic. Thus, the aims of the study are to investigate the pharmacokinetics of paclitaxel by UPLC-MS/MS in rats following intravenous infusion of paclitaxel and to explore whether pretreatment with JWXYS affects the pharmacokinetics and lymph distribution of paclitaxel. These results provide information crucial to conducting chemotherapy in combination with JWXYS.

## 2. Materials and Methods

### 2.1. Chemicals and Reagents.

The chemicals paclitaxel, docetaxel, and *tert*-Butyl methyl ether (TBME) were purchased from Sigma-Aldrich Chemicals (St. Louis, MO, USA). LC/MS grade solvents were obtained from J.T. Baker, Inc. (Phillipsburg, NJ, USA), and chromatographic reagents were obtained from Tedia Co., Inc. (Fairfield, OH, USA). Sodium chloride was purchased from E. Merck (Darmstadt, Germany). Triple deionized water (Millipore, Bedford, MA, USA) was used for all preparations. The pharmaceutical herbal product JWXYS manufactured in accordance with Good Manufacturing Practice (GMP) for Chinese Crude Drugs was obtained from pharmaceutical companies in Taiwan and has been used medicinally for patients. JWXYS consists of roots of *Angelica sinensis* (Oliv.) Diels, rhizomes of *Atractylodes macrocephala* Koidz., roots of *Paeonia lactiflora* Pall., roots of *Bupleurum chinensis* DC or *Bupleurum scorzonerifolium* Willd., sclerotia of the parasitic plant *Poria cocos* (Schw.) Wolf, roots and rhizomes of *Glycyrrhiza uralensis* Fisch., root barks of *Paeonia suffruticosa* Andr., ripe fruits of *Gardenia jasminoides* Ellis, rhizomes of *Zingiber officinale* Rosc., and stems and leaves of *Mentha haplocalyx* Briq., with a weight ratio of 4 : 4 : 4 : 4 : 4 : 2 : 2.5 : 2.5 : 4 : 2, respectively [17]. The pharmaceutical herbal product, JWXYS, was purchased from Sheng Chang Pharmaceutical Co., Ltd. (Taipei, Taiwan).

### 2.2. UPLC-MS/MS.

The UPLC-MS/MS analysis was performed using a Waters Acquity UPLC™ system (Waters, Manchester, UK) consisting of a binary solvent manager, an automatic liquid chromatographic sampler, and a Waters Xevo™ tandem quadrupole mass spectrometer equipped with an electrospray ionization (ESI) source. Separation was achieved using a Phenomenex Kinetex C18 analytical column (100 × 4.6 mm, length × inner diameter, particle size of 2.6 $\mu$m) maintained at 40°C in a column oven. The mobile phase consisted of triple deionized water and methanol (28 : 72; v/v) and the flow rate was set at 0.35 mL/min. The injection volume was 5 $\mu$L.

For operation in the MS/MS mode, the electrospray ion source was operated with polarity positive ion mode in a single run. The ESI parameters were set as follows:

source temperature: 150°C; desolvation temperature: 550°C; desolvation gas flow: 1000 L/h. The optimized cone voltages (CV) were 58 V for paclitaxel and 56 V for docetaxel. The multiple reaction monitoring (MRM) mode using specific precursor/product ion transitions was used for quantification. The molecular ions of paclitaxel and docetaxel were fragmented at collision energies of 28 and 26 eV using argon as the collision gas. Ion detection was performed by monitoring the transitions: $m/z$ 876.4 → 308.1 for paclitaxel and $m/z$ 830.4 → 549.2 for docetaxel. Docetaxel was used as the internal standard (IS) for positive ion mode analytes. A MassLynx 4.1 software data platform was used for spectral acquisition, spectral presentation, and peak quantification.

### 2.3. Animal Experiments.

All animal experimental protocols were reviewed and approved by the Institutional Animal Care and Use Committee (IACUC number: 1020716) of National Yang-Ming University. Male specific-pathogen-free Sprague-Dawley rats weighing $300 \pm 20$ g were obtained from the Laboratory Animal Center of the National Yang-Ming University, Taipei, Taiwan. Animals were provided free access to food (laboratory rodent diet 5P14, PMI Feeds, Richmond, IN) and water.

In accordance with published studies, the doses of paclitaxel and JWXYS for the animals were based on the human doses and were derived using the following conversion equation recommended by the US Food and Drug Administration guidelines: human equivalent dose (HED, mg/kg) = animal dose (mg/kg) × (animal $K_m$/human $K_m$) [18]. Clinically, paclitaxel is given as intravenous infusion for at least three hours, and the maximum daily dose of JWXYS for human is 12 g.

To investigate the herb-drug interaction effects of JWXYS on the pharmacokinetics of paclitaxel in rat plasma and lymph, paclitaxel was administered by intravenous infusion to rats with or without oral JWXYS at 1.23 g/kg for 7 days. The commercial pharmaceutical powdered JWXYS was weighed and suspended in sterile water at the dosing volume of 10 mL/kg. JWXYS at 1.23 g/kg was administered to each rat by oral gavage. At the 7th dose of JWXYS, rats were given 1 mL of olive oil by oral gavage thirty minutes preoperatively and then anesthetized with urethane (1 g/kg, IP) for mesenteric lymph duct, jugular vein, and femoral vein cannulation. The purpose of the oral dosing of olive oil 30 mins before operation was to facilitate identification of the lymph vessels [19, 20]. The procedure for the cannulation of the mesenteric lymph vessels was performed as previously described [21, 22]. The rats were administered 5 mg/kg of paclitaxel by intravenous infusion into the right femoral vein at the infusion rate of 2 mL/hour for 3 hours. Two hundred $\mu$L samples of blood were withdrawn from the cannula implanted in the jugular vein into heparin-rinsed vials at 0, 15, 30, 60, 120, 180, 185, 195, 210, 225, 240, 270, 300, 330, 360, 390, and 420 min. The lymph was collected into heparin-rinsed vials at 30 min intervals. The mesenteric lymph rate during the 24 h period following surgery averaged $2.4 \pm 1.1$ mL/h [19]. In order to compensate the loss of body fluid, the rats were intravenously infused with normal saline at an infusion rate of 2 mL/hour throughout the experiment according to the published literature [19, 20]. The plasma samples were immediately centrifuged at 6000 rpm for 10 min.

*2.4. Sample Preparation.* The biological samples were prepared by liquid-liquid extraction. The plasma and lymph samples (90 $\mu$L, resp.) spiked with 10 $\mu$L of docetaxel solution (IS, 2.5 $\mu$g/mL) were extracted by TBME for liquid-liquid extraction. Briefly, biological samples were extracted using 1 mL of TBME twice, vortexed for 5 min, and centrifuged at 13,000 rpm for 10 min. After centrifugation, the upper organic layer containing the paclitaxel was transferred to a new tube and evaporated to dryness using a vacuum pump. The dried residue was reconstituted with 100 $\mu$L of mobile phase (triple deionized water : methanol = 28 : 72) and analyzed by UPLC-MS/MS. If the paclitaxel concentration was in excess of 500 ng/mL, then the plasma and lymph samples were diluted by blank plasma and lymph samples at an appropriate ratio before analysis.

*2.5. Preparation of Standard Samples.* Stock solutions of paclitaxel and IS were prepared in methanol at a concentration of 1 mg/mL. The calibration curves were obtained from biological samples freshly spiked with IS and the stock solution of paclitaxel at concentration ranges of 5–500 ng/mL. The spiked biological samples were extracted following the sample preparation procedure described above.

*2.6. Method Validation.* The method validation assays for quantification of paclitaxel in rat plasma and lymphatic fluid were conducted based on the current US Food and Drug Administration (FDA) bioanalytical method validation guidelines [23]. Specificity, matrix effects, and recovery were evaluated. Biological samples were quantified using the ratio of the peak area of each analyte to that of the IS. Peak area ratios were plotted against analyte concentrations. All linear curves were required to have a coefficient of estimation of at least >0.995. Using the UPLC-MS/MS method described above, the intra- and interday variability were determined by quantitating six replicates at concentrations of 5, 10, 25, 50, 100, 250, and 500 ng/mL on the same day and on six consecutive days, respectively. The accuracy (% bias) and the relative standard deviation (RSD %) were calculated.

To evaluate matrix effect (ME) and recovery (RE), six different lots of blank plasma or lymph samples were extracted and then spiked with paclitaxel at three concentrations. The corresponding peak areas of paclitaxel in the spiked biological samples after extraction (A) were compared to those of the aqueous standards in mobile phase (B) at equivalent concentrations. The ratio (A/B × 100) is defined as the ME. The corresponding peak areas of paclitaxel in the spiked biological samples before extraction (C) were compared to those of paclitaxel in the spiked biological samples after extraction (A) at equivalent concentrations. The ratio (C/A × 100) is defined as the RE.

*2.7. Pharmacokinetic Data Analysis.* Pharmacokinetic calculations were performed on each individual data set by noncompartmental methods using WinNonlin Standard Edition, version 1.1 (Pharsight Corp., Mountain View, CA).

*2.8. Statistical Analysis.* Data were summarized as the mean ± SD or SEM. Comparison between two groups was performed using the unpaired Student's *t*-test. Statistical significance was set at $p < 0.05$.

# 3. Results

*3.1. Optimization of the UPLC-MS/MS Method.* For parameter optimization, a standard solution of paclitaxel or docetaxel was analyzed by direct injection in the spectrometer. A full scan in the positive mode with precursor-product combinations monitored in the MRM mode was used for analyte identification. Paclitaxel and the IS could be ionized under positive (ESI$^+$) electrospray ionization conditions. During initial infusion experiments with paclitaxel and docetaxel, the spectra revealed that both paclitaxel and docetaxel form Na$^+$ adducts. Under ESI$^+$ conditions, the precursor ions for paclitaxel and docetaxel were [paclitaxel + Na]$^+$ at *m/z* 876.4 and [docetaxel + Na]$^+$ at *m/z* 830.4, respectively. The MRM mode provided high selectivity and sensitivity for the quantification assay (Figure 1). The results of MS transitions demonstrate that the precursor ion of paclitaxel at *m/z* 876.4 [M + Na]$^+$ and its main product ion at *m/z* 308.1 and the precursor ion of docetaxel at *m/z* 830.4 [M + Na]$^+$ and its main product ion at *m/z* 549.2 were used to determine the analytes in the biological samples. Chromatographic conditions were optimized for good sensitivity, peak shape, and a relatively short run. Methanol provided the best peak shape and was selected as the organic phase. A mobile phase consisting of a water-methanol solution (isocratic elution) was used in the experiment.

*3.2. UPLC-MS/MS Method Validation of Paclitaxel in Rat Plasma and Lymph.* Assay specificity was assessed by comparing the chromatograms of blank plasma and lymph samples obtained from six rats with corresponding spiked plasma and lymph samples. Each blank plasma and lymph sample was tested using a liquid-liquid extraction procedure and UPLC-MS/MS conditions to ensure no interference of paclitaxel and IS from plasma and lymph. The results showed that no interference existed under the present analytical conditions (Figures 2(a) and 2(d)).

Figures 2(a) and 2(d) show the chromatograms of a blank plasma and lymph extract with mass transitions of *m/z* 876.4 → 308.1 for paclitaxel and *m/z* 830.4 → 549.2 for docetaxel (IS), illustrating a clean baseline with no interference peaks eluted within 10 min. Figures 2(b) and 2(e) show the chromatograms of a standard solution of paclitaxel (250 ng/mL) and IS (250 ng/mL) spiked in blank rat plasma and lymph. Figure 2(c) shows the chromatograms for a plasma sample containing paclitaxel (270 ng/mL) collected at 390 min after dosing with paclitaxel (5 mg/kg, i.v. infusion). Figure 2(f) shows the chromatograms for a lymph sample containing paclitaxel (245 ng/mL) collected from 330 to 360 min after dosing with paclitaxel (5 mg/kg, i.v. infusion). Each determination was completed within 10 min and no carry-over peaks were detected in the subsequent chromatograms of biological samples.

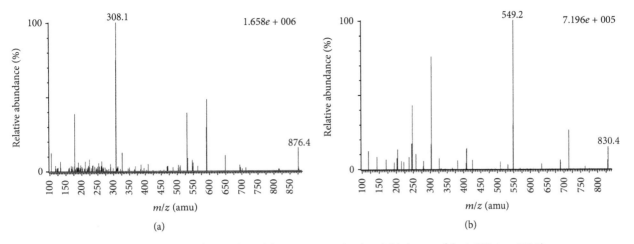

FIGURE 1: Mass spectra of (a) paclitaxel ($m/z$ 876.4 → 308.1) and (b) docetaxel ($m/z$ 830.4 → 549.2).

A 100% matrix effect value indicated that the response in the mobile phase and in the biological extracts was the same [20]. The mean matrix effects of paclitaxel and docetaxel (IS) in plasma were 106 ± 14 and 84 ± 5%, respectively; the mean matrix effects of paclitaxel and docetaxel (IS) in lymph were 80 ± 7 and 60 ± 5%, respectively (Table 1). The mean recovery for paclitaxel and IS in plasma was 85 ± 13 and 78 ± 4%, respectively; the mean recoveries for paclitaxel and IS in lymph were 84 ± 11 and 53 ± 5%, respectively (Table 1).

The calibration curve was constructed by plotting the peak area ratios of paclitaxel to the IS versus the concentrations of paclitaxel. The results demonstrated a linear response over the concentration ranges of 10–500 ng/mL, with a coefficient of estimation $r^2 > 0.995$. The data showed excellent reproducibility (Table 2). The limit of detection (LOD) and quantification (LOQ) were defined as the concentration of paclitaxel detected as a signal-to-noise (S/N) ratio of 3 and 10, respectively. The LOD and LOQ of paclitaxel in rat plasma and lymph were 5 ng/mL and the LOQ was 10 ng/mL. The intra- and interday precision (% RSD) and accuracy (% bias) values of paclitaxel in rat plasma and lymph were within 15% (Table 2). These results show that the UPLC-MS/MS method provides excellent quantitative analysis of paclitaxel in rat plasma and lymph extracts.

*3.3. Herb-Drug Interaction Effects of JWXYS on the Blood Pharmacokinetics of Paclitaxel.* The mean plasma concentration-time profiles of paclitaxel after intravenous infusion of paclitaxel at 5 mg/kg ($n = 11$) with or without pretreatment with JWXYS (1.23 g/kg, p.o. for 7 days) are illustrated in Figure 3(a) and the pharmacokinetic parameters are listed in Table 3. Following 7 days of pretreatment with oral JWXYS at 1.23 g/kg, the AUC and $C_{max}$ of paclitaxel in plasma were significantly reduced by approximately 1.5-fold, compared to paclitaxel alone (Table 3). Additionally, the elimination half-life ($T_{1/2}$) of paclitaxel in plasma was significantly prolonged 1.5-fold; the total body clearance (CL) increased by 43% and the volume of distribution (Vd) significantly increased 1.4-fold following coadministration with JWXYS. However, the

mean residence time (MRT) exhibited no changes with or without pretreatment with JWXYS.

*3.4. Herb-Drug Interaction Effects of JWXYS on the Lymph Pharmacokinetics of Paclitaxel.* The mean concentration-time profiles of paclitaxel in rat lymph ($n = 11$) after intravenous infusion of paclitaxel (5 mg/kg) with or without pretreatment with JWXYS (1.23 g/kg, p.o. for 7 days) are illustrated in Figure 3(b), and the pharmacokinetic parameters are illustrated in Table 3. As shown in Figure 3, the drug concentration versus time curve of paclitaxel in rat plasma and lymph after intravenous infusion of paclitaxel with or without pretreatment with JWXYS indicated that the amount of paclitaxel in rat lymph was lower than the amount of paclitaxel in rat plasma. Paclitaxel concentrations in plasma exceeded those in lymph by approximately 2.8-fold, with AUC values of 315 ± 38.2 min μg/mL in plasma and 113 ± 12.7 min μg/mL in lymph. The $C_{max}$ of paclitaxel in plasma was 3.6-fold greater than that in lymph.

Following 7 days of pretreatment with JWXYS, the AUC of paclitaxel in lymph was reduced by approximately 1.3-fold and the $C_{max}$ yielded similar results (Table 3). However, the $T_{1/2}$, Vd, CL, and MRT were not changed. The lymph absorption rate of paclitaxel ($AUC_{lymph}/AUC_{plasma+lymph} \times 100$) was 27 ± 3%, indicating that paclitaxel can be absorbed into the lymph system. However, pretreatment with JWXYS did not significantly affect the lymph absorption rate of paclitaxel (30 ± 2%) compared to paclitaxel alone. The biodistribution ($AUC_{lymph}/AUC_{plasma} \times 100$) of paclitaxel from plasma to lymph was 39 ± 5%; however, it increased to 45 ± 4% with JWXYS pretreatment. As shown in Figure 3, seven days of JWXYS at 1.23 g/kg significantly decreased the blood paclitaxel levels by approximately 30% and reduced the distribution of paclitaxel in rat lymph by around 24%.

## 4. Discussion

Although analytical methods have been reported for analysis of paclitaxel in biological matrices by high-performance

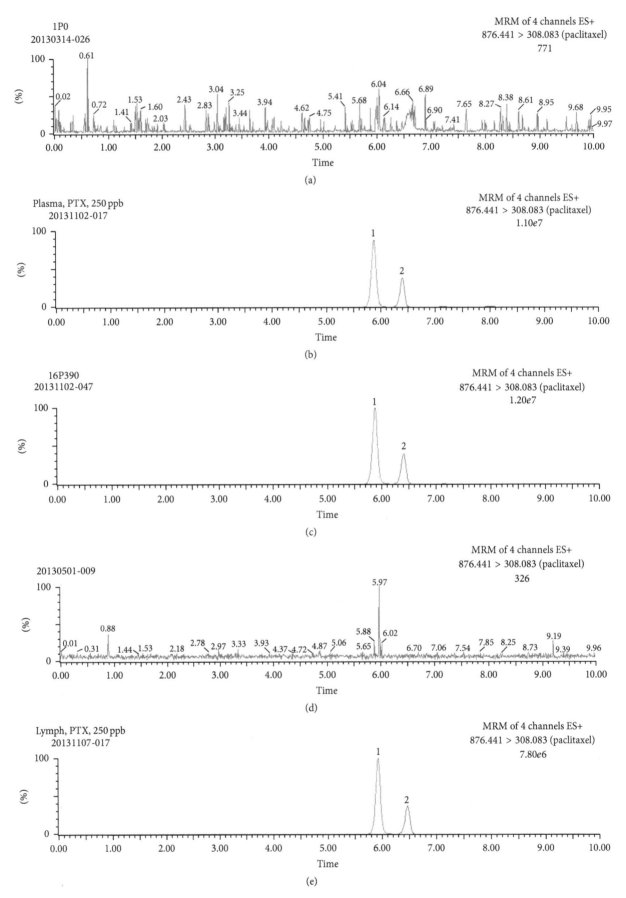

FIGURE 2: Continued.

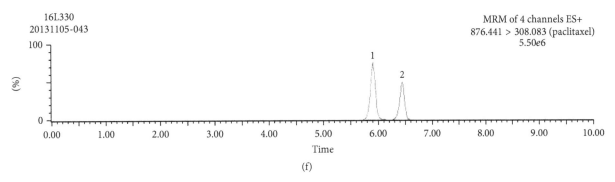

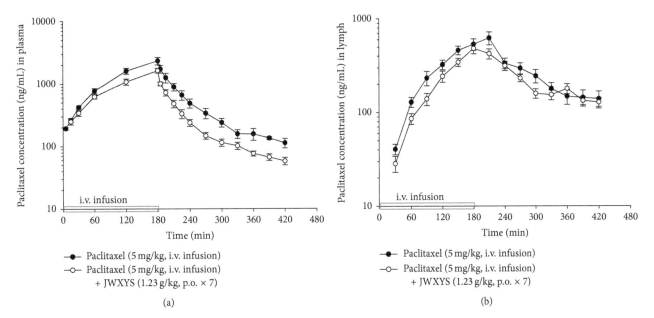

FIGURE 2: Representative chromatograms of paclitaxel in rat plasma and lymph. (a) Blank rat plasma; (b) blank rat plasma sample spiked with paclitaxel (250 ng/mL) and docetaxel (IS); (c) real rat plasma sample containing paclitaxel (270 ng/mL) collected at 390 min after administration of paclitaxel (5 mg/kg, i.v. infusion). (d) Blank rat lymph; (e) blank rat lymph sample spiked with paclitaxel (250 ng/mL) and docetaxel (IS); (f) real rat lymph sample containing paclitaxel (245 ng/mL) collected from 330 to 360 min after administration of paclitaxel (5 mg/kg, i.v. infusion). 1: paclitaxel; 2: docetaxel (IS, 250 ng/mL).

FIGURE 3: Mean concentration-time profiles of paclitaxel in rat plasma (a) and lymph (b) after intravenous infusion of paclitaxel (5 mg/kg) with or without JWXYS (1.23 g/kg, p.o. for 7 days) pretreatment. Each point represents mean ± SEM ($N = 11$).

liquid chromatography with UV [24, 25], and by tandem mass spectrometric detection [26, 27], there is no validated method for the determination of paclitaxel in rat lymph. The MS transitions of paclitaxel ($m/z$ 876.4 → 308.1) and docetaxel ($m/z$ 830.4 → 549.2) were in agreement with previous reports [27].

Numerous studies have indicated that the use of Chinese herbal medicines in combination with chemotherapy or radiotherapy for the treatment of cancer not only enhances the efficacy but also diminishes the side effects and complications induced by chemotherapy and radiotherapy treatments [5–9, 28]. Chinese herbal medicines, including Astragalus, Turmeric, Ginseng, TJ-41, PHY-906, Huachansu infection, and Kanglaite injection, are commonly used by patients for cancer treatment and/or for the reduction of toxicity associated with chemotherapy and radiotherapy [29]. Studies

on pharmacokinetic interactions between Chinese herbal medicines and Western medicines [5, 11, 13, 30] have been conducted, and the results suggest that oral administration of some phenolic substances might increase paclitaxel blood concentrations during chemotherapy. Because paclitaxel is a P-gp substrate, investigation on P-gp inhibition on the mesenteric lymphatic transport of paclitaxel has been reported [31]. The results demonstrated that pretreatment with a P-gp inhibitor, verapamil, increased the lymphatic transport of paclitaxel by 3.5-fold and absolute oral bioavailability by 1.8-fold.

The bioactive components, including ferulic acid [32], atractylenolide I-III [33], paeoniflorin [34], saikosaponins [35], polysaccharides and triterpenoids [36], glycyrrhizin [37], paeonol [38], geniposide [39], zingerone [40], and chlorogenic acid [41], were found in the individual herb of

TABLE 1: Matrix effect and recovery of paclitaxel and docetaxel in rat plasma and lymph.

| Nominal concentration (ng/mL) | Peak area | | | Matrix effect (%) | Recovery (%) |
|---|---|---|---|---|---|
| | Set 1 | Set 2 | Set 3 | | |
| *Plasma* | | | | | |
| Paclitaxel | | | | | |
| 10 | 36872 ± 4813 | 32992 ± 2473 | 24279 ± 2632 | 89 ± 7 | 74 ± 8 |
| 100 | 235603 ± 12101 | 269808 ± 27215 | 237379 ± 31147 | 115 ± 12 | 88 ± 12 |
| 500 | 1202318 ± 61512 | 1356123 ± 74986 | 1265995 ± 133390 | 113 ± 6 | 93 ± 10 |
| Average | | | | 106 ± 14 | 85 ± 13 |
| Docetaxel (IS) | | | | | |
| 250 | 465608 ± 9230 | 389823 ± 23305 | 302862 ± 16985 | 84 ± 5 | 78 ± 4 |
| *Lymph* | | | | | |
| Paclitaxel | | | | | |
| 10 | 30372 ± 3067 | 25645 ± 1935 | 20778 ± 2064 | 84 ± 6 | 81 ± 8 |
| 100 | 298923 ± 18866 | 246724 ± 5850 | 217499 ± 35420 | 83 ± 2 | 88 ± 14 |
| 500 | 2216455 ± 159883 | 1598223 ± 99812 | 1341908 ± 180573 | 72 ± 5 | 84 ± 11 |
| Average | | | | 80 ± 7 | 84 ± 11 |
| Docetaxel (IS) | | | | | |
| 250 | 465609 ± 9330 | 280022 ± 21317 | 147762 ± 12713 | 60 ± 5 | 53 ± 5 |

Data expressed as mean ± SD ($N = 6$). Matrix effect is expressed as the ratio of the mean peak area of an analyte spiked after extraction (set 2) to the mean peak area of the same analyte standard (set 1) multiplied by 100. A value of >100% indicates ionization enhancement, and a value of <100% indicates ionization suppression. Recovery was calculated as the ratio of the mean peak area of an analyte spiked before extraction (set 3) to the mean peak area of an analyte spiked after extraction (set 2) multiplied by 100.

TABLE 2: Intra- and interday precision (% RSD) and accuracy (% bias) of the UPLC-MS/MS method for determination of paclitaxel in rat plasma and lymph (6 days, 6 replicates per day).

| Nominal concentration (ng/mL) | Intraday | | | Interday | | |
|---|---|---|---|---|---|---|
| | Observed concentration (ng/mL) | Precision (% RSD) | Accuracy (% bias) | Observed concentration (ng/mL) | Precision (% RSD) | Accuracy (% bias) |
| *Plasma* | | | | | | |
| 10 | 9.58 ± 1.28 | 13.4 | −4.20 | 9.42 ± 1.36 | 14.4 | −5.77 |
| 25 | 23.9 ± 1.22 | 5.13 | −4.51 | 24.8 ± 2.11 | 8.50 | −0.88 |
| 50 | 49.5 ± 2.90 | 5.87 | −0.99 | 48.6 ± 3.25 | 6.69 | −2.88 |
| 100 | 102 ± 7.27 | 7.10 | 2.45 | 99.1 ± 2.46 | 2.48 | −0.89 |
| 250 | 259 ± 9.80 | 3.78 | 3.64 | 257 ± 7.19 | 2.80 | 2.76 |
| 500 | 495 ± 4.30 | 0.87 | −1.05 | 497 ± 4.17 | 0.84 | −0.62 |
| *Lymph* | | | | | | |
| 10 | 9.65 ± 1.25 | 12.9 | −3.49 | 9.21 ± 1.26 | 13.6 | −7.88 |
| 25 | 25.1 ± 2.67 | 10.6 | 0.28 | 25.1 ± 2.34 | 9.34 | 0.25 |
| 50 | 52.2 ± 3.04 | 5.83 | 4.34 | 52.4 ± 3.47 | 6.62 | 4.70 |
| 100 | 101 ± 4.32 | 4.30 | 0.58 | 101 ± 3.44 | 3.39 | 1.42 |
| 250 | 247 ± 10.5 | 4.26 | −1.32 | 248 ± 14.2 | 5.71 | −0.76 |
| 500 | 502 ± 4.94 | 0.99 | 0.33 | 498 ± 7.66 | 1.54 | −0.37 |

Data expressed as mean ± SD.

JWXYS. Studies on herb-drug interactions in pharmacokinetics based on metabolizing enzymes have been reported. For example, *in vitro* and *in vivo* studies showed that the potential components of *Angelica sinensis* (Oliv.) Diels roots, one of the major herbs in JWXYS, have the inhibitory effects on CYP3A4 [42]. It is known that lactones of Artemisia (ligustilide), n-butene acid lactones, ferulic acid, nicotinic acid, sucrose, amino acids, and sesquiterpene compounds are pharmacologically active components of *Angelica sinensis* (Oliv.) Diels [32]. Additionally, licorice root of *Glycyrrhiza*

TABLE 3: Pharmacokinetic parameters of paclitaxel (5 mg/kg, i.v. infusion) with or without JWXYS (1.23 g/kg, p.o. for 7 days) pretreatment.

| PK parameters | Paclitaxel (5 mg/kg, i.v. infusion) | Paclitaxel (5 mg/kg, i.v. infusion) + JWXYS (1.23 g/kg, p.o. × 7) |
|---|---|---|
| *Plasma* | | |
| $C_{max}$ (ng/mL) | 2355 ± 314 | 1630 ± 141[*] |
| $AUC_{0-420\,min}$ (min μg/mL) | 315 ± 38.2 | 209 ± 18.9[*] |
| $T_{1/2}$ (min) | 73.7 ± 12.2 | 111 ± 12.8[*] |
| Vd (L/kg) | 1.39 ± 0.15 | 2.00 ± 0.17[*] |
| CL (mL/min/kg) | 17.5 ± 1.95 | 25.1 ± 2.55[*] |
| MRT (min) | 68.6 ± 3.70 | 62.9 ± 1.71 |
| *Lymph* | | |
| $C_{max}$ (ng/mL) | 648 ± 94.3 | 494 ± 58.7 |
| $AUC_{0-420\,min}$ (min μg/mL) | 113 ± 12.7 | 89.8 ± 8.25 |
| $T_{1/2}$ (min) | 116 ± 17.6 | 122 ± 7.0 |
| Vd (L/kg) | 8.08 ± 1.59 | 10.0 ± 1.09 |
| CL (mL/min/kg) | 45.7 ± 8.17 | 48.3 ± 4.36 |
| MRT (min) | 119 ± 4.77 | 130 ± 4.34 |
| Biodistribution (%) | 39 ± 5 | 45 ± 4 |
| Lymph absorption rate (%) | 27 ± 3 | 30 ± 2 |

Data expressed as mean ± SEM ($N$ = 11). $C_{max}$: the peak plasma concentration of a drug after administration; AUC: area under the concentration versus time curve; $T_{1/2}$: elimination half-life; Vd: volume of distribution; CL: total body clearance; MRT: mean residence time; biodistribution, ($AUC_{lymph}/AUC_{plasma}$) × 100: the distribution of paclitaxel from plasma to lymph; lymph absorption rate, [($AUC_{lymph}/AUC_{plasma+lymph}$) × 100]: the lymph absorption rate of paclitaxel. [*]Significantly different from paclitaxel alone at $p < 0.05$.

*uralensis* Fisch. is another herbal component in JWXYS; its main active ingredient is glycyrrhizin [37]. *In vitro* studies have shown that isoflavone glabridin isolated from *Glycyrrhiza uralensis* Fisch could have CYP3A4 enzyme induction properties [42]. Furthermore, *in vivo* studies showed that repeated treatment with glycyrrhizae or glycyrrhizic acid could increase CYP3A4 substrate metabolism, and CYP3A4 was induced at both the mRNA and protein levels [42].

Our pharmacokinetic results demonstrate decreased blood and lymph paclitaxel concentrations following 7 days of pretreatment with JWXYS. However, pretreatment with JWXYS did not significantly influence the distribution and absorption rate of paclitaxel in lymph. The results suggest that orally administered JWXYS affects metabolizing enzymes as well as disturbing the distribution of paclitaxel into the circulation *in vivo*. The possible mechanism of interaction between JWXYS and paclitaxel could be increased metabolism of paclitaxel or affect transporter functions in the intestinal lymphatic system following oral administration of JWXYS; consequently, this would decrease paclitaxel levels in the peripheral and lymphatic system.

The lymphatic system plays an important role in fluid/macromolecular balance, lipid absorption, and immune functions. It is involved in various pathologic conditions such as inflammation, spread of cancer cells, and lymphedema [43]. The lymphatic system can also transport dietary lipids, fat-soluble vitamins, and water-insoluble drugs to the systemic circulation. Paclitaxel has been approved to treat metastatic breast cancer [44]; however, limited evidence shows that paclitaxel can gain access to the lymphatic system.

The only literature is the one in which Cai et al. has investigated the effects of lipid vehicle and P-gp inhibition on the mesenteric lymphatic transport of paclitaxel [31]. Few reports regarding the absorption of drugs into the lymphatic system [45–49] have been investigated due to practical difficulties in obtaining the lymphatic fluid. Studies on the determination of protein or water-insoluble compounds in lymph and plasma following intravenous or intestinal administration in rats have been reported [45–49]. The results suggest that, over a given dose range, a protein with a high molecular weight can be absorbed in both the portal vein blood stream and the thoracic duct lymph after intraduodenal administration of parotin [48]. Our pharmacokinetic results demonstrate that paclitaxel was detectable in rat lymph after intravenous infusion of paclitaxel; however, JWXYS significantly decreased blood paclitaxel levels by approximately 30%.

## 5. Conclusions

This is the first report to explore the herb-drug interaction effects of JWXYS on the pharmacokinetics of paclitaxel in rat peripheral and lymphatic systems. A validated UPLC-MS/MS method was applied for pharmacokinetic studies. The pharmacokinetic results demonstrate that pretreatment with JWXYS for 7 days significantly attenuated the distribution of paclitaxel in rat peripheral and lymphatic systems. Clinically, it is not practical to collect lymphatic fluid in patients following paclitaxel administration. These findings indicate that monitoring plasma levels of paclitaxel may help in assessing compliance and therapeutic effects and in dose optimization when coadministered with JWXYS.

## Competing Interests

The authors declare that there are no competing interests.

## Acknowledgments

Funding for this study was provided in part by research grants from the National Science Council (NSC102-2113-M-010-001-MY3) Taiwan and TCH10401-62-004 and TCH104-02 from Taipei City Hospital, Taipei, Taiwan.

## References

[1] M. Schmidt, "Chemotherapy in early breast cancer: when, how and which one?" *Breast Care*, vol. 9, no. 3, pp. 154–160, 2014.

[2] P. Ma and R. J. Mumper, "Paclitaxel nano-delivery systems: a comprehensive review," *Journal of Nanomedicine and Nanotechnology*, vol. 4, no. 2, Article ID 1000164, 2013.

[3] T. Iwamoto, "Clinical application of drug delivery systems in cancer chemotherapy: review of the efficacy and side effects of approved drugs," *Biological and Pharmaceutical Bulletin*, vol. 36, no. 5, pp. 715–718, 2013.

[4] V. Mandilaras, N. Bouganim, J. Spayne et al., "Concurrent chemoradiotherapy for locally advanced breast cancer—time for a new paradigm?" *Current Oncology*, vol. 22, no. 1, pp. 25–32, 2015.

[5] S. Y. K. Fong, Q. Gao, and Z. Zuo, "Interaction of carbamazepine with herbs, dietary supplements, and food: a systematic review," *Evidence-Based Complementary and Alternative Medicine*, vol. 2013, Article ID 898261, 15 pages, 2013.

[6] T. Makino, T. Inagaki, K.-I. Komatsu, and Y. Kano, "Pharmacokinetic interactions between Japanese traditional kampo medicine and modern medicine (IV). Effect of Kamisyoyosan and Tokisyakuyakusan on the pharmacokinetics of etizolam in rats," *Biological and Pharmaceutical Bulletin*, vol. 28, no. 2, pp. 280–284, 2005.

[7] S. Ohnishi and H. Takeda, "Herbal medicines for the treatment of cancer chemotherapy-induced side effects," *Frontiers in Pharmacology*, vol. 6, article 14, 2015.

[8] J.-N. Lai, C.-T. Wu, and J.-D. Wang, "Prescription pattern of Chinese herbal products for breast cancer in Taiwan: a population-based study," *Evidence-Based Complementary and Alternative Medicine*, vol. 2012, Article ID 891893, 7 pages, 2012.

[9] B.-R. Wang, Y.-L. Chang, T.-J. Chen et al., "Coprescription of Chinese herbal medicine and Western medication among female patients with breast cancer in Taiwan: analysis of national insurance claims," *Patient Preference and Adherence*, vol. 8, pp. 671–682, 2014.

[10] B. Rochat, "Role of cytochrome P450 activity in the fate of anticancer agents and in drug resistance: focus on tamoxifen, paclitaxel and imatinib metabolism," *Clinical Pharmacokinetics*, vol. 44, no. 4, pp. 349–366, 2005.

[11] J. Jin, H. Bi, J. Hu et al., "Effect of Wuzhi tablet (Schisandra sphenanthera extract) on the pharmacokinetics of paclitaxel in rats," *Phytotherapy Research*, vol. 25, no. 8, pp. 1250–1253, 2011.

[12] J. H. Park, J. H. Park, H. J. Hur, J. S. Woo, and H. J. Lee, "Effects of silymarin and formulation on the oral bioavailability of paclitaxel in rats," *European Journal of Pharmaceutical Sciences*, vol. 45, no. 3, pp. 296–301, 2012.

[13] R. Václavíková, S. Horský, P. Šimek, and I. Gut, "Paclitaxel metabolism in rat and human liver microsomes is inhibited by phenolic antioxidants," *Naunyn-Schmiedeberg's Archives of Pharmacology*, vol. 368, no. 3, pp. 200–209, 2003.

[14] J. H. Lee, A. Lee, J.-H. Oh, and Y.-J. Lee, "Comparative pharmacokinetic study of paclitaxel and docetaxel in streptozotocin-induced diabetic rats," *Biopharmaceutics and Drug Disposition*, vol. 33, no. 8, pp. 474–486, 2012.

[15] A. R. Tan, A. Dowlati, M. N. Stein et al., "Phase I study of weekly paclitaxel in combination with pazopanib and lapatinib in advanced solid malignancies," *British Journal of Cancer*, vol. 110, no. 11, pp. 2647–2654, 2014.

[16] X. Wang, L. Song, N. Li et al., "Pharmacokinetics and biodistribution study of paclitaxel liposome in Sprague-Dawley rats and Beagle dogs by liquid chromatography-tandem mass spectrometry," *Drug Research*, vol. 63, no. 11, pp. 603–606, 2013.

[17] C.-M. Lu, M.-L. Hou, L.-C. Lin, and T.-H. Tsai, "Chemical and physical methods to analyze a multicomponent traditional chinese herbal prescription using LC-MS/MS, electron microscope, and congo red staining," *Evidence-Based Complementary and Alternative Medicine*, vol. 2013, Article ID 952796, 10 pages, 2013.

[18] S. Reagan-Shaw, M. Nihal, and N. Ahmad, "Dose translation from animal to human studies revisited," *FASEB Journal*, vol. 22, no. 3, pp. 659–661, 2008.

[19] M. Boyd, V. Risovic, P. Jull, E. Choo, and K. M. Wasan, "A stepwise surgical procedure to investigate the lymphatic transport of lipid-based oral drug formulations: cannulation of the mesenteric and thoracic lymph ducts within the rat," *Journal of Pharmacological and Toxicological Methods*, vol. 49, no. 2, pp. 115–120, 2004.

[20] M. Ionac, "One technique, two approaches, and results: thoracic duct cannulation in small laboratory animals," *Microsurgery*, vol. 23, no. 3, pp. 239–245, 2003.

[21] C. H. Hsieh, M. L. Hou, L. Y. Wang, H. Tai, T. Tsai, and Y. Chen, "Local pelvic irradiation modulates pharmacokinetics of 5-fluorouracil in the plasma but not in the lymphatic system," *BMC Cancer*, vol. 15, no. 1, article 316, 2015.

[22] T.-H. Tsai, Y.-J. Chen, M.-L. Hou, L.-Y. Wang, H.-C. Tai, and C.-H. Hsieh, "Pelvic irradiation modulates the pharmacokinetics of cisplatin in the plasma and lymphatic system," *American Journal of Translational Research*, vol. 7, no. 2, pp. 375–384, 2015.

[23] D. Zimmer, "New US FDA draft guidance on bioanalytical method validation versus current FDA and EMA guidelines: chromatographic methods and ISR," *Bioanalysis*, vol. 6, no. 1, pp. 13–19, 2014.

[24] A. Jain, A. Gulbake, A. Jain et al., "Development and validation of the HPLC method for simultaneous estimation of paclitaxel and topotecan," *Journal of Chromatographic Science*, vol. 52, no. 7, pp. 697–703, 2014.

[25] S. S. Vasudev, F. J. Ahmad, R. K. Khar et al., "Validated HPLC method for the simultaneous determination of taxol and ellagic acid in a *Punica granatum* fruit extract containing combination formulation," *Pharmazie*, vol. 67, no. 10, pp. 834–838, 2012.

[26] J. Carlier, J. Guitton, L. Romeuf et al., "Screening approach by ultra-high performance liquid chromatography-tandem mass spectrometry for the blood quantification of thirty-four toxic principles of plant origin. Application to forensic toxicology," *Journal of Chromatography B: Analytical Technologies in the Biomedical and Life Sciences*, vol. 975, pp. 65–76, 2015.

[27] B. Liu, X. Gou, X. Bai et al., "Simultaneous determination of seven taxoids in rat plasma by UPLC-MS/MS and pharmacokinetic study after oral administration of Taxus yunnanensis

extracts," *Journal of Pharmaceutical and Biomedical Analysis*, vol. 107, pp. 346–354, 2015.

[28] J. A. Siddiqui, A. Singh, M. Chagtoo, N. Singh, M. Godbole, and B. Chakravarti, "Phytochemicals for breast cancer therapy: current status and future implications," *Current Cancer Drug Targets*, vol. 15, no. 2, pp. 116–135, 2015.

[29] F. Qi, A. Li, Y. Inagaki et al., "Chinese herbal medicines as adjuvant treatment during chemoor radio-therapy for cancer," *BioScience Trends*, vol. 4, no. 6, pp. 297–307, 2010.

[30] K. K. Kumar, L. Priyanka, K. Gnananath, P. R. Babu, and S. Sujatha, "Pharmacokinetic drug interactions between apigenin, rutin and paclitaxel mediated by P-glycoprotein in rats," *European Journal of Drug Metabolism and Pharmacokinetics*, vol. 40, no. 3, pp. 267–276, 2015.

[31] Q. Cai, X. Deng, Z. Li, D. An, T. Shen, and M. Zhong, "Effects of lipid vehicle and P-glycoprotein inhibition on the mesenteric lymphatic transport of paclitaxel in unconscious, lymph duct-cannulated rats," *Drug Delivery*, vol. 23, no. 1, pp. 147–153, 2014.

[32] L.-Y. Wang, Y.-P. Tang, X. Liu et al., "Effects of ferulic acid on antioxidant activity in Angelicae Sinensis Radix, Chuanxiong Rhizoma, and their combination," *Chinese Journal of Natural Medicines*, vol. 13, no. 6, pp. 401–408, 2015.

[33] G.-S. Shan, L.-X. Zhang, Q.-M. Zhao et al., "Metabolomic study of raw and processed *Atractylodes macrocephala* Koidz by LC-MS," *Journal of Pharmaceutical and Biomedical Analysis*, vol. 98, pp. 74–84, 2014.

[34] Y. Ji, T. Wang, Z.-F. Wei et al., "Paeoniflorin, the main active constituent of *Paeonia lactiflora* roots, attenuates bleomycin-induced pulmonary fibrosis in mice by suppressing the synthesis of type I collagen," *Journal of Ethnopharmacology*, vol. 149, no. 3, pp. 825–832, 2013.

[35] B. Y.-K. Law, J.-F. Mo, and V. K.-W. Wong, "Autophagic effects of Chaihu (dried roots of Bupleurum Chinese DC or Bupleurum scorzoneraefolium WILD)," *Chinese Medicine*, vol. 9, no. 1, article 21, 2014.

[36] J.-L. Ríos, "Chemical constituents and pharmacological properties of *Poria cocos*," *Planta Medica*, vol. 77, no. 7, pp. 681–691, 2011.

[37] X. Wang, H. Zhang, L. Chen, L. Shan, G. Fan, and X. Gao, "Liquorice, a unique 'guide drug' of traditional Chinese medicine: a review of its role in drug interactions," *Journal of Ethnopharmacology*, vol. 150, no. 3, pp. 781–790, 2013.

[38] C. H. Lau, C. M. Chan, Y. W. Chan et al., "Pharmacological investigations of the anti-diabetic effect of Cortex Moutan and its active component paeonol," *Phytomedicine*, vol. 14, no. 11, pp. 778–784, 2007.

[39] S. Cheng, L.-C. Lin, C.-H. Lin, and T.-H. Tsai, "Comparative oral bioavailability of geniposide following oral administration of geniposide, Gardenia jasminoides Ellis fruits extracts and Gardenia herbal formulation in rats," *Journal of Pharmacy and Pharmacology*, vol. 66, no. 5, pp. 705–712, 2014.

[40] B. Ahmad, M. U. Rehman, I. Amin et al., "A review on pharmacological properties of zingerone (4-(4-Hydroxy-3-methoxyphenyl)-2-butanone)," *The Scientific World Journal*, vol. 2015, Article ID 816364, 6 pages, 2015.

[41] W. J. Zhang, K. Yang, C. X. You et al., "Contact toxicity and repellency of the essential oil from *Mentha haplocalyx* Briq. against *Lasioderma serricorne*," *Chemistry & Biodiversity*, vol. 12, no. 5, pp. 832–839, 2015.

[42] C.-X. Liu, X.-L. Yi, D.-Y. Si, X.-F. Xiao, X. He, and Y.-Z. Li, "Herb-drug interactions involving drug metabolizing enzymes and transporters," *Current Drug Metabolism*, vol. 12, no. 9, pp. 835–849, 2011.

[43] A. A. Gashev, "Physiologic aspects of lymphatic contractile function: current perspectives," *Annals of the New York Academy of Sciences*, vol. 979, pp. 178–187, 2002.

[44] S. Binder, "Evolution of Taxanes in the treatment of metastatic breast cancer," *Clinical Journal of Oncology Nursing*, vol. 17, no. 1, pp. 9–14, 2013.

[45] A. C. Boileau, N. R. Merchen, K. Wasson, C. A. Atkinson, and J. W. Erdman Jr., "Cis-lycopene is more bioavailable than trans-lycopene in vitro and in vivo in lymph-cannulated ferrets," *Journal of Nutrition*, vol. 129, no. 6, pp. 1176–1181, 1999.

[46] I.-L. Chen, Y.-J. Tsai, C.-M. Huang, and T.-H. U. Tsai, "Lymphatic absorption of quercetin and rutin in rat and their pharmacokinetics in systemic plasma," *Journal of Agricultural and Food Chemistry*, vol. 58, no. 1, pp. 546–551, 2010.

[47] W. Faisal, C. M. O'Driscoll, and B. T. Griffin, "Bioavailability of lycopene in the rat: the role of intestinal lymphatic transport," *Journal of Pharmacy and Pharmacology*, vol. 62, no. 3, pp. 323–331, 2010.

[48] H. Manita, T. Sudo, and H. Asano, "Demonstration of parotin in thoracic duct lymph and portal vein blood upon intestinal administration in the rat," *Endocrinologia Japonica*, vol. 20, no. 5, pp. 463–474, 1973.

[49] Y.-J. Tsai and T.-H. Tsai, "Mesenteric lymphatic absorption and the pharmacokinetics of naringin and naringenin in the rat," *Journal of Agricultural and Food Chemistry*, vol. 60, no. 51, pp. 12435–12442, 2012.

# 5

# Gelam Honey Attenuates the Oxidative Stress-Induced Inflammatory Pathways in Pancreatic Hamster Cells

**Sher Zaman Safi,[1] Kalaivani Batumalaie,[1] Rajes Qvist,[1] Kamaruddin Mohd Yusof,[2] and Ikram Shah Ismail[1]**

[1]*Faculty of Medicine, Department of Medicine, University of Malaya, 50603 Kuala Lumpur, Malaysia*
[2]*Department of Molecular Biology and Genetics, Faculty of Arts and Science, Canik Basari University, Samsun, Turkey*

Correspondence should be addressed to Sher Zaman Safi; safi.nust@yahoo.com
and Kalaivani Batumalaie; kalaivanibatumalaie@gmail.com

Academic Editor: Abir El-Alfy

*Purpose.* Type 2 diabetes consists of progressive hyperglycemia and insulin resistance, which could result from glucose toxicity, inflammatory cytokines, and oxidative stress. In the present study we investigated the effect of Gelam honey and quercetin on the oxidative stress-induced inflammatory pathways and the proinflammatory cytokines. *Methods.* HIT-T15 cells were cultured and preincubated with the extract of Gelam honey (20, 40, 60, and 80 $\mu$g/mL), as well as quercetin (20, 40, 60, and 80 $\mu$M), prior to stimulation by 20 and 50 mM glucose. *Results.* HIT-T15 cells cultured under hyperglycemic condition showed a significant increase in the inflammatory pathways by phosphorylating JNK, IKK-$\beta$, and IRS-1 at Ser307 ($p < 0.05$). There was a significant decrease in the phosphorylation of Akt at Ser473 ($p < 0.05$). Pretreatment with Gelam honey and quercetin reduced the expression of phosphorylated JNK, IKK-$\beta$, and IRS-1, thereby significantly reducing the expression of proinflammatory cytokines like TNF-$\alpha$, IL-6, and IL-1$\beta$ ($p < 0.05$). At the same time there was a significant increase in the phosphorylated Akt showing the protective effects against inflammation and insulin resistance ($p < 0.05$). In conclusion, our data suggest the potential use of the extract from Gelam honey and quercetin in modulating the inflammation induced insulin signaling pathways.

## 1. Research Background

Diabetes is one of the most common noncommunicable diseases affecting millions of people globally [1, 2]. It is one of the most challenging health problems in many developing and industrialized countries and the exact cause is unknown. One of the foremost challenges we now face is to account mechanistically not only for the definition of hyperglycemia, but also for other physiological and biochemical abnormalities, which are the characteristics of the disease [3, 4].

Type 2 diabetes consists of progressive hyperglycemia, insulin resistance, and pancreatic $\beta$ cell failure. The pathogenesis of type 2 diabetes is complex and in most instances clearly requires defects in both $\beta$ cell function and insulin sensitivity, and together both of these abnormalities bring about hyperglycemia. Type 2 diabetes has a metabolic milieu, which is characterized by insulin resistance and chronic acute inflammation. In the last decade, a great deal of attention

has been focused on the understanding of insulin resistance which is an important contributor to the development and maintenance of hyperglycemia in type 2 diabetes [5, 6].

B cell dysfunction can result from glucose toxicity, inflammatory cytokines, oxidative stress, or lipotoxicity in the presence of excess glucose. Oxidative stress through the production of reactive oxygen species (ROS) has been proposed as the root cause underlying the development of insulin resistance, $\beta$ cell dysfunction, impaired glucose tolerance, and type 2 diabetes mellitus [3].

Oxidative stress is induced by reactive oxygen and nitrogen species produced by several biochemical pathways associated with hyperglycemia (glucose autooxidation, polyol pathway, prostanoid synthesis, and protein glycation) and is critically involved in the impairment of $\beta$ cell function during the development of type 2 diabetes [7, 8]. Reactive oxygen species can function as signaling molecules to activate a number of stress sensitive pathways and inflammatory pathways leading to the production of inflammatory markers such as IL-6 and TNF-$\alpha$ that impair insulin signaling through serine phosphorylation of IRS-1 [9].

Insulin is a pleiotropic hormone which has many functions that are exerted across a variety of insulin target tissues, through several intracellular signaling cascades. Insulin substrate (IRS-1) mediated insulin signaling regulates peripheral insulin action as well as pancreatic $\beta$ cell function by regulating proliferation, survival, and insulin secretion. The defects in insulin signaling pathway mainly involve IRS-1. Activation of the insulin receptor leads to tyrosine phosphorylation of IRS-1, thereby initiating signal transduction. Insulin receptor tyrosine kinases can signal through the phosphatidylinositol 3-kinase (PI3K) pathway, which is mainly responsible for the metabolic actions of insulin. The major target of PI3K is the serine threonine kinase Akt. It has been shown that the Akt dependent mechanism in the distal events of exocytosis is responsible for the defect in insulin secretion [7, 10].

This transient exposure of $\beta$ cells to oxidative stress interrupts the normal coupling of glucose metabolism to insulin secretion by activating stress signaling pathways and the inflammatory pathways [11]. Despite the multiplicity of inflammatory pathways, the development of insulin resistance is often due to the activation of jun-N-terminal kinase (JNK) and the IkappaB kinase (IKK-$\beta$). The JNK and IKK-$\beta$ pathways are activated by ROS and various other factors including the inflammatory cytokines such as TNF-$\alpha$, IL-6, and IL-1beta which are involved in the development of insulin resistance found in type 2 diabetes [12].

Reactive oxygen species and mitochondrial stress-induced [13] activation of JNK and IKK-$\beta$ promotes the phosphorylation of IRS-1 at serine sites that negatively regulate normal signaling through the insulin receptor/IRS-1 axis, as seen in the phosphorylation of IRS-1 at serine 307 (Ser307). It has been reported that serine phosphorylation of insulin receptor-1 (IRS-1) inhibits insulin stimulated tyrosine phosphorylation of IRS-1 leading to an increase in insulin resistance [10]. Therefore, one of the causes leading to a defect in insulin signaling can be attributed to serine phosphorylation of IRS-1 at serine 307 residues which activate the jun-N-terminal kinase (JNK) and IKK-$\beta$, thus providing a plausible mechanistic link between inflammation and insulin resistance [14].

Recently, protein kinase B (PKB and Akt) has been shown to function in the insulin signaling cascade by phosphorylating transcription factors which are responsible for the transcription and expression of genes, related to insulin synthesis and secretion. Previous studies have shown that inactivation of Akt can lead to insulin resistance, decreased $\beta$ cell mass, and impaired insulin secretion [15].

Numerous studies have shown that honey has antioxidant and scavenging properties, which prevents the oxidative damage caused by free radicals. The antioxidant property is due to the phenolic compounds which are present in the honey and it has been demonstrated that the biological activities correlate with the phenolic content of the honey [16]. The phenolic content of the Malaysian Gelam honey has been shown to have both anti-inflammatory and antioxidant properties [17]. Quercetin is one of the important components of Gelam honey that may be further elaborated in terms of its function and use as antidiabetic agent.

Therefore, the aim of our present study is to determine the effect of Gelam honey extract and quercetin on the JNK and IKK-$\beta$ inflammatory pathways and IRS-1 serine phosphorylation which causes insulin resistance and the Akt activated insulin signaling pathway, which improves insulin resistance.

## 2. Research Design and Methods

*2.1. Extraction of Phenolic Compounds from Honey by Solid Phase Extraction (SPE).* Gelam honey samples (Department of Agriculture, Parit Botak, Johor, Malaysia) were subjected to base hydrolysis and extracted with ethyl acetate as described by Wahdan [18] and Seo and Morr [19]. The recovered fractions were combined and dried under nitrogen gas.

*2.2. Determination of the Phenolic Content.* Phenolic compounds from the extract were assayed using Folin-Ciocalteu assay [20]. Briefly the extract (1 mL) was added to 10% Folin-Ciocalteu reagent (Sigma F9252) and 0.5% sodium carbonate. The contents were thoroughly mixed and allowed to stand for 2 hours. The absorbance of the blue color that developed after 2 hours was read at 765 nm. Results were expressed in micrograms of Gallic acid per gram of the extract, using a standard curve generated with Gallic acid (Sigma G7384).

*2.3. Determination of the Flavonoid Content.* The total flavonoid (TF) content was determined spectrophotometrically. Briefly 1 mL of honey extract or a standard solution of quercetin (Sigma Q4951) (10, 50, 100, 150, 200, and 250 $\mu$g/mL) in distilled water was added to a 10 mL volumetric flask containing 4 mL of double distilled water, 300 $\mu$L of $NaNO_2$ (5%, v/v), and 300 $\mu$L of 10% $AlCl_3$. The solution was allowed to stand at room temperature in the dark for 30 minutes and the absorbance was read at 430 nm. The TF content was determined using the standard curve of quercetin ($\mu$g/mL) and was expressed as $\mu$g of quercetin equivalents in 1 g of extract.

*2.4. Cell Culture.* HIT-T15 cells were cultured according to the instructions provided by ATCC (CRL-1777). On arrival the cells were cultured immediately in T-25 cm flask in the F12K medium (ATCC 30-2004) supplemented with 10% FBS and 1% penicillin and streptomycin at 37°C (5% $CO_2$ in air). Cells (3rd passage) were trypsinized and subcultured, following which they were incubated for 5 days until they reached 80% confluency.

*2.5. Treatment of HIT-T15 Cells with Quercetin and Gelam Honey Extract.* HIT-T15 cells ($5 \times 10^5$) were pretreated with Gelam honey extract (20, 40, 60, and 80 $\mu$g/mL) and quercetin (20, 40, 60, and 80 $\mu$M) for 24 hours, after which the medium was replaced with fresh medium. Following this glucose (Sigma G8769) (20 or 50 mM) was added and the cells were incubated for another 24 hours.

*2.6. Cell Lysate Preparation.* After treatment the cells were washed twice in PBS and lysed in mammalian cell lysis buffer (Sigma MCL-1 which was supplemented with protease and phosphatase inhibitors. Insoluble materials were eliminated by centrifugation (12,000 ×g, 10 min, 4°C), and the protein concentration in the supernatant was determined by Bradford assay (Bio-Rad Laboratories).

*2.7. Western Blot Analysis.* Thirty micrograms of protein extracts was loaded on 10% SDS-polyacrylamide gel and transferred to activated nitrocellulose membrane. The membranes were blocked with tris-buffered saline (TBS) containing 5% nonfat milk and incubated with pAkt (Ser473), pIRS-1 (Ser307), p-JNK, p-IKK-$\alpha/\beta$, IL-6, IL-1$\beta$, and TNF alpha primary antibodies (obtained from Santa Cruz Laboratories) overnight at 4°C with a concentration of 1:1000. $\beta$-actin was used as a loading control. After 3 times extensive washes in TBS (for 20–30 m each), membranes were incubated for 1 h at room temperature with the appropriate horseradish peroxidase-conjugated secondary antibodies. We use the concentration of 1:5000 for secondary antibodies. Then we visualized the film using chemiluminescence substrate according to the manufacturer's instructions (Amersham Life Sciences, Little Chalfont, UK). Quantitative analysis of the protein content was performed by Gel Documentation System (Biospectrum 410, UVP).

*2.8. Statistical Analyses.* Data were analyzed with one-way ANOVA using SPSS version 16.0 software. The results were expressed as the mean ± standard deviation value. $^*p < 0.05$ was considered to be statistically significant.

# 3. Results

*3.1. Total Phenolic and Flavonoid Content.* 10 g of liquefied fresh Malaysian Gelam honey (*Apis mellifera*) was extracted using ethyl acetate and the extract was found to contain 52 $\mu$g of Gallic acid per gram of extract of total phenolic content and 6.92 $\mu$g of quercetin per gram of extract of total flavonoid content.

In our previous paper [21] we demonstrated the presence of ROS by using 2'7'-dichlorodihydrofluorescein diacetate (DCFH-DA) reagent under hyperglycemic conditions and by the measurement of intracellular ROS in individual cells by image analysis. Our data showed the antioxidant effect of Gelam honey extract and the flavonoid compounds quercetin, luteolin, and chrysin in the cultured cells by significantly inhibiting the production of ROS in a dose dependent manner. Again our data showed the reduction of ROS in the single cells in a dose dependent manner after pretreatment with the honey extract and the flavonoids.

*3.2. Effect of Pretreatment with Quercetin and Gelam Honey Extract on Phospho-JNK Expression under Normal and Hyperglycemic Conditions.* HIT-T15 cells were pretreated with the quercetin at concentrations of 20, 40, 60, and 80 $\mu$M and Gelam honey extract at concentrations of 20, 40, 60, and 80 $\mu$g/mL for 24 hours, following which they were cultured with 20 mM (Figures 1(a), 1(c), and 1(e)) or 50 mM

(Figures 1(b), 1(d), and 1(f)) glucose to determine the phosphorylation of JNK. The data revealed that exposure of HIT-T15 cells to 20 and 50 mM glucose significantly increased the level of phospho-JNK expression compared to control. Pretreatment with quercetin and Gelam honey extract significantly ($p < 0.05$) reduced the ROS induced expression of phospho-JNK under 20 mM glucose (Figures 1(a), 1(c), and 1(e)) by 60% and 42% in a dose dependent manner. Pretreatment with quercetin and Gelam honey extract reduced the expression of phospho-JNK significantly ($p < 0.05$) by 64% and 50%, respectively, compared to the cells that were cultured with 50 mM glucose (Figures 1(b), 1(d), and 1(f)) alone. The phospho-JNK protein levels from each sample were normalized to their respective $\beta$-actin protein amounts ($^*p < 0.05$ and $^\#p < 0.005$ versus glucose treated group) (Figure 1).

*3.3. Effect of Pretreatment with Quercetin and Gelam Honey Extract on Phospho-IKK-$\beta$ Expression under Normal and Hyperglycemic Conditions.* HIT-T15 cells were pretreated with the quercetin at concentrations of 20, 40, 60, and 80 $\mu$M and Gelam honey extract at concentrations of 20, 40, 60, and 80 $\mu$g/mL for 24 hours, following which they were cultured with 20 mM (Figures 2(a), 2(c), and 2(e)) or 50 mM (Figures 2(b), 2(d), and 2(f)) glucose to determine the phosphorylation of IKK-$\beta$. The phosphorylation of IKK-$\beta$ was increased in HIT-T15 cells treated with 20 mM and 50 mM glucose alone as compared with control. Pretreatment with the quercetin and Gelam honey extract showed 55% and 44% decrease ($p < 0.05$) in the expression of phosphorylated IKK-$\beta$ in a dose dependent manner in the cells that were cultured in 20 mM (Figures 2(a), 2(c), and 2(e)) glucose. Pretreatment with quercetin and Gelam honey extract significantly ($p < 0.05$) decreased the expression of phosphorylated IKK-$\beta$ under 50 mM glucose (Figures 2(b), 2(d), and 2(f)) by 60% and 47% in a dose dependent manner. The phosphorylated IKK-$\beta$ protein levels from each sample were normalized to their respective $\beta$-actin protein amounts ($^*p < 0.05$ and $^\#p < 0.005$ versus glucose treated group) (Figure 2).

*3.4. Effect of Pretreatment with Quercetin and Gelam Honey Extract on IL-6 Expression under Normal and Hyperglycemic Conditions.* HIT-T15 cells were pretreated with the quercetin at concentrations of 20, 40, 60, and 80 $\mu$M and Gelam honey extract at concentrations of 20, 40, 60, and 80 $\mu$g/mL for 24 hours, following which they were cultured in 20 mM (Figures 3(a), 3(c), and 3(e)) or 50 mM (Figures 3(b), 3(d), and 3(f)) glucose to determine the expression of IL-6. The expression was increased in HIT-T15 cells treated with 20 mM and 50 mM glucose alone as compared with control. Pretreatment with the quercetin and Gelam honey extract showed 52% and 40% decrease ($p < 0.05$) in the expression of IL-6 in a dose dependent manner in the cells that were cultured in 20 mM glucose (Figures 3(a), 3(c), and 3(e)). Pretreatment with quercetin and Gelam honey extract significantly ($p < 0.05$) decreased the expression of IL-6 under 50 mM glucose (Figures 3(b), 3(d), and 3(f)) by 60% and 47% in a dose dependent manner. The IL-6 protein levels from each sample

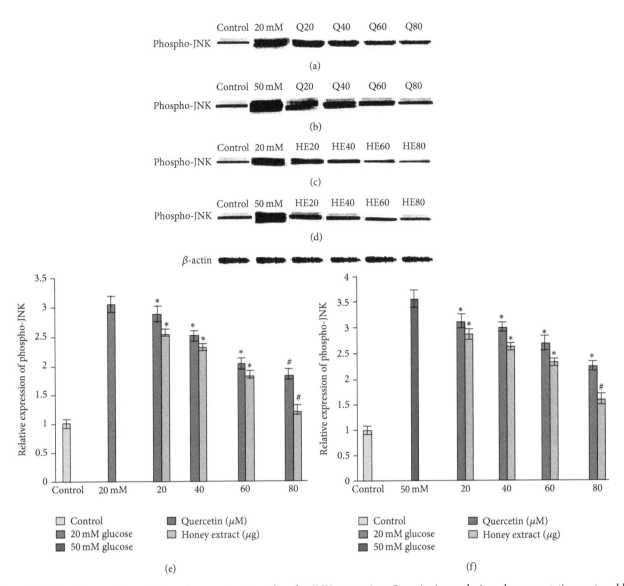

FIGURE 1: Effect of quercetin and Gelam honey extract on phospho-JNK expression. Quantitative analysis and representative western blot analysis of phospho-JNK in HIT-T15 cells pretreated with quercetin and honey extract in cells cultured in 20 mM ((a), (c), and (e)) and 50 mM ((b), (d), and (f)) glucose. The results were normalized with $\beta$-actin antibody. Data were analyzed with one-way ANOVA using SPSS version 16.0 software and are presented as the mean ± standard deviation and represent the mean of three different experiments. (e) $^*p < 0.05$ and $^\#p < 0.005$, quercetin and honey extract treated compared to the 20 mM glucose alone. (f) $^*p < 0.05$ and $^\#p < 0.005$, quercetin and honey extract treated compared to the 50 mM glucose alone.

were normalized to their respective $\beta$-actin protein amounts ($^*p < 0.05$ and $^\#p < 0.005$ versus glucose treated group).

*3.5. Effect of Pretreatment with Quercetin and Gelam Honey Extract on IL-1$\beta$ Expression under Normal and Hyperglycemic Conditions.* HIT-T15 cells were pretreated with the quercetin at concentrations of 20, 40, 60, and 80 $\mu$M and Gelam honey extract at concentrations of 20, 40, 60, and 80 $\mu$g/mL for 24 hours, following which they were then cultured with 20 or 50 mM glucose to determine the expression of IL-1$\beta$. IL-1$\beta$ in HIT-T15 cells was markedly increased following 20 mM (Figures 4(a), 4(c), and 4(e)) and 50 mM (Figures 4(b), 4(d), and 4(f)) glucose treatment, but the

trend was reversed after pretreatment with quercetin and Gelam honey extract. Pretreatment of the cells with different concentration of quercetin and honey extract for 24 hours significantly reduced the expression of IL-1$\beta$ up to 55% and 42%, respectively, compared to the cells that were cultured alone with 20 mM glucose (Figures 4(a), 4(c), and 4(e)). On the other hand, pretreatment with quercetin and honey extract reduced the expression of IL-1$\beta$ significantly ($p < 0.05$) up to 63% and 54%, respectively, compared to the cells that were cultured alone with 50 mM glucose (Figures 4(b), 4(d), and 4(f)). The IL-1$\beta$ protein levels from each sample were normalized to their respective $\beta$-actin protein amounts ($^*p < 0.05$ and $^\#p < 0.005$ versus glucose treated group), Figure 3.

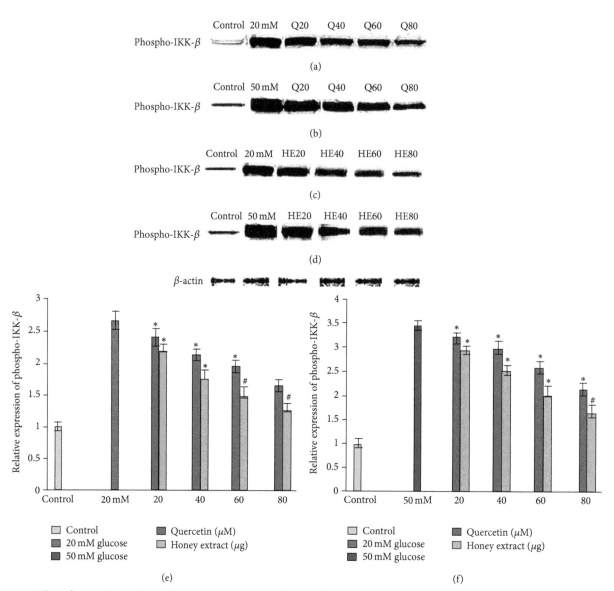

FIGURE 2: Effect of quercetin and Gelam honey extract on phospho-IKK-$\beta$ expression. Quantitative analysis and representative western blot analysis of phospho-IKK-$\beta$ in HIT-T15 cells pretreated with quercetin and honey extract in cells cultured in 20 mM ((a), (c), and (e)) and 50 mM ((b), (d), and (f)) glucose. The results were normalized with $\beta$-actin antibody. Data were analyzed with one-way ANOVA using SPSS version 16.0 software and are presented as the mean ± standard deviation and represent the mean of three different experiments. (e) $^*p < 0.05$ and $^\#p < 0.005$, quercetin and honey extract treated compared to the 20 mM glucose alone. (f) $^*p < 0.05$ and $^\#p < 0.005$, quercetin and honey extract treated compared to the 50 mM glucose alone.

*3.6. Effect of Pretreatment with Quercetin and Gelam Honey Extract on TNF Alpha Expression under Normal and Hyperglycemic Conditions.* HIT-T15 cells were pretreated with the quercetin at concentrations of 20, 40, 60, and 80 $\mu$M and Gelam honey extract at concentrations of 20, 40, 60, and 80 $\mu$g/mL for 24 hours, following which they were then cultured with 20 mM (Figures 5(a), 5(c), and 5(e)) or 50 mM (Figures 5(b), 5(d), and 5(f)) glucose to determine the TNF alpha. The TNF alpha was increased in HIT-T15 cells treated with 20 mM and 50 mM glucose alone as compared with control. Pretreatment with the quercetin and Gelam honey extract showed 43% and 55% decrease ($p < 0.05$) in the expression of TNF alpha in a dose dependent manner in the cells that were cultured in 20 mM glucose (Figures 5(a),

5(c), and 5(e)). Pretreatment with quercetin and Gelam honey extract significantly ($p < 0.05$) decreased the expression of TNF alpha in a dose dependent manner, in the cells cultured with 50 mM glucose (Figures 5(b), 5(d), and 5(f)) by 52% and 66%. The TNF alpha protein levels from each sample were normalized to their respective $\beta$-actin protein amounts ($^*p < 0.05$ and $^\#p < 0.005$ versus glucose treated group) (Figure 5).

*3.7. Effect of Pretreatment with Quercetin and Gelam Honey Extract on pIRS-1 (Ser307) Expression under Normal and Hyperglycemic Conditions.* HIT-T15 cells were pretreated with the quercetin at concentrations of 20, 40, 60, and 80 $\mu$M and Gelam honey extract at concentrations of 20, 40,

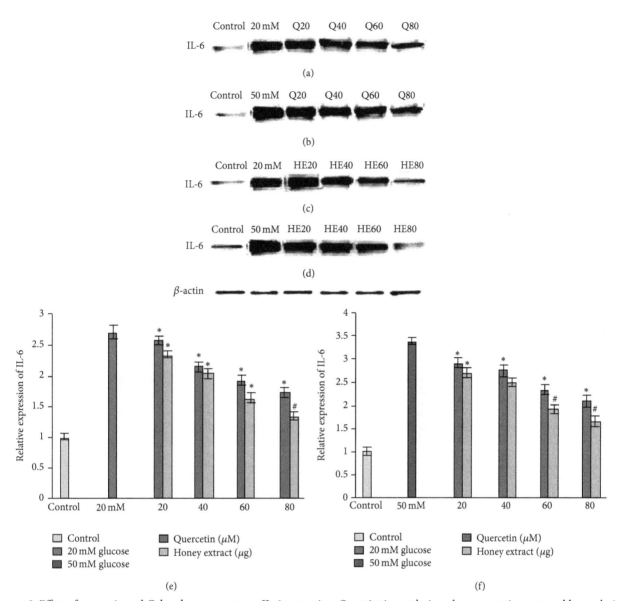

FIGURE 3: Effect of quercetin and Gelam honey extract on IL-6 expression. Quantitative analysis and representative western blot analysis of IL-6 in HIT-T15 cells pretreated with quercetin and honey extract in cells cultured in 20 mM ((a), (c), and (e)) and 50 mM ((b), (d), and (f)) glucose. The results were normalized with $\beta$-actin antibody. Data were analyzed with one-way ANOVA using SPSS version 16.0 software and are presented as the mean ± standard deviation and represent the mean of three different experiments. (e) $^{*}p < 0.05$ and $^{\#}p < 0.005$, quercetin and honey extract treated compared to the 20 mM glucose alone. (f) $^{*}p < 0.05$ and $^{\#}p < 0.005$, quercetin and honey extract treated compared to the 50 mM glucose alone.

60, and 80 μg/mL for 24 hours, following which they were then cultured with 20 mM (Figures 6(a), 6(c), and 6(e)) or 50 mM (Figures 6(b), 6(d), and 6(f)) glucose to determine the phosphorylation of IRS-1 (Ser307). The phosphorylation of IRS-1 (Ser307) was increased in HIT-T15 cells treated with 20 mM and 50 mM glucose alone as compared with control. Pretreatment with the quercetin and Gelam honey extract showed 49% and 55% decrease ($p < 0.05$) in the expression of pIRS-1 (Ser307) in a dose dependent manner in the cells that were cultured in 20 mM glucose (Figures 6(a), 6(c), and 6(e)). Pretreatment with quercetin and Gelam honey extract significantly ($p < 0.05$) decreased the expression of pIRS-1 (Ser307) in cells that were cultured in 50 mM

glucose (Figures 6(b), 6(d), and 6(f)) by 43% and 60% in a dose dependent manner. The pIRS-1 protein levels from each sample were normalized to their respective $\beta$-actin protein amounts ($^{*}p < 0.05$ and $^{\#}p < 0.005$ versus glucose treated group) (Figure 6).

### 3.8. Effect of Pretreatment with Quercetin and Gelam Honey Extract on pAkt (Ser473) Expression under Normal and Hyperglycemic Conditions. HIT-T15 cells were pretreated with the quercetin at concentrations of 20, 40, 60, and 80 μM and Gelam honey extract at concentrations of 20, 40, 60, and 80 μg/mL for 24 hours, following which they were then cultured with 20 or 50 mM glucose to determine the

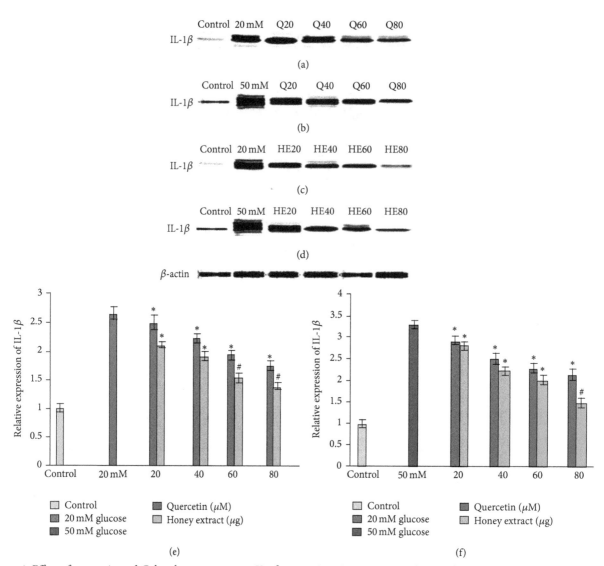

FIGURE 4: Effect of quercetin and Gelam honey extract on IL-1$\beta$ expression. Quantitative analysis and representative western blot analysis of IL-1$\beta$ in HIT-T15 cells pretreated with quercetin and honey extract in cells cultured in 20 mM ((a), (c), and (e)) and 50 mM ((b), (d), and (f)) glucose. The results were normalized with $\beta$-actin antibody. Data were analyzed with one-way ANOVA using SPSS version 16.0 software and are presented as the mean ± standard deviation and represent the mean of three different experiments. (e) $^*p < 0.05$ and $^\#p < 0.005$, quercetin and honey extract treated compared to the 20 mM glucose alone. (f) $^*p < 0.05$ and $^\#p < 0.005$ quercetin and honey extract treated compared to the 50 mM glucose alone.

phosphorylation of Akt (Ser473). There was no change in the Akt (Ser473) phosphorylation in HIT-T15 cells when treated with 20 mM glucose (Figures 7(a), 7(c), and 7(e)) but it was markedly reduced when the cells were treated with 50 mM (Figures 7(b), 7(d), and 7(f)) glucose. Pretreatment of the cells with different concentration of quercetin and honey extract for 24 hours significantly increased the expression of pAkt (Ser473) up to 38% and 70%, respectively, compared to the cells that were cultured alone with 20 mM glucose (Figures 7(a), 7(c), and 7(e)). On the other hand, pretreatment with quercetin and honey extract increased the expression of pAkt (Ser473) significantly ($p < 0.05$) up to 30% and 54%, respectively, compared to the cells that were cultured alone with 50 mM glucose (Figures 7(b), 7(d), and 7(f)). The cells that were exposed to Akt inhibitor VIII prevented the

quercetin and honey extract induced Akt Ser473 phosphorylation (Figure 7). The pAkt protein levels from each sample were normalized to their respective $\beta$-actin protein amounts ($^*p < 0.05$ and $^\#p < 0.005$ versus glucose treated group) (Figure 7).

## 4. Discussion

In our previous study we investigated the antioxidant effect of the Malaysian Gelam honey and some of its flavonoid components (chrysin, luteolin, and quercetin) individually, on pancreatic hamster cells (HIT-T15) cultured under hyperglycemic conditions. Our data demonstrated that the cultured cells, pretreated with the extract of the Gelam honey and the different flavonoid components (quercetin,

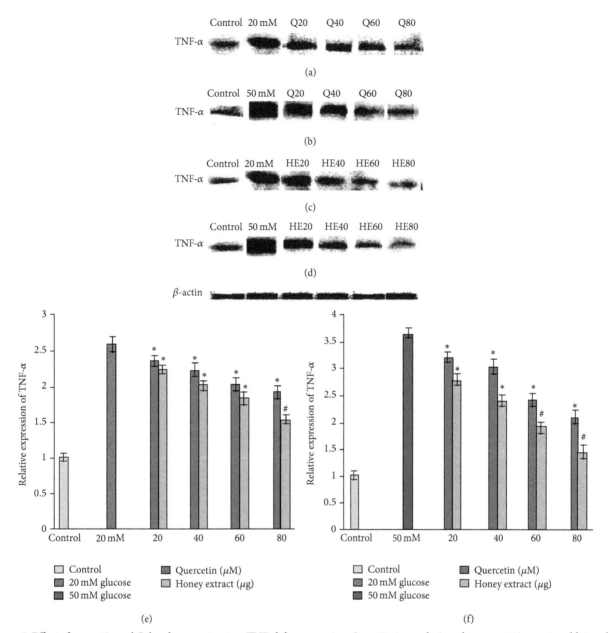

FIGURE 5: Effect of quercetin and Gelam honey extract on TNF alpha expression. Quantitative analysis and representative western blot analysis of TNF alpha in HIT-T15 cells pretreated with quercetin and honey extract in cells cultured in 20 mM ((a), (c), and (e)) and 50 mM ((b), (d), and (f)) glucose. The results were normalized with $\beta$-actin antibody. Data were analyzed with one-way ANOVA using SPSS version 16.0 software and are presented as the mean ± standard deviation and represent the mean of three different experiments. (e) $^*p < 0.05$ and $^#p < 0.005$, quercetin and honey extract treated compared to the 20 mM glucose alone. (f) $^*p < 0.05$ and $^#p < 0.005$, quercetin and honey extract treated compared to the 50 mM glucose alone.

luteolin, and chrysin) at varying concentrations for 24 hours, protected the $\beta$ cell from oxidative damage caused by ROS induced by hyperglycemia [21]. Furthermore, we investigated the effect of Gelam honey extract and quercetin on the stress activated NF-$\kappa$B and MAPK pathways and IRS-1 serine phosphorylation causing insulin resistance and the Akt activated insulin signaling pathway, causing increase in insulin content. Our data demonstrated that the Gelam honey extract and quercetin had the best protective effect against hyperglycemia induced oxidative stress by improving the insulin content and insulin resistance [22].

The floral source of Gelam honey is *Melaleuca cajuputi*. This was the only source of Gelam honey that was used in Kamaruddin et al. laboratory and different students worked on the different aspects of this honey. They were the first to establish the detection of the phenolic compounds in Gelam honey found in Malaysia using HPLC [23]. Chromatogram of phenolic acid and flavonoids detected in Malaysian Gelam honey, using HPLC-UV absorption (1) 290 nm and (2) 340 nm, is shown in the paper of the same group [24]. In our previous study we used three different flavonoids: chrysin, luteolin, and quercetin [21, 22]. This shows that the quercetin

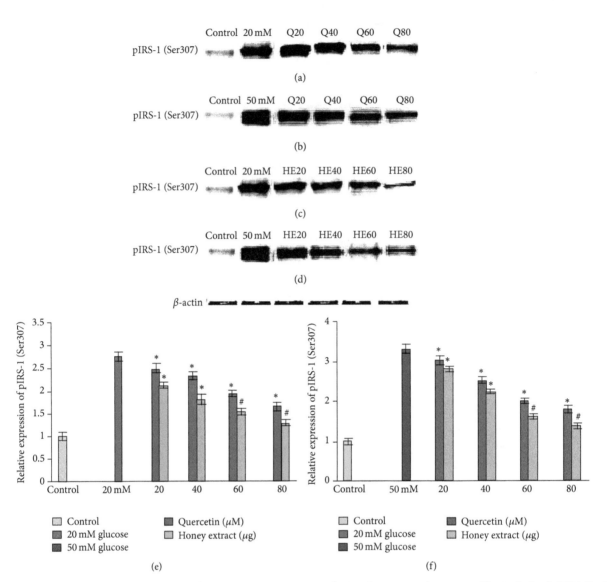

FIGURE 6: Effect of quercetin on pIRS-1 (Ser307) expression. Quantitative analysis and representative western blot analysis of pIRS-1 (Ser307) in HIT-T15 cells pretreated with quercetin and Gelam honey extract in cells cultured in 20 mM ((a), (c), and (e)) and 50 mM ((b), (d), and (f)) glucose. The results were normalized with $\beta$-actin antibody. Data were analyzed with one-way ANOVA using SPSS version 16.0 software and are presented as the mean ± standard deviation and represent the mean of three different experiments. (e) $^*p < 0.05$ and $^#p < 0.005$, quercetin and honey extract treated compared to the 20 mM glucose alone. (f) $^*p < 0.05$ and $^#p < 0.005$ quercetin and honey extract treated compared to the 50 mM glucose alone.

was the most effective amongst the three flavonoids. The work on caffeic acid on the same Gelam honey has already been published by the above-mentioned group [25, 26].

Therefore, in our present study, we determined the effect of Gelam honey extract and quercetin on the oxidative stress activated JNK and IKK-$\beta$ inflammatory pathways and IRS-1 serine phosphorylation causing insulin resistance and the Akt activated insulin signaling pathway, which attenuates the inflammation, thereby increasing insulin sensitivity.

Several studies have demonstrated that flavonoids may reduce hyperglycemia and exert protective effects against nonenzymatic glycation of proteins in animals [27, 28]. The flavonoid quercetin in particular has been reported to have anti-inflammatory properties in diabetic animal models,

by protecting the retinal cell apoptosis in diabetes [29]. Under diabetic conditions, hyperglycemia induced ROS and inflammatory cytokines presumably lead to the activation of the JNK and IKK-$\beta$ pathways. It has been shown that IKK and JNK control the major inflammatory response pathways in hyperglycemia and that they are activated by oxidative stress [30, 31].

Yuan et al. [32] demonstrated that reduced signaling through the IKK-$\beta$ pathway inhibition by sodium salicylate in obese mice is accompanied by improved insulin sensitivity. Again the study showed that phosphorylation of IKK-$\beta$ was increased in diabetes, but the blockade of NF-$\kappa$B, oxidative stress, and the genetic deletion of TNF-$\alpha$ attenuated phosphorylation of IKK-$\beta$, suggesting

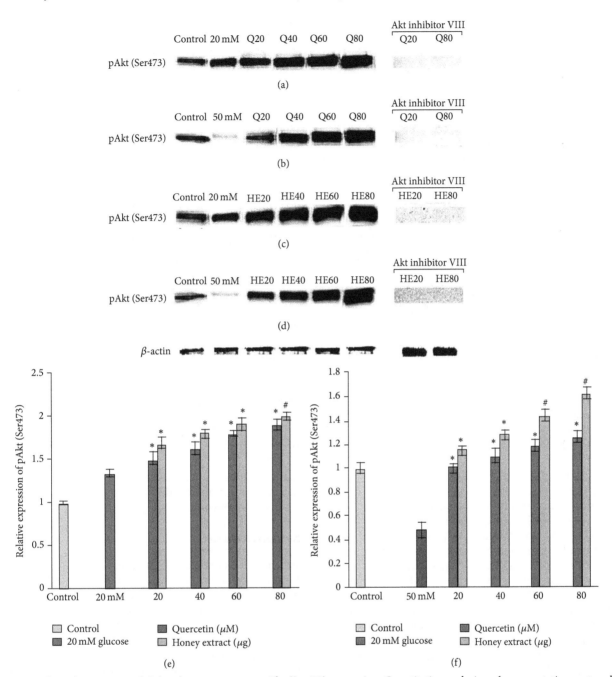

FIGURE 7: Effect of quercetin and Gelam honey extract on pAkt (Ser473) expression. Quantitative analysis and representative western blot analysis of pAkt (Ser473) in HIT-T15 cells pretreated with quercetin and honey extract in cells cultured in 20 mM ((a), (c), and (e)) and 50 mM ((b), (d), and (f)) glucose. An increase in the level of pAkt (Ser473) was observed after pretreatment with quercetin and honey extract. Akt inhibitor VIII prevented the expression of Akt Ser473 phosphorylation induced by quercetin and honey extract. The results were normalized with $\beta$-actin antibody. Data were analyzed with one-way ANOVA using SPSS version 16.0 software and are presented as the mean ± standard deviation and represent the mean of three different experiments. (e) $^*p < 0.05$ and $^\#p < 0.005$, quercetin and honey extract treated compared to the 20 mM glucose alone. (f) $^*p < 0.05$ and $^\#p < 0.005$, quercetin and honey extract treated compared to the 50 mM glucose alone.

that the phosphorylation of IKK-$\beta$ is increased in diabetic mice by the activation of oxidative stress and TNF-$\alpha$ [33].

The increase in free fatty acids, inflammatory cytokines, and oxidative stress under diabetic conditions activates the JNK pathway which causes insulin resistance and pancreatic $\beta$ cell dysfunction [34]. It has been reported that the JNK pathway was abnormally activated in the liver, muscle, and adipose tissue in obese type 2 diabetic mice and that the insulin resistance was substantially reduced when the mice were homozygous for a targeted mutation in the JNK1 gene.

Our data showed that exposure of HIT-T15 cells to 20 and 50 mM glucose caused a significant increase in the level of phosphorylated JNK (Figure 1) and phosphorylated IKK-$\beta$

(Figure 2) expressions compared to the control. Pretreatment with quercetin and Gelam honey extract significantly ($p <$ 0.05) reduced the ROS induced inflammatory pathway of phosphorylated JNK (Figure 1) and phosphorylated IKK-$\beta$ (Figure 2) when treated with 20 and 50 mM glucose. This gives further support to the fact that oxidative stress induced by high glucose activates the major inflammatory pathways.

It has been shown that hyperglycemia is proinflammatory and is normally restrained by the anti-inflammatory effect of insulin secreted in response to that stimulus [35]. Hyperglycemia induced by glucose clamping in normal subjects showed a significant increase in the circulating levels of interleukin- (IL-) 6, IL-18, Il-1$\beta$, and tumor necrosis factor-$\alpha$ (TNF-$\alpha$). These effects were more sustained in patients with impaired glucose tolerance as well as in those after consecutive pulses of intravenous glucose, which were annulled by glutathione, implicating an oxidative mechanism [31]. Interestingly enough, these cytokines have been implicated in insulin resistance (TNF-$\alpha$, IL-6, and IL-1$\beta$), atherosclerotic plaque destabilization (IL-18), and future cardiovascular events (IL-6, IL-18, IL-1$\beta$, and TNF-$\alpha$). So, an increased oxidative stress may be a likely mechanism linking stress hyperglycemia to increased inflammatory cytokine production [31, 34]. Several cross-sectional studies showed that insulin resistance and type 2 diabetes are associated with higher levels of C-reactive protein (CRP), interleukin-6 (IL-6), interleukin-1$\beta$, and tumor necrosis factor-$\alpha$ (TNF-$\alpha$), which are markers of subclinical systemic inflammation [35]. Furthermore, various longitudinal studies have shown that elevated levels of CRP, IL-1$\beta$, IL-6, and TNF-$\alpha$ predict the development of type 2 diabetes [35].

Our data supported the above statement by showing that TNF-$\alpha$, IL-6, and IL-1$\beta$ expressions (Figures 3, 4, and 5) in HIT-T15 cells were markedly increased following 20 and 50 mM glucose treatment but were reversed after pretreatment with quercetin and Gelam honey extract. In addition, our data showed that the expression of TNF-$\alpha$, IL-6, and IL-1$\beta$ (Figures 3, 4, and 5) was decreased.

Our previous data demonstrated that Akt (Ser473) phosphorylation was increased after pretreatment with quercetin and honey extract (REF). Effect of Gelam honey on the oxidative stress induced signaling pathways in pancreatic hamster cells [22].

In the year 2001 it was reported that mice lacking the pAkt (Ser473) protein were insulin resistant, with impaired insulin secretion [36]. It was shown that Akt (Ser473) is necessary for normal pancreatic $\beta$ cell function including a novel regulatory role for Akt signaling in insulin secretion [37]. Several studies reported that a decrease in insulin secretion and insulin resistance induced by hyperglycemia has been associated with decreased Akt activity [38–41].

In our previous papers [21, 22] we showed that the cells cultured under 20 mM glucose did not show any changes at the level of the Akt phosphorylation while under 50 mM the Akt (serine 473) phosphorylation was reduced significantly. The phosphorylation was increased significantly after pretreatment with quercetin and honey extract. Akt inhibitor VIII prevented the expression of Akt Ser473 phosphorylation induced by quercetin and honey extract. When we studied

the insulin content our data demonstrated that there was a significant increase in the insulin content ($p < 0.05$) when the cells cultured under 20 mM glucose were pretreated with quercetin and honey extract, but there was a significant decrease in the insulin content ($p < 0.05$) when the cells were treated with Akt inhibitor VIII, before pretreating with quercetin and Gelam honey extract when the cells were cultured in 50 mM glucose, and there was a significant increase in the insulin content ($p < 0.05$ and $p < 0.005$) when the cells were pretreated with quercetin and Gelam honey extract. A significant decrease was seen ($p < 0.05$ and $p < 0.005$) when the cells were treated with Akt inhibitor VIII before pretreating with quercetin and Gelam honey extract.

Thus, our data demonstrated the protective effects of Akt against $\beta$ cell dysfunction and insulin resistance, which was further supported by the fact that Akt inhibitor increased the insulin resistance by decreasing the quantity of insulin secreted.

It has been shown that activation of the IKK-$\beta$ and JNK pathways increases IRS-1 serine phosphorylation which leads to suppression of insulin signaling and that suppression of the IKK pathway decreases insulin resistance and ameliorates glucose intolerance in diabetic mice [29]. Our data which supports the above statement showed that phosphorylation of IRS-1 (Ser307) was increased in HIT-T15 cells treated with 20 and 50 mM glucose alone as compared with control. Pretreatment with the quercetin and Gelam honey extract significantly decreased ($p < 0.05$) the expression of pIRS-1 (Ser307) (Figure 6) in a dose dependent manner in the cells that were cultured in 20 and 50 mM glucose (Figure 6). Our data suggest that there is decrease in phosphorylation of IRS-1(Ser307) (Figure 6).

## 5. Conclusion

In conclusion our data suggest the potential use of the extract from Gelam honey in treating diabetes, by modulating the inflammatory pathways. The data provide further support to the role of inflammation in $\beta$ cell dysfunction and insulin resistance. In addition, since stress-induced JNK and IKK pathways are involved in the development of insulin resistance, inflammation, and $\beta$ cell dysfunction, it is possible that such pathways could be a therapeutic target for type 2 diabetes.

## Disclosure

Sher Zaman Safi and Kalaivani Batumalaie are both first authors of this paper in which the western blotting was performed by Kalaivani Batumalaie.

## Conflict of Interests

The authors declare no conflict of interests in this work.

## Authors' Contribution

Sher Zaman Safi contributed to conception and design of the study. Rajes Qvist performed revision of paper. Kalaivani

Batumalaie is the student who did the experiments of WB. Ikram Shah Ismail is Head of the Diabetic Group and revised the paper. Sher Zaman Safi and Kalaivani Batumalaie have contributed equally to this work.

## Acknowledgments

The authors would like to thank the University of Malaya for their financial support, Grants nos. RG516-13HTM and RG528-13HTM. The authors are also thankful to the IPPP for supporting the postdoctoral fellowship.

## References

[1] S. Wild, G. Roglic, A. Green, R. Sicree, and H. King, "Global prevalence of diabetes: estimates for the year 2000 and projections for 2030," *Diabetes Care*, vol. 27, no. 5, pp. 1047–1053, 2004.

[2] S. Z. Safi, R. Qvist, K. Chinna, M. A. Ashraf, D. Paramasivam, and I. S. Ismail, "Gene expression profiling of the peripheral blood mononuclear cells of offspring of one type 2 diabetic parent," *International Journal of Diabetes in Developing Countries*, pp. 1–13, 2015.

[3] A. F. Amos, D. J. McCarty, and P. Zimmet, "The rising global burden of diabetes and its complications: estimates and projections to the year 2010," *Diabetic Medicine*, vol. 14, no. 5, pp. S7–S85, 1997.

[4] S. Z. Safi, H. Shah, G. O. S. Yan, and R. Qvist, "Insulin resistance provides the connection between hepatitis C virus and diabetes," *Hepatitis Monthly*, vol. 15, no. 1, Article ID e23941, 2015.

[5] S. E. Shoelson, J. Lee, and A. B. Goldfine, "Inflammation and insulin resistance," *The Journal of Clinical Investigation*, vol. 116, no. 7, pp. 1793–1801, 2006.

[6] S. Z. Safi, R. Qvist, S. Kumar, K. Batumalaie, and I. S. B. Ismail, "Molecular mechanisms of diabetic retinopathy, general preventive strategies, and novel therapeutic targets," *BioMed Research International*, vol. 2014, Article ID 801269, 18 pages, 2014.

[7] D. Giugliano, A. Ceriello, and G. Paolisso, "Oxidative stress and diabetic vascular complications," *Diabetes Care*, vol. 19, no. 3, pp. 257–267, 1996.

[8] S. Z. Safi, R. Qvist, G. O. S. Yan, and I. S. B. Ismail, "Differential expression and role of hyperglycemia induced oxidative stress in epigenetic regulation of $\beta$1, $\beta$2 and $\beta$3-adrenergic receptors in retinal endothelial cells," *BMC Medical Genomics*, vol. 7, article 29, 2014.

[9] N. Sattar, C. G. Perry, and J. R. Petrie, "Type 2 diabetes as an inflammatory disorder," *The British Journal of Diabetes and Vascular Disease*, vol. 3, no. 1, pp. 36–41, 2003.

[10] V. Aguirre, E. D. Werner, J. Giraud, Y. H. Lee, S. E. Shoelson, and M. F. White, "Phosphorylation of Ser[307] in insulin receptor substrate-1 blocks interactions with the insulin receptor and inhibits insulin action," *Journal of Biological Chemistry*, vol. 277, no. 2, pp. 1531–1537, 2002.

[11] N. Li, T. Brun, M. Cnop, D. A. Cunha, D. L. Eizirik, and P. Maechler, "Transient oxidative stress damages mitochondrial machinery inducing persistent $\beta$-cell dysfunction," *The Journal of Biological Chemistry*, vol. 284, no. 35, pp. 23602–23612, 2009.

[12] V. T. Samuel and G. I. Shulman, "Mechanisms for insulin resistance: common threads and missing links," *Cell*, vol. 148, no. 5, pp. 852–871, 2012.

[13] S. Z. Safi, K. Batumalaie, M. Mansor et al., "Glutamine treatment attenuates hyperglycemia-induced mitochondrial stress and apoptosis in umbilical vein endothelial cells," *Clinics*, vol. 70, no. 8, pp. 569–576, 2015.

[14] B. Draznin, "Molecular mechanisms of insulin resistance: Serine phosphorylation of insulin receptor substrate-1 and increased expression of p85$\alpha$: the two sides of a coin," *Diabetes*, vol. 55, no. 8, pp. 2392–2397, 2006.

[15] E. Bernal-Mizrachi, S. Fatrai, J. D. Johnson et al., "Defective insulin secretion and increased susceptibility to experimental diabetes are induced by reduced Akt activity in pancreatic islet $\beta$ cells," *The Journal of Clinical Investigation*, vol. 114, no. 7, pp. 928–936, 2004.

[16] M. A. Mamary, A. A. Meeri, and M. A. Habori, "Antioxidant activities and total phenolics of different types of honey," *Nutrition Research*, vol. 22, no. 9, pp. 1041–1047, 2002.

[17] A. Aljadi and M. Kamaruddin, "Evaluation of phenolic contents and antioxidant capacities of two Malaysian floral honeys," *Food Chemistry*, vol. 85, no. 4, pp. 513–518, 2004.

[18] H. A. L. Wahdan, "Causes of the antimicrobial activity of honey," *Infection*, vol. 26, no. 1, pp. 26–31, 1998.

[19] A. Seo and C. V. Morr, "Improved high-performance liquid chromatographic analysis of phenolic acids and iso-flavonoids from soybean protein products," *Journal of Agricultural and Food Chemistry*, vol. 32, no. 3, pp. 530–533, 1984.

[20] S. Z. Hussein, K. M. Yusoff, S. Makpol, and Y. A. Yusof, "Antioxidant capacities and total phenolic contents increase with gamma irradiation in two types of Malaysian honey," *Molecules*, vol. 16, no. 8, pp. 6378–6395, 2011.

[21] B. Kalaivani, Q. Rajes, M. Y. Kamaruddin, S. I. Ikram, and D. S. Shamala, "The antioxidant effect of the Malaysian Gelam honey on pancreatic hamster cells cultured under hyperglycemic conditions," *Clinical and Experimental Medicine*, vol. 14, no. 2, pp. 185–195, 2014.

[22] B. Kalaivani, Z. S. Sher, M. Y. Kamaruddin, S. I. Ikram, D. S. Shamala, and Q. Rajes, "Effect of Gelam honey on the oxidative stress-induced signaling pathways in pancreatic hamster cells," *International Journal of Endocrinology*, vol. 2013, Article ID 367312, 10 pages, 2013.

[23] A. M. Aljadi and K. M. Yusoff, "Isolation and identification of phenolic acids in Malaysian honey with anti-bacterial properties," *Turkish Journal of Medical Sciences*, vol. 33, pp. 229–236, 2003.

[24] S. Z. Hussein, K. M. Yusoff, S. Makpol, and Y. A. M. Yusof, "Antioxidant capacities and total phenolic contents increase with gamma irradiation in two types of Malaysian honey," *Molecules*, vol. 16, no. 8, pp. 6378–6395, 2011.

[25] M. Kassim, M. Mansor, T. A. Kamalden et al., "Caffeic acid Phenethyl ester (CAPE): scavenger of peroxynitrite in vitro and in sepsis models," *Shock*, vol. 42, no. 2, pp. 154–160, 2014.

[26] M. Kassim, M. Mansor, A. Suhaimi, G. Ong, and K. M. Yusoff, "Gelam honey scavenges peroxynitrite during the immune response," *International Journal of Molecular Sciences*, vol. 13, no. 9, pp. 12113–12129, 2012.

[27] O. Coskun, M. Kanter, A. Korkmaz, and S. Oter, "Quercetin, a flavonoid antioxidant, prevents and protects streptozotocin-induced oxidative stress and $\beta$-cell damage in rat pancreas," *Pharmacological Research*, vol. 51, no. 2, pp. 117–123, 2005.

[28] N. Y. Nuraliev and G. A. Avezov, "The efficacy of quercetin in alloxan diabetes," *Experimental and Clinical Pharmacology*, vol. 55, no. 1, pp. 42–44, 1992.

[29] I. Jessica, B. Maia, G. Muraya, and G. Carlos, "Quercetin ameliorates hyperglycemia-induced inflammation and apoptosis in the retina and lateral geniculate nucleus in a rat model of type 2 diabetes mellitus," *The FASEB Journal*, vol. 28, no. 1, article 688.8, 2014.

[30] E. Katherine, M. Raffaele, and G. Dario, "Stress hyperglycemia, inflammation, and cardiovascular events," *Diabetes Care*, vol. 26, no. 5, pp. 1650–1651, 2003.

[31] S. Kumar, S. Z. Safi, R. Qvist, and I. S. Ismail, "Effect of agonists of adenosine receptors on inflammatory markers in human Muller cells," *Current Science*, vol. 106, no. 4, pp. 582–586, 2014.

[32] M. Yuan, N. Konstantopoulos, J. Lee et al., "Reversal of obesity- and diet-induced insulin resistance with salicylates or targeted disruption of $Ikk\beta$," *Science*, vol. 293, no. 5535, pp. 1673–1677, 2001.

[33] H. Kaneto, N. Katakami, M. Matsuhisa, and T. Matsuoka, "Role of reactive oxygen species in the progression of Type 2 diabetes and atherosclerosis," *Mediators of Inflammation*, vol. 2010, Article ID 453892, 11 pages, 2010.

[34] H. Kaneto, Y. Nakatani, D. Kawamori, T. Miyatsuka, and T.-A. Matsuoka, "Involvement of oxidative stress and the JNK pathway in glucose toxicity," *The Review of Diabetic Studies*, vol. 1, no. 4, pp. 165–174, 2004.

[35] D. R. Nathalie, P. Rita, D. Jingzhong et al., "Diabetes, hyperglycemia, and inflammation in older individuals: the health, aging and body composition study," *Diabetes Care*, vol. 29, no. 8, pp. 1902–1908, 2006.

[36] H. Cho, J. Mu, J. K. Kim et al., "Insulin resistance and a diabetes mellitus-like syndrome in mice lacking the protein kinase Akt2 (PKB$\beta$)," *Science*, vol. 292, no. 5522, pp. 1728–1731, 2001.

[37] E. Bernal-Mizrachi, S. Fatrai, J. D. Johnson et al., "Defective insulin secretion and increased susceptibility to experimental diabetes are induced by reduced Akt activity in pancreatic islet $\beta$ cells," *The Journal of Clinical Investigation*, vol. 114, no. 7, pp. 928–936, 2004.

[38] P. Gual, Y. Le Marchand-Brustel, and J.-F. Tanti, "Positive and negative regulation of insulin signaling through IRS-1 phosphorylation," *Biochimie*, vol. 87, no. 1, pp. 99–109, 2005.

[39] D. A. Glauser and W. Schlegel, "The emerging role of FOXO transcription factors in pancreatic $\beta$ cells," *Journal of Endocrinology*, vol. 193, no. 2, pp. 195–207, 2007.

[40] A. D. Kohn, S. A. Summers, M. J. Birnbaum, and R. A. Roth, "Expression of a constitutively active Akt Ser/Thr kinase in 3T3-L1 adipocytes stimulates glucose uptake and glucose transporter 4 translocation," *The Journal of Biological Chemistry*, vol. 271, no. 49, pp. 31372–31378, 1996.

[41] K. K. Y. Cheng, K. S. L. Lam, D. Wu et al., "APPL1 potentiates insulin secretion in pancreatic $\beta$ cells by enhancing protein kinase Akt-dependent expression of SNARE proteins in mice," *Proceedings of the National Academy of Sciences of the United States of America*, vol. 109, no. 23, pp. 8919–8924, 2012.

# 6

# Traditional Therapies Used to Manage Diabetes and Related Complications in Mauritius: A Comparative Ethnoreligious Study

**M. Fawzi Mahomoodally,[1] A. Mootoosamy,[1] and S. Wambugu[2]**

[1]Department of Health Sciences, Faculty of Science, University of Mauritius, 230 Réduit, Mauritius
[2]Department of Veterinary Anatomy and Physiology, University of Nairobi, Nairobi 30197 00100, Kenya

Correspondence should be addressed to M. Fawzi Mahomoodally; f.mahomoodally@uom.ac.mu

Academic Editor: Andrea Pieroni

Religious communities from Mauritius still rely on traditional therapies (TT) for primary healthcare. Nonetheless, there is still a dearth of scientific information on TT used by the different religious groups to manage diabetes and related complications (DRC). This study aimed to gather ethnomedicinal knowledge on TT used by the different religious groups against DRC. Diabetic patients ($n = 95$) and traditional healers ($n = 5$) were interviewed. Fifty-two plant species belonging to 33 families and 26 polyherbal formulations were documented to manage DRC. The most reported DRC was hypertension ($n = 36$). Leaves (45.2%) and juice (36%) were the most cited mode of preparation of herbal recipes. Plants which scored high relative frequency of citation were *Citrus aurantifolia* (0.55) and *Morinda citrifolia* (0.54). The cultural importance index showed that *Ocimum tenuiflorum, Cardiospermum halicacabum, Camellia sinensis,* and *Ophiopogon japonicas* were the most culturally important plants among Hindu, Muslim, Christian, and Buddhist community, respectively. Hindu and Muslim community showed the highest similarity of medicinal plants usage (Jaccard index = 95.8). Seven animal species distributed over 4 classes were recorded for the management of DRC. Plants and animals recorded as TT should be submitted to scientific studies to confirm safety and efficacy in clinical practice and to identify pharmacologically active metabolites.

## 1. Background

Diabetes mellitus, generally termed as diabetes, is a chronic metabolic disorder of the endocrine system characterised by abnormalities in carbohydrates, protein, and fat metabolism [1–3]. The incidence of diabetes mellitus continues to soar exponentially in both developed and developing countries leading to an increase in the cost of management/treatment of the disease and its related complications. Diabetes mellitus is a global epidemic currently affecting more than 371 million people and the death toll from the disease rose to 1.5 million in 2012 [4, 5]. The World Health Organisation has argued that diabetes will be the 7th leading cause of death in 2030 [6].

Diabetes mellitus is one of the most important health issues in Mauritius with a prevalence of 24.5% in 2015 [7]. The International Diabetes Federation reported that in 2015 there were 220,000 cases of diabetes in Mauritius and the number of cases of diabetes in adults that are undiagnosed was found to be 113100 [7]. Alterations in carbohydrates, protein, and fat metabolism entail an increase in blood glucose level which causes long-term devastating complications in many organs of the body [8]. Prolonged uncontrolled hyperglycemic level leads to macrovascular complications (coronary artery disease, peripheral arterial disease, and stroke) and to microvascular complications (diabetic nephropathy, neuropathy, and retinopathy) [9]. Complications related to diabetes are the major cause of disability and mortality among the Mauritian diabetic population.

Nowadays, diabetes is managed with oral hypoglycemic agents and insulin. Though the efficacy of these treatments is irrefutable, they have to be given throughout the lifetime of the patient and entail numerous potential

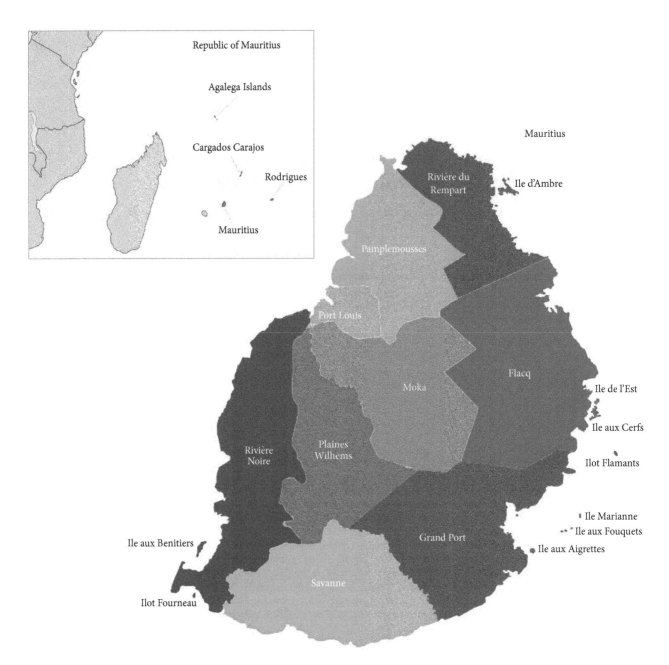

FIGURE 1: Map of Mauritius indicting the study area (spread over 9 main districts).

side effects, namely, hypoglycemic coma and hepatorenal disturbances [10, 11]. Hence, there is a growing interest in traditional therapies mostly because of the less frequent side effects associated with them as compared to conventional medicines.

Mauritius is a tropical island located in the southern hemisphere in the middle of the Indian Ocean. Mauritius is bestowed with a rich variety of medicinal flora, fauna, and cultural diversity. The volcanic island of Mauritius lies in the middle of the Indian Ocean (Figure 1) with coordinates $57°30'$ east and $20°20'$ south. Mauritius has an area of 1,865 km$^2$ and

about 43% of the area is allocated to agriculture. Mauritius enjoys a mild tropical climate, characterised by a warm humid summer between November and April and a cool dry winter between June and September whereby October and May are the transition months. Mean summer temperature is 24.7°C and mean winter temperature is 20.4°C [12]. Mauritius has a rich heritage of indigenous and endemic plants. During the past, allopathic medicine was not easily available for the local population and the use of traditional medicine was therefore necessary in order to alleviate signs and symptoms of diseases. Nowadays, healthcare facilities are within the reach of everybody; nonetheless, traditional medicine continues to remain active in the lives of the local population.

The multicultural society of Mauritius encompasses descendants of Indian indentured labourers, Chinese shop-keepers, African slaves, and British and French colonisers. The Indo-Mauritians community (Hindus and Muslims) represents the majority of the population followed by the Christian community and the Sino-Mauritians community. The Hindu community is subdivided into several distinct religious and sociocultural groups. The main religious groups are the Hindi or Bhojpuri speaking people constituting 40.2% of the total population and 76.5% of all Hindus. The Tamils are the second largest ethnic community (13.9%), while Telugus (5.6%) and Marathis (4%) represent smaller minorities within the overall Hindu community. The Hindus have a common language (Bhojpuri), the same regional origin (Uttar Pradesh and Bihar), and religious practices and rituals [13]. The official language in Mauritius is the English language but "Creole" is the native language of the island and is mostly used in infor-mal settings. Mauritius is reputed worldwide for the peaceful harmony which prevails in the island among the different great religions of the world, namely, Hinduism, Christianity, Islam, and Buddhism. In Mauritius, traditional therapies are paramount to panoply of ailments treatment/management offering profound therapeutic benefits and the indigenous communities rely heavily on them to meet their medical needs. Though allopathic medicine is the primary form of healthcare in Mauritius, some patients prefer traditional medicine for the treatment/management of a number of human diseases. The rising costs of synthetic drugs have fueled the interest of the local population in traditional medicine usage, thereby reintroducing such therapies as a novel emerging form of health aid. Mauritius is endowed with a number of tropical rainforests which are rich repositories of a diverse range of invaluable medicinal plants and animal species. Recently, Mauritius has become the arena of a number of ethnopharmacological field studies conducted by various workers which have emphasised mostly medicinal plants and animals among the Mauritian population and have led to several publications [14, 15]. Nonetheless, none of these studies have addressed the patterns of similarity and dissimilarity of medicinal plants and animals usage among the different religious communities present in the island. Heinrich et al. [16] reported that most studies on medicinal plants focus on the role of these plants within one particular ethnic group and little emphasis has been given to the comparison of medicinal plant species among various cultures. Moreover, an analysis of medicinal plants usage must be carried out in order to understand the patterns of use intra- and interculturally. However, studies on cross-cultural analysis of medicinal plants usage are lacking in Mauritius. Therefore, the current study specifically seeks to bring in the limelight of the scientific community the documentation of traditional remedies used among the diabetic patients in Mauritius. We also attempted to identify the most culturally important medicinal plants and animals in each religious group, compare the use of plant and animal species interculturally, and examine how the different religious groups present in the island value tradi-tional remedies in their daily lives in their quest for sound health.

## 2. Methods

*2.1. Data Collection.* The project was approved by the Faculty of Science, University of Mauritius, Mauritius. A total of 100 key informants (27 Hindus, 24 Muslims, 26 Christians, and 23 Buddhists) were interviewed from June to August, 2015. Data was collected from key informants, through face-to-face interviews, using a semistructured questionnaire (supplementary file in Supplementary Material available online at http://dx.doi.org/10.1155/2016/4523828). Traditional information was sought from diabetic patients older than 30 years based on the assumption that the mature population is better versed in traditional knowledge. Moreover, partic-ipants should be users of traditional medicine and formally diagnosed to be diabetic by their treating physician. During the course of the study, 12 field trips were carried out in different regions of the island. The interview was performed in "Creole," the native language of the Mauritian population. The questionnaire developed for the survey consisted of both close- and open-ended questions. Participants were informed about the purpose of the survey and a prior informed consent form was dully signed by the participants before the interview was carried out. The traditional healers were interviewed using the same questionnaire. The interviews were performed in health centers, home visits, markets, and Chinese shops (Figure 2). Figure 1 illustrates the different regions where the survey was carried out.

The questionnaire comprised three main parts: Parts A, B, and C. Part A consisted of demographic data which included age, gender, level of education, occupation, income, and religious belief. Part B of the questionnaire consisted of information about the herbal remedies used to manage diabetes and related complications, the local vernacular name of the plant, the method of preparation, the dosage, the route of administration, and the duration of treatment. Part C was based on animal-based remedy used to man-age diabetes and related complications, the local vernac-ular name of the animal, the method of preparation, the dosage, the route of administration, and the duration of treatment.

*2.2. Collection and Identification of Medicinal Plants.* During the field visits, when a remedy was mentioned by the traditional healer or diabetic patient, where possible, the participant was encouraged to show us a sample of the remedy which was collected *in situ* and photographed. The collected sample was then identified by local botanist. Our local repository database was updated whereby plant samples were assigned a collection number for future reference and data mining. Data obtained during the survey was cross-checked (local names/scientific names) according to a locally published book by Gurib-Fakim and Brendler [17]. Scientific names of plant species were identified according to the Inter-national Plant Name Index (IPNI: http://www.ipni.org/).

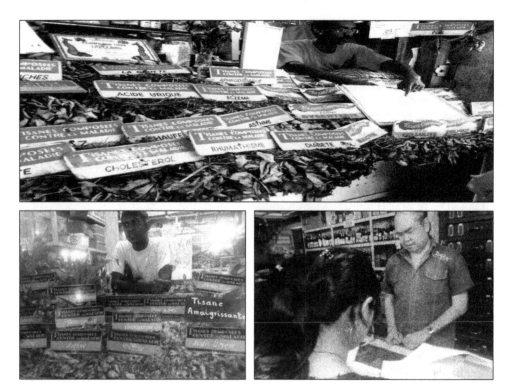

FIGURE 2: Interview with traditional healers.

*2.3. Ailments Categories.* Based on the information obtained from the key informants in the study area, all the reported ailments were classified into 9 categories based on published scientific literature from Riaz [18], ADA [19], Yadav et al. [20], Ginsberg et al. [21], and Bodansky et al. [22]. The categories were diabetic angiopathy, diabetic nephropathy, eye diseases, diabetic neuropathy, infections and wounds, hypertension, skin complications, diabetic dyslipidemia, and diabetes.

*2.4. Data Analysis and Ethnobotanical Indexes.* The indigenous medicinal information of plant and animal species was analyzed using different quantitative indexes.

*2.4.1. Relative Frequency of Citation.* Relative frequency of citation is calculated as follows: relative frequency of citation = FC/N, where FC is the number of informants mentioning the use of the species and $N$ is the number of informants participating in the survey. This index theoretically varies from 0 to 1. According to Sharma et al. [23], when relative frequency of citation is 0, it means that nobody refers to the plant/animal as useful, and when relative frequency of citation is 1, it means that all informants in the survey refer to the plant/animal as useful.

*2.4.2. Cultural Importance Index.* Culturally important species as medicines are identified by the cultural importance index (CII) [24]. The CII was used to determine the most

culturally important plant/animal species in each religious group. It can be calculated by the following formula:

$$CII = \sum_{u=u_1}^{u_{NC}} \sum_{i=i_1}^{i_n} \frac{UR_{ui}}{N}, \qquad (1)$$

where NC is the total number of different illness categories (of each $i$ species), UR is the total number of use reports for each species, and $N$ is the total number of informants in each religious group. The cultural importance index is the sum of the proportion of informants that mention each of the use-categories for a given species. The maximum value of the index equals the total number of different use-categories (NC), which would occur if all informants in a religious group would mention the use of a species in all use-categories. This index was used to estimate the cultural significance of each plant/animal species [24] and to determine to what extent each plant/animal species is present in the memory of the informants belonging to each religious group.

*2.4.3. Jaccard Similarity Index.* The Jaccard similarity index adapted from Güzel et al. [25] was used to determine the degree of similarity of medicinal plants' use among the different religious groups. The Jaccard similarity index is calculated as follows: Jaccard similarity index = $C \times 100/A + B - C$, where $A$ is the number of plant species reported by religious group A, $B$ is the number of plant species reported by the religious group B, and $C$ is the number of plant species reported by both A and B [25].

TABLE 1: Demographic data of the informants ($N = 100$).

| Variable | Categories | Frequency ($n = 100$) |
|---|---|---|
| Age (years) | 30–39 | 2 |
| | 40–49 | 17 |
| | 50–59 | 27 |
| | 60–69 | 41 |
| | 70–79 | 8 |
| | ≥80 | 5 |
| Sex | Male | 38 |
| | Female | 62 |
| Level of education | No formal education | 7 |
| | Primary | 64 |
| | Secondary | 20 |
| | Tertiary | 9 |
| Occupation | Retired | 36 |
| | Nongovernment officer | 25 |
| | Housewife | 18 |
| | Government officer | 16 |
| | Traditional healer | 2 |
| | Ayurvedic medicine practitioner | 2 |
| | Traditional Chinese medicine practitioner | 1 |
| Monthly household income | <Rs 5000 | 2 |
| | Rs 5001–10000 | 48 |
| | Rs 10001–20000 | 40 |
| | Rs 20001–30000 | 8 |
| | >Rs 30001 | 2 |
| Religion | Hindu | 27 |
| | Muslim | 24 |
| | Christian | 26 |
| | Buddhist | 23 |
| Diabetes related complications | Hypertension | 36 |
| | High level of cholesterol | 27 |
| | Neuropathic pain | 25 |
| | Cardiovascular diseases | 12 |
| | Cataracts | 9 |
| | Urinary tract infections | 7 |
| | Renal failure | 5 |
| | Foot ulcers | 4 |
| | Gangrene | 3 |
| | Infected wounds | 3 |
| | Stress | 2 |
| | Dry skin | 2 |
| | Erectile dysfunction | 1 |
| | Hearing loss | 1 |
| | Memory loss | 1 |
| | Depression | 1 |

# 3. Results and Discussion

*3.1. Demographic Profile of the Participants.* The demographic characteristics of the participants were determined and documented through face-to-face interviews using semistructured questionnaire (Tables 1 and 2). A total of 100 randomly selected informants (38 males and 62 females) were interviewed as summarized in Tables 1 and 2. Our finding resembled the study of Ishola et al. [26] where the majority of traditional medicine users were female since they were typically in charge of preparing herbal preparations in the domestic setting. According to Hardy [27], women are the

TABLE 2: Age and gender distribution within each religious community.

| Religious community | Age | Number of participants | Gender | Number of participants |
|---|---|---|---|---|
| Hindu | 30–39 | 1 | Male | 12 |
|  | 40–49 | 3 | Female | 15 |
|  | 50–59 | 8 |  |  |
|  | 60–69 | 7 |  |  |
|  | 70–79 | 6 |  |  |
|  | ≥80 | 2 |  |  |
| Muslim | 30–39 | 0 | Male | 11 |
|  | 40–49 | 4 | Female | 13 |
|  | 50–59 | 3 |  |  |
|  | 60–69 | 14 |  |  |
|  | 70–79 | 2 |  |  |
|  | ≥80 | 1 |  |  |
| Christian | 30–39 | 1 | Male | 10 |
|  | 40–49 | 4 | Female | 16 |
|  | 50–59 | 7 |  |  |
|  | 60–69 | 13 |  |  |
|  | 70–79 | 0 |  |  |
|  | ≥80 | 1 |  |  |
| Buddhist | 30–39 | 0 | Male | 5 |
|  | 40–49 | 6 | Female | 18 |
|  | 50–59 | 9 |  |  |
|  | 60–69 | 7 |  |  |
|  | 70–79 | 0 |  |  |
|  | ≥80 | 1 |  |  |

main source of conservation and dissemination of traditional knowledge. Ethnographic investigations revealed that the greatest contribution in terms of traditional information was provided by interviewees belonging to the age group 60–69 years old ($N = 41$). They were followed by informants belonging to the age category 50–59 years old ($N = 27$). This information implies that the young generation neglects traditional medicine practice which might lead to the rapid loss of valuable traditional knowledge regarding the use of medicinal plants [28]. There exist several reasons which might account for the loss of traditional knowledge in the study area: (1) holders of empirical knowledge have died before passing on this knowledge to the younger generation, (2) the younger generation believes more in the efficacy of allopathic medicine, and (3) given the free cost of healthcare facilities provided by the Mauritian government in public hospitals, allopathic medicine is more accessible to the population.

Moreover, the results revealed that the majority of the participants studied till the primary level only ($N = 64$). Our finding is in accordance with the work of Gakuya et al. [29] where elder people with little formal education possess more knowledge concerning the use of medicinal plants. It was also noted that the majority of the informants were retired

($N = 36$) and had a monthly household income of Rs 5001–10000 (1 US$ ≈ Rs 36.00) ($N = 48$). The retirement age in Mauritius is 60 years and above. Nonetheless, some of the participants were found to continue working though they reached the retirement age. The traditional health practitioners ($N = 5$) were found to play vital roles in the study area whereby the indigenous communities rely on them for the provision of herbal medicines. The traditional health practitioners were found to be key custodians of traditional information on the medicinal use of plant and animal species. Their practice of healing involved panoply of methodologies which are considered trustworthy among the indigenous community in the study area. Traditional health practitioners in Mauritius were willing to share their valuable traditional knowledge in order to prevent extinction of this cultural heritage.

In order to allow better comparison of medicinal plants and animals use among the four religious groups present in the study area, the number of participants surveyed in each religious group was approximately equal: 27, 24, 26, and 23 for the Hindu, Muslim, Christian, and Buddhist religious group, respectively. The most common diabetes related complications reported by the informants were hypertension ($N = 36$) followed by high level of cholesterol (27), neuropathic pain ($N = 25$), and cardiovascular diseases ($N = 12$). According to the American Diabetes Association, in type 2 diabetes, hypertension is often present as part of the metabolic syndrome of insulin resistance, while in type 1 diabetes, hypertension may reflect the onset of diabetic nephropathy [30].

*3.2. Herbal Remedies Used to Manage Diabetes and Related Complications.* The present research revealed the ethnobotanical use of 52 plant species belonging to 33 families used to manage diabetes and related complications. Information on medicinal plants obtained from the four religious groups, namely, Hindu, Muslim, Christian, and Buddhist, was arranged alphabetically according to their botanical families along with their ethnomedicinal uses (Table 3).

*3.3. Source of Medicinal Plants.* Informants obtained the medicinal plants from three main sources: gathering from the wild (39%), harvesting from home gardens (37%), and purchasing from the herbalists' store (24%). Our result is in agreement with the work of Singh et al. [31] where the majority of medicinal plants used in the preparation of herbal remedies are obtained from the wild. Indigenous people also cultivate medicinal plants in home garden where medicinal plants are grown in small areas surrounding the house. Moreover, medicinal plants are also grown in clay pots. One informant reported that effective medicinal plants are cultivated close to the house to allow easy accessibility. On the other hand, medicinal plants which are considered rare by the informants and which are not easily available are purchased from the herbalists' store.

*3.4. Forms of Medicinal Plants.* It was found that the informants showed no particular preference for using either fresh

TABLE 3: List of medicinal plants and polyherbal formulations with their related information used against diabetes and related complications reported by the informants.

| Family | Scientific name of plant (identification number) | Local name of plant | Indication | Part of plant used | Method of preparation and administration | RFC | $CII_H$ | $CII_M$ | $CII_C$ | $CII_B$ |
|---|---|---|---|---|---|---|---|---|---|---|
| Acanthaceae | Graptophyllum pictum (L.) Griff. (AM15) | Lait de vierge | Type 2 diabetes | L | Prepare a decoction with 3 leaves and drink 2 cups daily for 1 week. | 0.16 | 0.02 | 0.04 | 0.10 | 0.00 |
| Alismataceae | Alisma plantago-aquatica subsp. orientale (Sam) Sam. (AM09) | — | High level of cholesterol | — | Sold as a Chinese tea against cholesterol. Prepare an infusion with the teabags which contain Alisma orientalis (Rhizoma alismatis), Radix angelicae sinensis, Herba artemisiae capillaris, Hawthorn berry, Rhizoma atractylodis macrocephalae, Semen ziziphi spinosae, and Chinese tea. Drink 1 cup daily. | 0.12 | 0.00 | 0.00 | 0.03 | 0.09 |
| Amaryllidaceae | Allium cepa L. (AM04) | Zoiyon/oignon | Type 1 diabetes | B | Prepare a decoction with the bulb and drink 1 cup daily for 1 week. | 0.48 | 0.28 | 0.12 | 0.17 | 0.03 |
|  |  |  | Type 2 diabetes | B | Prepare a decoction with the bulb and drink 1 cup daily for 1 week. |  |  |  |  |  |
|  |  |  | Type 2 diabetes | B | Prepare juice with the bulb and add 1 teaspoon of honey. Drink 1 cup daily for 3 months. |  |  |  |  |  |
|  |  |  | High level of cholesterol | B | Prepare a decoction with the bulb and drink 1 cup daily for 1 week. |  |  |  |  |  |
|  |  |  | Renal failure | B | Prepare a decoction with the bulb and drink 1 cup daily for 1 week. |  |  |  |  |  |
|  |  |  | Hearing loss | B | Crush and press the bulb to obtain the juice and mix 30 g of the juice with 30 g of water. Heat and instill 3-4 drops in the affected ear. |  |  |  |  |  |
|  |  |  | Erectile dysfunction | B | Prepare juice with the bulb and add 1 teaspoon of honey. Drink 1 cup daily for 3 months. |  |  |  |  |  |
|  |  |  | Cataract | B | Prepare a decoction with the bulb and add 2 teaspoons of honey. Allow it to cool and use it as an eyebath daily. |  |  |  |  |  |
|  | Allium sativum L. (AM39) | L'ail | Type 2 diabetes | B | Prepare a decoction with 2-3 cloves and drink 1 cup thrice per week. | 0.42 | 0.24 | 0.09 | 0.22 | 0.06 |
|  |  |  | Cataract | B | Prepare a decoction with 2-3 cloves and drink 1 cup thrice per week. |  |  |  |  |  |
|  |  |  | Renal failure | B | Consume 2-3 raw cloves daily for 1 week. |  |  |  |  |  |
|  |  |  | Hypertension | B | Swallow 2 small cloves with a cup of water thrice per week. |  |  |  |  |  |
|  |  |  | Wound | B | Crush and press the bulb to obtain juice and apply the juice on the wound daily till healing. |  |  |  |  |  |
|  |  |  | Ulcer | B | Crush and press the bulb to obtain juice and apply the juice on the ulcer daily till healing. |  |  |  |  |  |
| Anacardiaceae | Mangifera indica L. (AM20) | Mangue | Type 2 diabetes | L | Prepare an infusion of the leaves and drink 1 cup twice per week. | 0.31 | 0.17 | 0.03 | 0.10 | 0.01 |
| Annonaceae | Annona muricata L. (AM29) | Coronsol | Hypertension | L | Prepare an infusion of the leaves and drink 1 cup twice per week. | 0.16 | 0.07 | 0.03 | 0.06 | 0.00 |

TABLE 3: Continued.

| Family | Scientific name of plant (identification number) | Local name of plant | Indication | Part of plant used | Method of preparation and administration | RFC | $CII_H$ | $CII_M$ | $CII_C$ | $CII_B$ |
|---|---|---|---|---|---|---|---|---|---|---|
| Aphloiaceae | Aphloia theiformis* (Vahl) Benn. (AM51) | Fandamane | Cataract | L | Prepare an infusion with the leaves and wash the eyes with it daily. | 0.18 | 0.08 | 0.02 | 0.10 | 0.00 |
| | | | Type 2 diabetes | L | Prepare an infusion of the leaves and drink 1 cup twice per week. | | | | | |
| Apiaceae | Apium graveolens L. (AM07) | Céleri | Type 2 diabetes | L | Prepare a decoction with the leaves and drink 1 cup twice per week. | 0.37 | 0.12 | 0.08 | 0.19 | 0.03 |
| | | | Hypertension | L | Prepare a decoction with the leaves and drink 1 cup twice per week. | | | | | |
| | Coriandrum sativum L. (AM11) | Cotomili | Type 2 diabetes | L | Prepare an infusion with the leaves and drink 1 cup twice per week. | 0.18 | 0.05 | 0.02 | 0.11 | 0.00 |
| | | | High level of cholesterol | L | Prepare a decoction with the leaves and drink 1 cup twice per week. | | | | | |
| | Petroselinum crispum (Mill.) Nyman ex A.W. Hill. (AM52) | Persil | High level of cholesterol | L | Prepare a soup with the leaves together with Apium graveolens L. and Allium ampeloprasum var. porrum. Consume it twice per week. | 0.27 | 0.12 | 0.07 | 0.16 | 0.01 |
| | | | Type 2 diabetes | L | Prepare a decoction with the leaves and drink 1 cup twice per week. | | | | | |
| | | | Renal failure | L | Prepare a decoction with the leaves and drink 1 cup twice per week. | | | | | |
| | | | Hypertension | L | Prepare juice with the leaves together with Daucus carota and Apium graveolens L. Drink 1 cup twice per week. | | | | | |
| Apocynaceae | Catharanthus roseus L. G.Don (AM17) | Saponnaire (blanc) | Type 2 diabetes | L | Prepare an infusion with 7 leaves in 2 cups of hot water. Drink 1 cup thrice per week. | 0.18 | 0.04 | 0.05 | 0.08 | 0.01 |
| Arecaceae | Cocos nucifera L. (AM21) | Coco | Cataract | Fr | Instill 2 drops of oil in the eye twice per day. | 0.23 | 0.08 | 0.02 | 0.12 | 0.00 |
| | | | Type 2 diabetes | Fr | Prepare a decoction with the young fruits and drink 1 cup thrice per week. | | | | | |
| | | | Renal failure | Fr | Drink 1 cup of the fruit water four times per week. | | | | | |
| | | | Renal failure | R | Prepare a decoction of the root and drink 1 cup twice per week. | | | | | |
| Asparagaceae | Ophiopogon japonicus (Thunb.) Ker Grawl. (AM22) | — | Type 2 diabetes | — | Sold as Chinese antidiabetic tea. Prepare an infusion with the tea bags which contain Ophiopogon japonicas (Radix ophiopogonis), fragrant solomonseal rhizome, Chinese yam, Hawthorn berry, Radix puerariae, and white tea. Drink 1 cup daily. | 0.13 | 0.00 | 0.00 | 0.02 | 0.11 |

TABLE 3: Continued.

| Family | Scientific name of plant (identification number) | Local name of plant | Indication | Part of plant used | Method of preparation and administration | RFC | $CII_H$ | $CII_M$ | $CII_C$ | $CII_B$ |
|---|---|---|---|---|---|---|---|---|---|---|
| Asteraceae | Bidens pilosa L. (AM31) | Lavilbag | Type 2 diabetes | L | Prepare a decoction of 3 leaves and drink 1 cup twice per week. | 0.28 | 0.14 | 0.07 | 0.10 | 0.04 |
| | | | Hypertension | L | Prepare a decoction of 3 leaves and drink 1 cup twice per week. | | | | | |
| | | | Type 2 diabetes | L | Prepare an infusion with 10 g of leaves in 1 L of water and drink 1 cup twice/thrice per week. | | | | | |
| | | | High level of cholesterol | L | Prepare an infusion of the leaves and drink 1 cup twice per day for 1 week. | | | | | |
| | Cynara cardunculus L. (AM24) | Artichaut | High level of cholesterol | L | Prepare juice with the leaves and drink 1 cup daily for 1 week. | 0.31 | 0.10 | 0.06 | 0.15 | 0.07 |
| | | | Atherosclerosis | L | Prepare an infusion of the leaves and drink 1 cup twice per day for 1 week. | | | | | |
| | | | Atherosclerosis | L | Prepare juice with the leaves and drink 1 cup twice per day for 1 week. | | | | | |
| | | | Type 2 diabetes | L | Prepare a decoction of the leaves and drink 1 cup twice per week. | | | | | |
| | Sigesbeckia orientalis L. (AM05) | Herbe de flacq | Type 2 diabetes | L | Prepare a decoction of the leaves together with Aphloia theiformis, Faujasiopsis flexuosa, Rubus alceifolius, Ravenala madagascariensis, and Rhizophora mucronata. Drink 1 cup twice per week. | 0.34 | 0.17 | 0.09 | 0.08 | 0.00 |
| Brassicaceae | Brassica oleracea L. (AM33) | Li chou | Cardiovascular disease | L | Prepare juice with the leaves and drink 1 cup daily for 1 week. | | | | | |
| | | | Type 2 diabetes | L | Prepare juice with the leaves and drink 1 cup daily for 1 week. | | | | | |
| | | | Wound | L | Apply the leaves as a cataplasm on the wound. | | | | | |
| | | | Cataract | L | Crush and press the leaves to obtain juice and instill 3–4 drops in each eye 2 hours daily till healing. | 0.37 | 0.13 | 0.11 | 0.17 | 0.02 |
| | | | Hearing loss | L | Prepare juice with the leaves and mix equal amount of the juice with equal amount of the juice of Citrus medica L. fruit. Instill 2 drops in the ears daily before going to bed. | | | | | |
| Bromeliaceae | Ananas comosus (L.) Merr. (AM30) | Anana | Renal failure | Fr | Consume ripe fruit twice per week. | 0.15 | 0.03 | 0.01 | 0.13 | 0.00 |
| | | | Cardiovascular disease | Fr | Prepare juice with the fruit and water and drink 1 cup twice per week. | | | | | |
| Caricaceae | Carica papaya L. (AM45) | Papaya | Hypertension | Fr | Consume ripe fruit half an hour before breakfast thrice per week. | | | | | |
| | | | High level of cholesterol | Fr | Crush and press the raw fruit to obtain milky liquid and drink 1 teaspoon twice per week. | 0.21 | 0.07 | 0.08 | 0.05 | 0.02 |
| | | | Cardiovascular disease | Fr | Prepare juice with the fruit together with Daucus carota. Drink 1 cup thrice per week. | | | | | |

TABLE 3: Continued.

| Family | Scientific name of plant (identification number) | Local name of plant | Indication | Part of plant used | Method of preparation and administration | RFC | $CII_H$ | $CII_M$ | $CII_C$ | $CII_B$ |
|---|---|---|---|---|---|---|---|---|---|---|
| | Cucumis sativus L. (AMI0) | Concombre | Type 1 diabetes | Fr | Prepare juice with the fruit and water and drink 1 cup on alternative days. | 0.14 | 0.02 | 0.01 | 0.12 | 0.01 |
| | | | Type 2 diabetes | Fr | Prepare juice with the fruit and water and drink 1 cup on alternative days. | | | | | |
| | | | Type 2 diabetes | Fr | Prepare a decoction with the peels in water and drink 1 cup daily for 1 week. | | | | | |
| | Cucurbita maxima Duchesne (AM01) | Giromon | Cataract | Fl | Crush and press the flower to obtain juice. Apply juice as compress externally on the eyes. | 0.23 | 0.02 | 0.07 | 0.14 | 0.01 |
| | | | Renal failure | Se | Seeds are dried in bright sunlight for 1 day and eaten raw the following day. Seeds should be consumed thrice per week. | | | | | |
| | | | Wound | Fr | Prepare juice with the fruit and apply it on wound till healing. | | | | | |
| | Lagenaria siceraria (Molina) Standl. (AM41) | Calebasse | Type 2 diabetes | Fr | Prepare a decoction of the peels in water by allowing it to boil for 20 minutes. Drink 1 cup for 3 days. | 0.32 | 0.14 | 0.09 | 0.09 | 0.07 |
| | | | High level of cholesterol | L | Prepare a decoction with the leaves and drink 1 cup twice per week. | | | | | |
| | | | Hypertension | L | Prepare a decoction with the leaves and drink 1 cup twice per week. | | | | | |
| | | | Hypertension | L | Crush and press 3–5 leaves to obtain juice and drink it twice per week. | | | | | |
| | | | Cardiovascular disease | L | Prepare juice with the leaves together with Swertia chirayita and honey. Drink 1 cup twice per week. | 0.17 | 0.03 | 0.05 | 0.11 | 0.00 |
| Cucurbitaceae | Luffa acutangula (L.) Roxb. (AM08) | Patole | Type 2 diabetes | L | Eat 2-3 leaves twice per week. | | | | | |
| | | | Type 2 diabetes | L | Extract the liquid by crushing the leaves and drink 1 teaspoon twice per week. | | | | | |
| | | | Type 2 diabetes | Fr | Extract the liquid by crushing the fruit and drink 1-2 teaspoons twice per week. | | | | | |
| | | | Type 2 diabetes | Se | Dry the seeds in bright sunlight during the day and at night allow them to soak in a cup of water and drink it the next morning on an empty stomach. | | | | | |
| | | | Type 2 diabetes | L | Prepare juice with 3 leaves and add Piper nigrum. Drink it once per week. | | | | | |
| | Momordica charantia L. (AM03) | Margose | Type 2 diabetes | Fr | Prepare juice with the fruit together with Phaseolus vulgaris L., Malus domestica, and Aloe barbadensis. Drink 1 cup once per week. | 0.46 | 0.23 | 0.09 | 0.11 | 0.05 |
| | | | Type 2 diabetes | Fr | Prepare juice with the fruit together with the fruit of Phyllanthus emblica and the fruit of Syzygium cumini. Drink 1 cup twice per week. | | | | | |
| | | | Type 2 diabetes | Fr | Prepare juice with the fruit together with Phaseolus vulgaris L. and drink 1 cup twice per week. | | | | | |
| | | | Type 2 diabetes | Fr | Prepare juice with the fruit together with Cucumis sativus and drink 1 cup twice per week. | | | | | |
| | | | High level of cholesterol | Fr | Prepare juice with the fruit together with the fruit of Phyllanthus emblica and the fruit of Syzygium cumini. Drink 1 cup twice per week. | | | | | |
| | Tamarindus indica L. (AM37) | Tamarin | Hypertension | Fr | Prepare juice with the pulp and water and drink 1 cup twice per day for 1 day. | 0.39 | 0.12 | 0.09 | 0.18 | 0.02 |
| | | | Pain | L | Prepare a foot bath with a decoction of the leaves mixed with 1 teaspoon of salt. | | | | | |
| Fabaceae | Trigonella foenum-graecum L. (AM18) | Methi | Type 2 diabetes | Se | Prepare a decoction with the seeds and drink 1 cup thrice per week. | 0.43 | 0.23 | 0.06 | 0.22 | 0.01 |
| | | | High level of cholesterol | Se | Soak the seeds in 1 glass of water for 1 night and drink it the next morning on an empty stomach. | | | | | |
| | | | Erectile dysfunction | Se | Prepare a decoction with 1 teaspoon of seeds and 2 cups of water. Drink 1 cup on an empty stomach in the morning daily for 1 week. | | | | | |

TABLE 3: Continued.

| Family | Scientific name of plant (identification number) | Local name of plant | Indication | Part of plant used | Method of preparation and administration | RFC | $CII_H$ | $CII_M$ | $CII_C$ | $CII_B$ |
|---|---|---|---|---|---|---|---|---|---|---|
| | | | Type 2 diabetes | L | Crush and press the leaves to obtain juice and drink 2 teaspoons twice per week. | | | | | |
| | | | Type 2 diabetes | L | Consume 2 raw leaves twice per week. | | | | | |
| | | | Hypertension | L | Crush and press the leaves to obtain juice and drink 2 teaspoons twice per week. | | | | | |
| | | | Cataract | L | Crush 2 leaves and press to obtain juice and take 1 drop of the juice in the eye daily. | | | | | |
| Lamiaceae | Ocimum tenuiflorum L. (AM26) | Tulsi | Cataract | L | Crush and press 3-4 leaves to obtain juice and add 2 teaspoons of honey. Instill 2 drops of the mixture in the eye each night for 5 days. | 0.48 | 0.39 | 0.15 | 0.16 | 0.02 |
| | | | Erectile dysfunction | L | Prepare a decoction with 3 leaves together with 3 leaves of Piper betle and drink 1 cup twice per week. | | | | | |
| | | | Wound | L | Crush and press the leaves to obtain juice and mix the juice with the oil of Cocos nucifera that has previously been heated and apply it on the wound. | | | | | |
| | | | High level of cholesterol | L | Crush and press 3 leaves to obtain juice and add 2 teaspoons of honey and drink twice per week. | | | | | |
| | Prunella vulgaris L. (AM28) | — | Hypertension | — | Sold as Chinese antihypertensive tea. Prepare an infusion with the tea bags which contain Prunella vulgaris L. (Selfheal spike), Ramulus uncariae cumuncis, Fructus leonuri, and Chinese oolong tea. Drink 1 cup daily. | 0.09 | 0.00 | 0.00 | 0.01 | 0.08 |
| Lauraceae | Persea americana Mill. (AM34) | Avocat | Cataract | Fr | Prepare juice with 2 cups of yoghurt, 1/2 a cup of the fruit, and 1/2 a cup of water and drink 1 cup once per week. | 0.21 | 0.08 | 0.04 | 0.11 | 0.00 |
| | | | High level of cholesterol | Fr | Prepare juice with 2 cups of yoghurt, 1/2 a cup of the fruit, and 1/2 a cup of water and drink 1 cup once per week. | | | | | |

TABLE 3: Continued.

| Family | Scientific name of plant (identification number) | Local name of plant | Indication | Part of plant used | Method of preparation and administration | RFC | $CII_H$ | $CII_M$ | $CII_C$ | $CII_B$ |
|---|---|---|---|---|---|---|---|---|---|---|
| Linaceae | Linum usitatissimum Linnaeus. (AM40) | Grain de lin | Type 2 diabetes | Se | Soak the seeds in a cup of water at night and drink it the next morning on an empty stomach. Drink it thrice per week. | | | | | |
| | | | Renal failure | Se | Soak the seeds in a cup of water at night and drink it the next morning on an empty stomach. Drink it thrice per week. | 0.34 | 0.16 | 0.13 | 0.08 | 0.01 |
| | | | High level of cholesterol | Se | Soak the seeds in a cup of water at night and drink it the next morning on an empty stomach. Drink it thrice per week. | | | | | |
| Meliaceae | Azadirachta indica A. Juss (AM16) | Neem, lila perche | Type 2 diabetes | L | Prepare a decoction of the leaves and drink 1 cup twice per week. | | | | | |
| | | | Type 2 diabetes | L | Crush the leaves and make small balls with them and allow them to dry in the sun. The following day, swallow 2 balls with 1 glass of water twice per week. | 0.46 | 0.21 | 0.12 | 0.09 | 0.04 |
| Moraceae | Artocarpus heterophyllus Lam. (AM36) | Zack | Type 2 diabetes | Fr | Prepare a decoction with the young fruits and drink 1 cup daily for 1 week. | 0.19 | 0.07 | 0.02 | 0.08 | 0.02 |
| Moringaceae | Moringa oleifera Lam. (AM42) | Brède mouroungue | Type 2 diabetes | L | Crush and press the leaves to obtain juice. Mix it with milk and drink 1 cup twice per week. | | | | | |
| | | | High level of cholesterol | L | Crush and press the leaves to obtain juice. Mix it with milk and drink 1 cup twice per week. | 0.26 | 0.12 | 0.06 | 0.16 | 0.00 |
| | | | Hypertension | R | Prepare a decoction with the root and drink 1 cup twice per week. | | | | | |
| | | | Hypertension | St | Prepare a decoction with the stem and drink 1 cup twice per week. | | | | | |
| | Eucalyptus globulus Labill. (AM32) | Eucalyptus | Type 2 diabetes | L | Prepare an infusion with 2-3 leaves and drink 1 cup twice per week. | 0.13 | 0.05 | 0.00 | 0.08 | 0.00 |
| | | | | L | Prepare an infusion with 3 leaves and drink 1 cup daily for 1 week. | | | | | |
| | Psidium guajava L. (AM50) | Goyave | | Fr | Consume rip fruit thrice per week. | 0.38 | 0.17 | 0.04 | 0.15 | 0.02 |
| | | | Type 2 diabetes | Fr | Prepare a juice of the fruit and drink 1 cup daily for 1 week. | | | | | |
| Myrtaceae | | | | L | Prepare a decoction with the leaves and drink 1 cup daily for 1 week. | | | | | |
| | | | | Fr | Consume 10 ripe fruits thrice per week. | | | | | |
| | | | | Fr | Prepare juice with 1 cup of the fruits and 2 cups of water. Drink 1 cup twice per week. | | | | | |
| | Syzygium cumini L. Skeels (AM06) | Jamblon | Type 2 | Se | Prepare a decoction with the seeds and drink 1 cup twice per week. | 0.49 | 0.19 | 0.14 | 0.13 | 0.03 |
| | | | | Fr | Sold as an Ayurvedic preparation known as "Karela jamun" which contains Syzygium cumini and Momordica charantia. Drink 5–10 ml of the preparation with 1/2 a glass of water twice per day. | | | | | |
| | | | | Fr | Sold as an Ayurvedic preparation known as "Yesaka" which contains Phyllanthus emblica, Terminalia chebula, Terminalia bellerica, Syzygium cumini, Picrorhiza kurroa, Swertia chirata, Tinospora cordifolia, Gymnema sylvestre, Momordica charantia, Curcuma longa, Salacia chinensis Linn., and Melia azadirachta. Drink 1 tablespoon twice per day. | | | | | |

TABLE 3: Continued.

| Family | Scientific name of plant (identification number) | Local name of plant | Indication | Part of plant used | Method of preparation and administration | RFC | $CII_H$ | $CII_M$ | $CII_C$ | $CII_B$ |
|---|---|---|---|---|---|---|---|---|---|---|
| Oleaceae | Olea europaea L. (AM02) | Zolive | Hypertension | L | Prepare an infusion of the leaves and drink 1 cup daily for 1 week. | 0.24 | 0.10 | 0.04 | 0.13 | 0.02 |
| | | | Cardiovascular disease | L | Prepare an infusion of the leaves and drink 1 cup daily for 1 week. | | | | | |
| | | | Type 2 diabetes | L | Prepare an infusion of the leaves and drink 1 cup daily for 1 week. | | | | | |
| Phyllanthaceae | Phyllanthus emblica L. (AM13) | Amla | Type 2 diabetes | — | Sold as an Ayurvedic preparation called "Triphala" containing Phyllanthus emblica, Bellirica myrobalan, and Chebulic myrobalan. Drink 1 tablespoon daily. | 0.52 | 0.25 | 0.14 | 0.16 | 0.06 |
| | | | Type 2 diabetes | — | Sold as an Ayurvedic preparation known as "Amla karela" which contains Phyllanthus emblica and Momordica charantia. Drink 10–30 ml of the preparation daily in 100 ml of water. | | | | | |
| | | | Type 2 diabetes | Fr | Consume raw fruits thrice per week. | | | | | |
| | | | Type 2 diabetes | Fr | Prepare juice with 1 cup of fruits and 1 cup of water and add 1 teaspoon of honey to the juice (optional). Drink 1 cup thrice per week. | | | | | |
| | | | High level of cholesterol | Fr | Prepare juice with 1 cup of fruits and 1 cup of water and drink 1 cup thrice per week. | | | | | |
| Poaceae | Avena sativa L. (AM35) | Oatmeal | Type 2 diabetes | Gr | The grains are soaked in 1 cup of water during the night and drunk in the morning on an empty stomach. | 0.32 | 0.19 | 0.08 | 0.13 | 0.02 |
| | | | High level of cholesterol | Gr | The grains are soaked in 1 cup of water during the night and drunk in the morning on an empty stomach. | | | | | |
| | | | Dry skin | Gr | The grains are crushed into fined powders and mixed with 1 tablespoon of almond oil to form a paste and applied on wet skin after bath. Leave it for 10 minutes then rinse it with water. | | | | | |
| Primulaceae | Lysimachia christinae Hance (AM19) | — | Urinary tract infection | L | Prepare a decoction of the leaves and drink 1 cup daily for 1 week. | 0.05 | 0.00 | 0.00 | 0.00 | 0.05 |
| Rhizophoraceae | Rhizophora mucronata* Lam. (AM25) | Manglier | Type 2 diabetes | R | Prepare an infusion of the roots and drink 1 cup twice per week. | 0.39 | 0.16 | 0.04 | 0.19 | 0.00 |
| Rosaceae | Crataegus laevigata Poir. DC. (AM38) | Aubépine | Cataract | L | Prepare an infusion of the leaves and wash the eye with it. | 0.32 | 0.14 | 0.06 | 0.17 | 0.00 |
| | | | High level of cholesterol | L | Prepare an infusion of the leaves and drink 1 cup twice per week. | | | | | |
| | | | Hypertension | Fl | Prepare an infusion with 1 teaspoon of flower and drink 2 cups per day twice per week. | | | | | |
| | | | Atherosclerosis | Fl | Prepare an infusion with 1 teaspoon of flower and drink 2 cups per day twice per week. | | | | | |
| | Rubus alceifolius Poir. (AM14) | Piquant loulou | Type 2 diabetes | L | Prepare a decoction with the leaves and drink 1 cup twice per week. | 0.36 | 0.11 | 0.09 | 0.14 | 0.02 |

TABLE 3: Continued.

| Family | Scientific name of plant (identification number) | Local name of plant | Indication | Part of plant used | Method of preparation and administration | RFC | $CII_H$ | $CII_M$ | $CII_C$ | $CII_B$ |
|---|---|---|---|---|---|---|---|---|---|---|
| Rubiaceae | *Morinda citrifolia* L. (AMI2) | Noni | Type 2 diabetes | Fr | The fruit is peeled, crushed, and pressed to obtain the juice. Drink 1 cup thrice per week. | 0.54 | 0.24 | 0.19 | 0.25 | 0.07 |
| | | | High level of cholesterol | Fr | The fruit is peeled, crushed, and pressed to obtain the juice. Drink 1 cup thrice per week. | | | | | |
| | *Vangueria madagascariensis* J.F.Gmel. (AM27) | Vavangue | Hypertension | L | Prepare an infusion with the leaves and drink 1 cup twice per week. | 0.37 | 0.12 | 0.08 | 0.19 | 0.02 |
| | | | Pain | L | Apply warm oil on the painful area and bind it with the leaves. | | | | | |
| | | | Type 2 diabetes | L | Prepare a decoction of the leaves and drink 1 cup twice per week. | | | | | |
| | | | Hypertension | L | Prepare a decoction of the leaves and drink 1 cup twice per week. | | | | | |
| Rutaceae | *Citrus aurantifolia* (Christm.) Swingle (AM49) | Limon | Hypertension | Fr | Peel and press the fruit to obtain the juice and drink 1 cup. | | | | | |
| | | | Type 2 diabetes | Fr | Prepare juice with the fruit together with 1 clove of *Allium sativum*, 1 teaspoon of honey, and 1 cup of water. Drink 1 cup twice per week. | | | | | |
| | | | Renal failure | L | Peel and press the fruit to obtain juice and drink 1 cup twice per week. | | | | | |
| | | | Renal failure | Fr | Peel and prepare juice with the pulp and add 1 teaspoon of honey. Drink thrice per week in the morning. | 0.55 | 0.24 | 0.10 | 0.23 | 0.05 |
| | | | Cardiovascular disease | L | Prepare an infusion with 4 leaves and drink 1 cup thrice per week. | | | | | |
| | | | Cardiovascular disease | Fr | Prepare juice with the fruit together with 1 clove of *Allium sativum* L., 1 teaspoon of honey, and 1 cup of water. Drink 1 cup twice per week. | | | | | |
| | | | Cataract | Fr | Prepare juice with the pulp and add 2 teaspoons of honey and use it as an eyebath daily. | | | | | |
| | | | Type 2 diabetes | Fr | Prepare a decoction of the peels in water and drink 1 cup thrice per week. | | | | | |
| | *Citrus maxima* (Burm.) Osbeck (AM47) | Pamplemousse | High level of cholesterol | Fr | Prepare a decoction of the peels in water and drink 1 cup thrice per week. | 0.48 | 0.20 | 0.18 | 0.19 | 0.02 |
| | | | High level of cholesterol | Fr | Prepare juice with the fruit together with *Daucus carota* and 2 cm of *Zingiber officinale* root. Drink 1 cup once per week. | | | | | |
| | *Murraya koenigii* (L.) Spreng (AM44) | Carripoulet | Hypertension | L | Prepare an infusion with 3 leaves and drink 1 cup twice per week. | 0.18 | 0.09 | 0.03 | 0.05 | 0.01 |
| Sapindaceae | *Cardiospermum halicacabum* L. (AM23) | Pocpoc | Gangrene | L | Prepare an infusion of the leaves together with *Senna alexandrina* Mill. and *Senna alata* L. Drink 1 cup twice per week. | 0.21 | 0.08 | 0.09 | 0.05 | 0.00 |
| | | | Wound | L | Crush the leaves and apply them on the wound as a poultice. | | | | | |
| | | | Type 2 diabetes | L | Prepare a decoction of the leaves and drink 1 cup twice per week. | | | | | |
| Theaceae | *Camellia sinensis* L. Kuntze (AM48) | Thé vert | Cataract | L | Prepare an infusion with the tea bags and wash the eye with it. | | | | | |
| | | | Type 2 diabetes | L | Prepare an infusion with the tea bags and drink 1 cup twice per week. | 0.45 | 0.26 | 0.12 | 0.27 | 0.08 |
| | | | Hypertension | L | Prepare an infusion with the tea bags and drink 1 cup twice per week. | | | | | |
| | | | High level of cholesterol | L | Prepare an infusion with the tea bags and drink 1 cup twice per week. | | | | | |
| | | | High level of cholesterol | L | Prepare an infusion with the teabags together with *Cinnamomum verum*. Drink 1 cup twice per week at night. | | | | | |

TABLE 3: Continued.

| Family | Scientific name of plant (identification number) | Local name of plant | Indication | Part of plant used | Method of preparation and administration | RFC | $CII_H$ | $CII_M$ | $CII_C$ | $CII_B$ |
|---|---|---|---|---|---|---|---|---|---|---|
| Verbenaceae | *Aloysia citriodora* Palau (AM45) | Verveine | Cardiovascular disease | W | Prepare an infusion with 1 teaspoon of the plant in 1 cup of hot water. Allow it to infuse for 10 minutes and drink 1 cup thrice per week. | 0.09 | 0.02 | 0.00 | 0.07 | 0.00 |
| Xanthorrhoeaceae | *Aloe vera* (L.) Burm.f. (AM46) | Aloe vera | Type 2 diabetes | L | Gel is removed from the leaf pulp and 2 tablespoons are eaten daily in the morning for 1 week. | | | | | |
| | | | Type 2 diabetes | L | Sold as an Ayurvedic juice. 10 ml taken twice daily after meal. | | | | | |
| | | | High level of cholesterol | L | Prepare a mixture with 2 tablespoons of the gel removed from the leaf pulp, 1 cup of yoghurt, and 1/2 a cup of water. Mix all in a juicer and drink 1 cup of the juice obtained twice per week. | 0.53 | 0.17 | 0.15 | 0.23 | 0.06 |
| | | | Gangrene | L | Prepare a footbath with the decoction of the leaf mixed with 1 teaspoon of salt and 1 teaspoon of vinegar. Soak foot for 30–45 minutes daily for 1 week. | | | | | |

RFC: relative frequency of citation, $CII_H$: cultural importance index among the Hindu community, $CII_M$: cultural importance index among the Muslim community, $CII_C$: cultural importance index among the Christian community, and $CII_B$: cultural importance index among the Buddhist community. *Plant part used:* R, root; L, leaf; Fr, fruit; Se, seeds; W, whole plant; B, bulb; St, stem; Fl, flower; Gr, grain. *List of endemic plants.

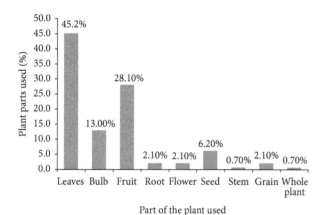

FIGURE 3: Plant parts employed in herbal remedies by the participants.

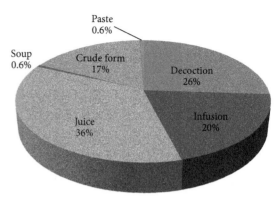

FIGURE 4: Forms of herbal preparations.

or dried plants in the preparation of herbal remedies. They reported that the use of either fresh or dried plants in herbal recipes did not make any difference in the efficacy of the herbal remedies. However, the traditional healers reported that they preferred dried plants which should be kept in open air and not in closed container. Furthermore, drying enabled indigenous people to use medicinal plants during off season. This is supported by the work of Tahraoui et al. [32] whereby plant parts are dried in shade and stored in a house room free of humidity and sunlight for their use during unavailability. Similarly, Lingaraju et al. [33] reported that, in the absence of fresh materials, the dried ones were prescribed in the preparation of herbal remedies. Previous studies had shown that there were quantitative and qualitative differences in the essential oil contents of fresh and dry plant materials [34, 35]. Ishola et al. [26] reported that dry plant materials might not be as potent as freshly collected herbs since some of their enzymes may have been denatured or the heat labile compounds could have been destroyed.

*3.5. Parts of Medicinal Plants Used in the Preparation of Herbal Remedies.* In the current investigation, different parts of medicinal plants were documented in the preparation of indigenous herbal medicines to manage diabetes and related complications. Whole plant in addition to different parts of the same plant including leaf, bulb, fruit, root, flower, seed, stem, and grain was used in the preparation of herbal remedies for the management of diabetes and related complications (Figure 3). Leaf was the most frequently used plant parts (45.2%), followed by fruit (28.1%), bulb (13%), seed (6.2%), root (2.1%), flower (2.1%), grain (2.1%), stem (0.7%), and whole plant (0.7%). These observations resonate with finding obtained by Sadeghia and Mahmood [36] in which the part of the plant most commonly used was leaves. According to Tuttolomondo et al. [37], greater accessibility of the aboveground parts of the plants in natural ecosystems and the greater abundance of leaves compared to other plant parts may explain the higher use-frequency of these plant parts in traditional medicine. Leaves are the most favored parts in the preparation of herbal medicines since they contain

a high concentration of pharmacologically active secondary metabolites which are valuable in phytotherapy [38, 39]. The result of the present study showed that whole plant is not commonly used in the preparation of herbal remedies because its removal will threaten the conservation of the plant species and hence impair sustainability of indigenous flora in the study area. The result of the study deviates from the work of Cheikhyoussef et al. [40] who observed that roots are mostly used in the preparation of herbal remedies. From the current study, the root of *Rhizophora mucronata*, an endemic plant, was reported to be used against type 2 diabetes. According to Flatie et al. [41], roots contain high concentration of bioactive substances. Nonetheless, frequent harvesting of roots has a negative influence on the survival of the plant species and is therefore discouraged. Different parts of a plant species may contain different types and concentrations of pharmacologically active constituents resulting in distinct pharmacological activities. In the present work, the fruit of *Cucurbita maxima* was reported to be used against type 2 diabetes, and in wound healing, its leaves were used against cataract while its seeds were used against renal failure. The phytochemical analysis of an ethanolic extract of *Cucurbita maxima* seeds revealed the presence of tannins, carbohydrates, glycosides, alkaloids, volatile oils, saponins, proteins, and flavonoids [42].

*3.6. Method of Preparation of Herbal Remedies.* Various preparation modes of herbal medicines like juice, decoction, infusion, crude form, paste, and soup were used by the indigenous community in Mauritius (Figure 4). The most common modes of preparation were juice (36%) followed by decoction (26%) and infusion (20%). Similar finding was reported by Malla et al. [43] in western Nepal where juice was the most commonly used preparation method for administering medicinal plants. Most of the reported herbal preparations are made with water as dilution media. This finding is in line with previous work [44], where water was mostly used as solvent medium in the preparation of herbal remedies. Decoctions are usually prepared by boiling plant parts in water until the amount of water is reduced to half its original amount. According to a study conducted by Zhang et al. [45], on heating various biological reactions

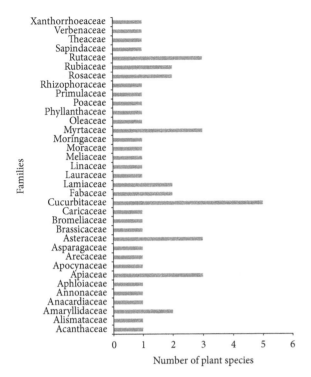

FIGURE 5: Representative botanical families.

are accelerated resulting in many active compounds, hence accounting for the effectiveness of herbal remedies prepared by decoction.

### 3.7. Administration of Herbal Remedies.
Regarding the means of administration, oral ingestion (87.1%) was the preferred mode of administration of herbal remedies followed by external use (12.9%). This is in agreement with the finding of Sadeghia and Mahmood [36] where herbal remedies are mostly administered orally. It was reported that the predominance of oral route for administration of herbal remedies can be attributed to the ease of administration without using costly and complex accessories [46].

### 3.8. Botanical Families.
The predominantly quoted medicinal plant families were Cucurbitaceae with five species, followed by Apiaceae, Asteraceae, Myrtaceae, and Rutaceae with three species each and Amaryllidaceae, Fabaceae, Lamiaceae, Rosaceae, and Rubiaceae with two species each. The remaining 23 families were each represented by one species (Figure 5). The Cucurbitaceae family encompasses 800 species distributed mainly in tropical and subtropical regions of the world [47]. The most plausible reason for the predominance of the Cucurbitaceae family in the study area could be due to the large group of plant species belonging to this family which are medicinally valuable due to their phytochemical profile. Moreover, the high citations of the Cucurbitaceae family may be because of the high availability of plant species belonging to this family in the study area. Further, plants belonging to the Cucurbitaceae family contain a group of active secondary metabolites, namely, triterpenoid, which

are well known for their bitterness [47], hence justifying their use in the management of diabetes in the present study. It was noted from the current investigation that some of the informants believed that type 2 diabetes is caused by excess sugar in the blood; hence, bitter plants are used to neutralise the excess sugar. In an ethnopharmacological survey conducted in Congo by Katemo et al. [48], it was reported that bitter plants are prescribed to control blood sugar level. Some of the bitter plants recorded from the present study used to manage diabetes with high relative frequency of citation include *Aloe vera* (0.53), *Phyllanthus emblica* (0.52), *Azadirachta indica* (0.46), and *Momordica charantia* (0.46). *Phyllanthus emblica* has been shown to contain an array of bioactive components like quercetin, phyllaemblic compounds, gallic acid, tannins, flavonoids, pectin, vitamin C, terpenoids, and alkaloids which possesses useful biological activities [49–51]. According to Walia and Boolchandani [52], *Phyllanthus emblica* contain high vitamin C content which is effective in controlling diabetes and tannins which has the capacity to enhance glucose uptake and inhibit adipogenesis. The majority of the informants (92%) responded that after consumption of the herbal remedy they felt an improvement in their health state.

### 3.9. Relative Frequency of Citation.
Relative frequency of citation was calculated to ascertain the most commonly occurring medicinal plants used for the management of diabetes and related complications and thus aids in the selection of plants for further phytochemical and pharmacological studies. *Citrus aurantifolia* (0.55) was the predominant plant species which exhibited the highest relative frequency of citation demonstrating its importance in indigenous phytotherapy. It is followed by *Morinda citrifolia* (0.54), *Aloe vera* (0.53), *Phyllanthus emblica* (0.52), and *Syzygium cumini* (0.49). Plant species with high relative frequency of citation reflected their popularity due to their strong healing power and they were easily available and affordable in the study area. According to Kpodar et al. [46], other reasons why plant species are cited frequently might be (1) the trust that the indigenous community have in these plants as medicine and (2) the relatively high cost of synthetic drugs. Based on these results, such plants should be focused on for the investigation of bioactive phytochemical constituents and other pharmacological activities. It is important to note that the plants with high relative frequency of citation have been previously screened for their pharmacological activities. Unripen juices of *Citrus aurantifolia* showed antioxidant activities *in vitro* [53]. Moorthy and Reddy [54] reported that the ethanolic extract of the roots of *Morinda citrifolia* lowered blood pressure in an anesthetized dog. An experimental investigation carried out by Alam et al. [55] demonstrated that leaves of *Syzygium cumini* contain the bioactive compounds lupeol, 12-oleanen-3-ol-3$\beta$-acetate, stigmasterol, and $\beta$-sitosterol which possess potential antidiabetic activities, hence supporting the traditional use of the leaves for treating diabetes. Some of the plant species reported, namely, *Lysimachia christinae* (0.05), *Prunella vulgaris* (0.09), and *Aloysia citriodora* (0.09), scored low relative frequency of citation since they have

TABLE 4: Culturally most important plant and animal species used against diabetes and related complications.

| Religious groups | Hindu | Muslim | Christian | Buddhist |
|---|---|---|---|---|
| Plant species | Ocimum tenuiflorum (0.39) | Cardiospermum halicacabum (0.09) | Camellia sinensis (0.27) | Ophiopogon japonicas (0.11) |
| | Allium cepa (0.28) | Carica papaya (0.08) | Morinda citrifolia (0.25) | Alisma plantago-aquatica (0.09) |
| | Phyllanthus emblica (0.25) | | Aloe vera (0.23) | Prunella vulgaris (0.08) |
| | Allium sativum (0.24) | | Apium graveolens (0.19) | Lysimachia christinae (0.05) |
| | Citrus aurantifolia (0.24) | | Rhizophora mucronata (0.19) | |
| | Momordica charantia (0.23) | | Vangueria madagascariensis (0.19) | |
| | Trigonella foenum-graecum (0.23) | | Tamarindus indica (0.18) | |
| | Azadirachta indica (0.21) | | Brassica oleracea (0.17) | |
| | Citrus maxima (0.20) | | Crataegus laevigata (0.17) | |
| | Avena sativa (0.19) | | Moringa oleifera (0.16) | |
| | Syzygium cumini (0.19) | | Petroselinum crispum (0.16) | |
| | Mangifera indica (0.17) | | Cynara cardunculus (0.15) | |
| | Psidium guajava (0.17) | | Cucurbita maxima (0.14) | |
| | Sigesbeckia orientalis (0.17) | | Rubus alceifolius (0.14) | |
| | Linum usitatissimum (0.16) | | Ananas comosus (0.13) | |
| | Bidens pilosa (0.14) | | Olea europaea (0.13) | |
| | Lagenaria siceraria (0.14) | | Cocos nucifera (0.12) | |
| | Murraya koenigii (0.09) | | Cucumis sativus (0.12) | |
| | Annona muricata (0.07) | | Coriandrum sativum (0.11) | |
| | | | Luffa acutangula (0.11) | |
| | | | Persea americana (0.11) | |
| | | | Aphloia theiformis (0.10) | |
| | | | Graptophyllum pictum (0.10) | |
| | | | Artocarpus heterophyllus (0.08) | |
| | | | Catharanthus roseus (0.08) | |
| | | | Eucalyptus globules (0.08) | |
| | | | Aloysia citriodora (0.07) | |
| Animal species | Anguilla japonica (0.02) | | Salmo salar (0.08) | Rattus rattus (0.02) |
| | | | Apis mellifera (0.03) | |
| | | | Tenrec ecaudatus (0.03) | |
| | | | Helix aspersa (0.02) | |
| | | | Periplaneta americana (0.02) | |

been reported by few informants only. Low relative frequency of citation values of these plants imply that traditional knowledge about their use is on the verge of extinction. Furthermore, they were found to be scarce in the study area due to deforestation and urbanization. Since Lysimachia christinae is not native to Mauritius, many informants were unaware of this medicinal plant. The traditional Chinese medicine practitioner reported that this plant is imported in its dried form from China. Lysimachia christinae contains flavonoid and phenolic compounds which possess promising pharmacological activities in vivo [56].

3.10. Cultural Importance Index. The cultural importance index showed that Ocimum tenuiflorum (0.39), Cardiospermum halicacabum (0.09), Camellia sinensis (0.27), and Ophiopogon japonicas (0.11) are the most culturally important plant species among the Hindu, Muslim, Christian, and Buddhist community, respectively (Table 4). The high cultural importance index of these plants indicates their importance in their respective culture because of their medicinal properties and versatility. These plant species have been used since time immemorial and the medicinal knowledge of these plants has been transmitted from one generation to the next within the

TABLE 5: Jaccard similarity index for the different religious groups of Mauritius regarding the number of medicinal plants used to manage diabetes and related complications.

|           | Hindu | Muslim | Christian | Buddhist |
|-----------|-------|--------|-----------|----------|
| Hindu     | —     | 95.8   | 94.1      | 63.5     |
| Muslim    | 95.8  | —      | 90.2      | 66.0     |
| Christian | 94.1  | 90.2   | —         | 69.2     |
| Buddhist  | 63.5  | 66.0   | 69.2      | —        |

specific religious group. According to Tardío and Pardo-de-Santayana [57], the cultural importance index is an efficient tool for highlighting those species with a high agreement for the culture of the study area and hence recognises the shared knowledge of these people. From Table 4, it is evident that plant species which scored very low cultural importance index value in a particular religious group imply that little cultural importance is given to these plant species in traditional medicine in that particular religious group. Tuttolomondo et al. [37] reported that plants with low cultural importance index value indicate that the local populations had little trust in them concerning their use in the treatment of certain pathologies or indicate a fall in traditional plant knowledge regarding medicinal uses of these plants which is an evidence of an ongoing process of cultural erosion. Cultural and religious preferences also influence the use of medicinal plants [58]. Some of the documented medicinal plants were found to play important roles in religious ceremonies among the Hindu community. *Ocimum sanctum* is considered as sacred by the Hindu community. The holy basil worship is done every morning in every Hindu community household in order to keep the family members healthy. Moreover, *Azadirachta indica* and *Mangifera indica* were reported to play fundamental role in "Durga pooja," a prayer dedicated to goddess "Durga."

*3.11. Jaccard Similarity Index.* In the current investigation, the Christian community provided us with the highest number of medicinal plants (51) followed by the Hindu (48), Muslim (46), and the Buddhist (37) community. As depicted in Table 5, the Hindu community and the Muslim community showed the highest similarity of medicinal plants usage with Jaccard similarity index value of 95.8. The Hindu and Muslim community are both descendants of Indian indentured labourers who were recruited by the British Empire to work on sugar cane, banana, tea, and coffee plantations. They came from the same village in eastern Uttar Pradesh and western Bihar in northern India and arrived to Mauritius in the same ships [59]. It was observed that the Hindu and Muslim community in Mauritius commonly spoke the "Bhojpuri" dialect which is an amalgam of Creole and Hindi language. Moreover, certain traditions were found to be similar among these two religious groups. For instance, the use of henna to decorate women's hands during weddings was found to be similar among both religious groups. The high degree of similarity of medicinal plants usage between these two

communities implies that there has been an exchange of traditional information between these two cultures on the use of medicinal plant species to manage diabetes and related complications. The Hindu community and the Buddhist community showed the least similarity of medicinal plants usage with Jaccard similarity index value of 63.5. The reason for this least similarity is most likely because the Buddhist community have their own system of healing which is distinct to that of the Hindu community. Moreover, the Buddhist community commonly purchased medicinal plants from herbal stores which are imported from China and some of plants employed by the Buddhist community are unknown by the other three religious communities. Moreover, the Buddhist community was observed to be quite reticent to share their traditional knowledge with people not belonging to their cultural group. According to Güzel et al. [25], detailed anthropological studies should be carried out in order to identify factors affecting ethnomedicinal similarities and differences amongst different cultural groups.

*3.12. Ailment Categories.* The reported ailments were grouped into 9 broad categories of diseases (Table 6). The ailment categories treated by the greatest number of medicinal plants were diabetes with 40 listed plant species, followed by diabetic dyslipidemia and hypertension with 19 plant species each. The reasons for this may be due to high prevalence of diabetes in the study area as reported earlier, hence the need to search for more hypoglycemic plants. The efficacy demonstrated by some of the antidiabetic plants identified in this study has previously been documented in either *in vivo* or *in vitro* studies. Ethanolic leaf extract of *Azadirachta indica* was found to normalize blood glucose level in streptozotocin-induced diabetic rats [60]. *Syzygium cumini* bark extract lowered blood glucose level in streptozotocin-induced diabetic albino Wistar rats [61]. Aqueous leaf extract of *Graptophyllum pictum* was found to have hypoglycemic effect which is comparable to metformin in alloxan-induced diabetic Wistar rats [62]. Aqueous alcohol extract of the aerial parts of *Bidens pilosa* lowered blood glucose in db/db mice, a type 2 diabetes mouse model [63]. However, herbal medicinal practices may vary among different groups of people in different parts of the world. For example, *Trigonella foenum-graecum* was reported to be used against diabetes, high level of cholesterol, and erectile dysfunction in Mauritius but in Iran it is used against gynaecological problems [36]. The result revealed that 63.5% of the plant species enlisted were employed for the management of more than one kind of disease. This finding is in agreement with previous result described by Yousuf et al. [64] and Gupta et al. [65] where most plant species used by indigenous people have multiple uses.

*3.13. Cross-Cultural Comparison of Medicinal Plants among the Different Religious Groups.* Though the four religious groups in Mauritius possess different cultures and traditions, it was observed that they have common knowledge about the majority of the reported medicinal plant species. Thirty-three plants species were used commonly among the four religious

TABLE 6: The use of plant-based remedies and animal-based remedies by illness categories.

| Illness categories | Ethnomedicinal applications | Plant species | Animal species |
|---|---|---|---|
| Diabetic angiopathy | Atherosclerosis, cardiovascular disease | *Cynara cardunculus, Brassica oleracea, Ananas comosus, Carica papaya, Luffa acutangula, Olea europaea, Crataegus laevigata, Citrus aurantifolia,* and *Aloysia citriodora* | — |
| Diabetic nephropathy | Renal failure | *Allium cepa, Allium sativum, Petroselinum crispum, Cocos nucifera, Ananas comosus, Cucurbita maxima, Linum usitatissimum,* and *Citrus aurantifolia* | *Tenrec ecaudatus* |
| Diabetic neuropathy | Pain, erectile dysfunction, and hearing loss | *Allium cepa, Brassica oleracea, Tamarindus indica, Trigonella foenum-graecum, Ocimum tenuiflorum,* and *Morinda citrifolia* | *Anguilla japonica* |
| Eye diseases | Cataracts | *Allium cepa, Allium sativum, Aphloia theiformis, Cocos nucifera, Brassica oleracea, Cucurbita maxima, Ocimum tenuiflorum, Persea americana, Crataegus laevigata, Citrus aurantifolia,* and *Camellia sinensis* | *Helix aspersa Apis mellifera* |
| Diabetic dyslipidemia | High level of cholesterol | *Alisma plantago-aquatica, Allium cepa, Petroselinum crispum, Cynara cardunculus, Carica papaya, Lagenaria siceraria, Momordica charantia, Trigonella foenum-graecum, Ocimum tenuiflorum, Persea americana, Linum usitatissimum, Moringa oleifera, Phyllanthus emblica, Avena sativa, Crataegus laevigata, Morinda citrifolia, Citrus maxima, Camellia sinensis,* and *Aloe vera* | — |
| Hypertension | Hypertension | *Allium sativum, Annona muricata, Apium graveolens, Petroselinum crispum, Bidens pilosa, Carica papaya, Lagenaria siceraria, Luffa acutangula, Tamarindus indica, Ocimum tenuiflorum, Prunella vulgaris, Moringa oleifera, Olea europaea, Crataegus laevigata, Morinda citrifolia, Vangueria madagascariensis, Citrus aurantifolia, Murraya koenigii,* and *Camellia sinensis* | — |
| Infections and wounds | Ulcers, gangrene, urinary tract infection, and wound healing | *Allium sativum, Brassica oleracea, Cucurbita maxima, Ocimum tenuiflorum, Lysimachia christinae, Cardiospermum halicacabum,* and *Aloe vera* | *Periplaneta americana Rattus rattus* |
| Diabetes | Type 1 diabetes, type 2 diabetes | *Graptophyllum pictum, Allium cepa, Allium sativum, Mangifera indica, Aphloia theiformis, Apium graveolens, Coriandrum sativum, Petroselinum crispum, Catharanthus roseus, Cocos nucifera, Ophiopogon japonicas, Bidens pilosa, Cynara cardunculus, Sigesbeckia orientalis, Brassica oleracea, Cucumis sativus, Cucurbita maxima, Lagenaria siceraria, Momordica charantia, Trigonella foenum-graecum, Ocimum tenuiflorum, Linum usitatissimum, Azadirachta indica, Artocarpus heterophyllus, Moringa oleifera, Eucalyptus globules, Psidium guajava, Syzygium cumini, Olea europaea, Phyllanthus emblica, Avena sativa, Rhizophora mucronata, Rubus alceifolius, Morinda citrifolia, Vangueria madagascariensis, Citrus aurantifolia, Citrus maxima, Cardiospermum halicacabum, Camellia sinensis,* and *Aloe vera* | *Salmo salar* |
| Skin complications | Dry skin | *Avena sativa* | — |

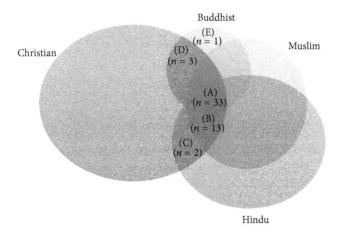

FIGURE 6: Venn diagram representing the overlap of plant species cited by participants from Hindu, Muslim, Christian, and Chinese communities in Mauritius. (A) Plant species common to Hindu, Muslim, Christian, and Buddhist religious group (*Allium cepa, Allium sativum, Mangifera indica, Apium graveolens, Petroselinum crispum, Catharanthus roseus, Bidens pilosa, Cynara cardunculus, Brassica oleracea, Carica papaya, Cucumis sativus, Cucurbita maxima, Lagenaria siceraria, Momordica charantia, Tamarindus indica, Trigonella foenum-graecum, Ocimum tenuiflorum, Linum usitatissimum, Azadirachta indica, Artocarpus heterophyllus, Psidium guajava, Syzygium cumini, Olea europaea, Phyllanthus emblica, Avena sativa, Rubus alceifolius, Morinda citrifolia, Vangueria madagascariensis, Citrus aurantifolia, Citrus maxima, Murraya koenigii, Camellia sinensis,* and *Aloe vera*). (B) Plant species common to Hindu, Muslim, and Christian religious group only (*Graptophyllum pictum, Annona muricata, Aphloia theiformis, Coriandrum sativum, Cocos nucifera, Sigesbeckia orientalis, Ananas comosus, Luffa acutangula, Persea americana, Moringa oleifera, Rhizophora mucronata, Crataegus laevigata,* and *Cardiospermum halicacabum*). (C) Plant species common to Hindu and Christian religious group only (*Eucalyptus globules, Aloysia citriodora*). (D) Plant species common to Christian and Buddhist religious group only (*Alisma plantago-aquatica, Ophiopogon japonicas,* and *Prunella vulgaris*). (E) Plant species common to Buddhist religious group only (*Lysimachia christinae*).

groups, whereas 13 plant species were common among the Hindu, Muslim, and Christian religious groups only, 2 plants were common between Hindu and Christian communities only, 3 plants were common between the Christian and Buddhist communities only, and 1 plant was used exclusively by the Buddhist community (Figure 6). A high correspondence between the uses of the same medicinal plant species among the four religious groups was surprising. The possible reason accounting for the high similarity of plant species used to manage diabetes and related complications among the four religious groups might be due to the frequent cross-cultural exchange of traditional knowledge on medicinal plants between them to manage these ailments. Moreover, the four religious groups live in close proximity to each other and share similar flora. Lingaraju et al. [33] reported that different ethnic groups influence each other in the adoption and usage of certain medicinal plant species. According to Masevhe et al. [66], the use of plant species by different cultural

groups may also indicate their potential pharmacological efficacy. Medicinal plants are not selected at random but exhibit a considerable degree of patterning within one culture [16]. Moreover, plants are selected and used in a consistent manner because of their culturally perceived effectiveness [67, 68]. According to Heinrich et al. [16], the parallel use of plant taxa among different ethnic groups may be due to (1) coincidence (a random selection of similar species), (2) similar criteria for selecting plants, and (3) shared information on the potential usefulness of a plant. Therefore, medicinal plant species which are used in parallel among the four religious groups require further pharmacological, toxicological, and phytochemical analysis for the discovery of potential novel drugs to manage diabetes and related complications.

*3.14. Animal-Based Remedies Used to Manage Diabetes and Related Complications.* In this study, a total of 7 medicinal animal species distributed over 4 classes were recorded for the management of diabetes and related complications (Table 7). Among them, Actinopterygii, Insecta, and Mammalia occupied the most cited classes with two species each. Our present analysis reveals that various parts of animal species were selected as medicinal materials. Whole animal (71.4%) was mostly recorded in the preparation of animal-based remedies followed by honey (14.3%) and skin (14.3%). The result depicts that animal-based remedies were mainly taken in the raw form (57.1%). Our finding is comparable to that of Vijayakumar et al. [69] where medicinal animal species are mostly taken as raw for the treatment of ailments. Based on relative frequency of citation, the most frequently cited medicinal animal species was *Salmo salar* (0.12). *Salmo salar* was found to be commonly used against diabetes in the study area since it contains a polyunsaturated compound, namely, omega-3. Malasanos and Stacpoole [70] reported that omega-3 fatty acids reduce serum lipids and lipoproteins, impair platelet aggregation, increase cell membrane fluidity, and lower blood pressure in diabetic subjects. Further studies are required to confirm the presence of bioactive compounds in these animal remedies reported in the current study. With regard to the administration routes of the animal-based remedies, external application (57.1%) was the most commonly used route of administration. It was observed that certain animal species were used exclusively in a specific religious group. For instance, *Tenrec ecaudatus* was reported to be used against renal failure by the Christian community only. This can be explained by the fact that *Tenrec ecaudatus* is regarded as impure by the Hindu and Muslim community and their religious values forbid them from consuming the meat of this animal. In addition, animal-based remedies were found to be more prominent among the Christian community as compared to the other three religious groups. It is fundamental to carry out studies to evaluate the safety, efficacy, and optimal dosage of the reported animal-based remedies in order to validate their traditional use and ensure proper treatment outcomes.

TABLE 7: Inventory of animal species used to manage diabetes and related complications.

| Class | Scientific name | Local name | Indication | Part used | Method of preparation and administration | RFC | $CII_H$ | $CII_M$ | $CII_C$ | $CII_B$ |
|---|---|---|---|---|---|---|---|---|---|---|
| Actinopterygii | *Salmo salar* | Saumon | Type 2 diabetes | Whole body | A dish of the whole body is prepared and it is taken once per week. | 0.12 | 0.04 | 0.00 | 0.08 | 0.00 |
| | *Anguilla japonica* | Anguille | Neuropathic pain | Skin | The skin is peeled and dried in bright sunlight. The dried skin is then placed in a bottle of oil. Massage the painful area daily using this oil. | 0.03 | 0.02 | 0.00 | 0.01 | 0.00 |
| Gastropoda | *Helix aspersa* | Courpa | Cataract | Whole body | The whole body is crushed to obtain white liquid and 2 drops of the liquid are instilled in the eye. | 0.02 | 0.00 | 0.00 | 0.02 | 0.00 |
| Insecta | *Apis mellifera* | Mouche di miel | Cataract | Honey | A small amount is instilled in the eye daily. | 0.04 | 0.01 | 0.00 | 0.03 | 0.00 |
| | *Periplaneta americana* | Cancrela | Gangrene | Whole body | Prepare an infusion with 4 cockroaches and 1 handful of *Petroselinum crispum*. Filter in a cloth and drink 1 cup daily. | 0.03 | 0.00 | 0.00 | 0.02 | 0.01 |
| Mammalia | *Tenrec ecaudatus* | Tang | Renal failure | Whole body | A dish of the body is prepared using *Cinnamomum verum*, *Syzygium aromaticum*, *Murraya koenigii* L., and 1 cup of white wine. The dish is taken once per week. | 0.03 | 0.00 | 0.00 | 0.03 | 0.00 |
| | *Rattus rattus* | Le rat | Wound | Whole body | The animal is placed in a bottle of coconut oil for 1-2 days and the oil is then applied on the wound. | 0.02 | 0.00 | 0.00 | 0.00 | 0.02 |

RFC: relative frequency of citation, $CII_H$: cultural importance index among the Hindu community, $CII_M$: cultural importance index among the Muslim community, $CII_C$: cultural importance index among the Christian community, and $CII_B$: cultural importance index among the Buddhist community.

# 4. Conclusion

To the best of our knowledge, this is the first cross-cultural investigation on traditional therapies used to manage diabetes and related complications in Mauritius. The panoply of information gathered in the present study demonstrates the important recognition of herbal and animal-based remedies among diabetic patients and traditional healers for the management of diabetes and related complications. The high popularity of *Citrus aurantifolia* demonstrates its importance in the study area for the management of diabetes and related complications. However, there is a tendency of using particular types of plants excessively in traditional medicine for its therapeutic effects without concerning its vulnerability to extinction. Hence, appropriate measures should be taken in order to preserve important plant species and emphasis should be placed on the judicious use of medicinal plants. Interviews with individuals from different religious background revealed intra- and interculturally important medicinal plants. Though cultural divergence exists among the 4 religious groups of the island, a high degree of similarity of medicinal plants usage among them has been observed. The possible reason for the high correspondence of the use of the same medicinal plant species is due to the frequent cross-cultural exchange of traditional knowledge on medicinal plants. Nonetheless, the use of certain medicinal plants and animal species has been found to be confined in only a particular religious group. According to Mustafa et al. [71], cross-cultural studies could be important for proposing culturally sensitive ways of using plant natural resources in future sustainable economic development initiatives. Culturally important plant species such as *Ocimum tenuiflorum*, *Cardiospermum halicacabum*, *Camellia sinensis*, and *Ophiopogon japonicas* should be subjected to detailed screenings for pharmacologically active metabolites for the discovery of new therapeutic agents. As a concluding note, the present study reflects the rich cultural heritage in terms of ethnomedicinal knowledge possessed by the different religious groups in Mauritius. However, this knowledge is in jeopardy due to the lack of interest shown by the younger generation. Therefore, we keenly emphasise the importance of transmitting this precious knowledge which is vanishing at an alarming rate in order to safeguard our cultural heritage.

# Competing Interests

The authors declare that they have no competing interests.

# Authors' Contributions

M. Fawzi Mahomoodally, A. Mootoosamy, and S. Wambugu designed the study and contributed to discussion regarding the study and to the preparation of the paper. A. Mootoosamy conducted the field work. All authors read and approved the final paper.

# Acknowledgments

The authors express their gratefulness to all the participants who were willing to share their precious knowledge during the course of field study and the University of Mauritius for financial support.

# References

[1] M. Jung, M. Park, H. C. Lee, Y.-H. Kan, E. S. Kang, and S. K. Kim, "Antidiabetic agents from medicinal plants," *Current Medicinal Chemistry*, vol. 13, no. 10, pp. 1203–1218, 2006.

[2] R. M. O'Brien and D. K. Granner, "Regulation of gene expression by insulin," *Physiological Reviews*, vol. 76, no. 4, pp. 1109–1161, 1996.

[3] International Diabetes Federation, *Types of Diabetes*, International Diabetes Federation, Brussels, Belgium, 2011.

[4] International Diabetes Federation, *IDF Diabetes Atlas Update 2012*, International Diabetes Federation, Brussels, Belgium, 2012.

[5] World Health Organization, *Global Health Estimates: Deaths by Cause, Age, Sex and Country, 2000–2012*, World Health Organization, Geneva, Switzerland, 2014.

[6] C. D. Mathers and D. Loncar, "Projections of global mortality and burden of disease from 2002 to 2030," *PLoS Medicine*, vol. 3, no. 11, pp. 2011–2030, 2006.

[7] International Diabetes Federation, *Mauritius*, International Diabetes Federation, Brussels, Belgium, 2015.

[8] F. Qamar, S. Afroz, Z. Feroz, S. Siddiqui, and A. Ara, "Evaluation of hypoglycemic effect of *Cassia italic*," *Journal of Basic and Applied Sciences*, vol. 7, no. 1, pp. 61–64, 2011.

[9] M. J. Fowler, "Microvascular and macrovascular complications of diabetes," *Clinical Diabetes*, vol. 26, no. 2, pp. 77–82, 2008.

[10] M. H. Eshrat, "Effect of *Coccinia indica* (L.) and *Abroma augusta* (L.) on glycemia, lipid profile and on indicators of end-organ damage in streptozotocin induced diabetic rats," *Indian Journal of Clinical Biochemistry*, vol. 18, no. 2, pp. 54–63, 2003.

[11] F. Mustaffa, J. Indurkar, N. I. M. Ali et al., "A review of Malaysian medicinal plants with potential antidiabetic activity," *Journal of Pharmacy Research*, vol. 4, no. 11, pp. 4217–4224, 2011.

[12] Mauritius Meteorological Services, "Climate of Mauritius," March 2016, http://metservice.intnet.mu/climate-services/climate-of-mauritius.php.

[13] O. Hollup, "The disintegration of caste and changing concepts of Indian ethnic identity in Mauritius," *Ethnology*, vol. 33, no. 4, pp. 297–316, 1994.

[14] V. Chintamunnee and M. F. Mahomoodally, "Herbal medicine commonly used against non-communicable diseases in the tropical island of Mauritius," *Journal of Herbal Medicine*, vol. 2, no. 4, pp. 113–125, 2012.

[15] M. F. Mahomoodally and Z. D. Hossain, "Traditional medicines for common dermatological disorders in Mauritius," *TANG*, vol. 3, no. 4, pp. 31.1–31.8, 2013.

[16] M. Heinrich, A. Ankli, B. Frei, C. Weimann, and O. Sticher, "Medicinal plants in Mexico: Healers' consensus and cultural importance," *Social Science and Medicine*, vol. 47, no. 11, pp. 1859–1871, 1998.

[17] A. Gurib-Fakim and T. Brendler, *Medicinal and Aromatic Plants of Indian Ocean Islands*, Medpharm Scientific, Stuttgart, Germany, 2004.

[18] S. Riaz, "Diabetes mellitus," *Scientific Research and Essays*, vol. 4, no. 5, pp. 367–373, 2009.

[19] American Diabetes Association (ADA), Complications, January 2014, http://www.diabetes.org/living-with-diabetes/complications/.

[20] R. Yadav, P. Tiwari, and E. Dhanaraj, "Risk factors and complications of type 2 diabetes in Asians," *CRIPS*, vol. 9, no. 2, pp. 8–12, 2008.

[21] H. N. Ginsberg, Y.-L. Zhang, and A. Hernandez-Ono, "Regulation of plasma triglycerides in insulin resistance and diabetes," *Archives of Medical Research*, vol. 36, no. 3, pp. 232–240, 2005.

[22] H. J. Bodansky, A. G. Cudworth, R. A. F. Whitelocke, and J. H. Dobree, "Diabetic retinopathy and its relation to type of diabetes: review of a retinal clinic population," *British Journal of Ophthalmology*, vol. 66, no. 8, pp. 496–499, 1982.

[23] U. K. Sharma, S. Pegu, D. Hazarika, and A. Das, "Medico-religious plants used by the Hajong community of Assam, India," *Journal of Ethnopharmacology*, vol. 143, no. 3, pp. 787–800, 2012.

[24] C. Leto, T. Tuttolomondo, S. La Bella, and M. Licata, "Ethnobotanical study in the Madonie Regional Park (Central Sicily, Italy). Medicinal use of wild shrub and herbaceous plant species," *Journal of Ethnopharmacology*, vol. 146, no. 1, pp. 90–112, 2013.

[25] Y. Güzel, M. Güzelşemme, and M. Miski, "Ethnobotany of medicinal plants used in Antakya: a multicultural district in Hatay Province of Turkey," *Journal of Ethnopharmacology*, vol. 174, article 9657, pp. 118–152, 2015.

[26] I. O. Ishola, I. A. Oreagba, A. A. Adeneye, C. Adirije, K. A. Oshikoya, and O. O. Ogunleye, "Ethnopharmacological survey of herbal treatment of malaria in Lagos, Southwest Nigeria," *Journal of Herbal Medicine*, vol. 4, no. 4, pp. 224–234, 2014.

[27] M. L. Hardy, "Herbs of special interest to women," *Journal of the American Pharmaceutical Association*, vol. 40, no. 2, pp. 234–242, 2000.

[28] M. F. Kadir, M. S. Bin Sayeed, N. I. Setu, A. Mostafa, and M. M. K. Mia, "Ethnopharmacological survey of medicinal plants used by traditional health practitioners in Thanchi, Bandarban Hill Tracts, Bangladesh," *Journal of Ethnopharmacology*, vol. 155, no. 1, pp. 495–508, 2014.

[29] D. W. Gakuya, S. M. Itonga, J. M. Mbaria, J. K. Muthee, and J. K. Musau, "Ethnobotanical survey of biopesticides and other medicinal plants traditionally used in Meru central district of Kenya," *Journal of Ethnopharmacology*, vol. 145, no. 2, pp. 547–553, 2013.

[30] American Diabetes Association, "Hypertension management in adults with diabetes," *Diabetes Care*, vol. 27, supplement 1, pp. S65–S67, 2004.

[31] A. G. Singh, A. Kumar, and D. Tewari, "An ethnobotanical survey of medicinal plants used in Terai forest of western Nepal," *Journal of Ethnobiology and Ethnomedicine*, vol. 8, article 19, 2012.

[32] A. Tahraoui, J. El-Hilaly, Z. H. Israili, and B. Lyoussi, "Ethnopharmacological survey of plants used in the traditional treatment of hypertension and diabetes in south-eastern Morocco (Errachidia province)," *Journal of Ethnopharmacology*, vol. 110, no. 1, pp. 105–117, 2007.

[33] D. P. Lingaraju, M. S. Sudarshana, and N. Rajashekar, "Ethnopharmacological survey of traditional medicinal plants in tribal areas of Kodagu district, Karnataka, India," *Journal of Pharmacy Research*, vol. 6, no. 2, pp. 284–297, 2013.

[34] F. Sefidkon, K. Abbasi, and G. B. Khaniki, "Influence of drying and extraction methods on yield and chemical composition of the essential oil of *Satureja hortensis*," *Food Chemistry*, vol. 99, no. 1, pp. 19–23, 2006.

[35] O. O. Okoh, A. P. Sadimenko, O. T. Asekun, and A. J. Afolayan, "The effects of drying on the chemical components of essential oils of *Calendula officinalis* L.," *African Journal of Biotechnology*, vol. 7, no. 10, pp. 1500–1502, 2008.

[36] Z. Sadeghia and A. Mahmood, "Ethno-gynecological knowledge of medicinal plants used by Baluch tribes, southeast of Baluchistan, Iran," *Revista Brasileira de Farmacognosia*, vol. 24, no. 6, pp. 706–715, 2014.

[37] T. Tuttolomondo, M. Licata, C. Leto et al., "Popular uses of wild plant species for medicinal purposes in the Nebrodi Regional Park (North-Eastern Sicily, Italy)," *Journal of Ethnopharmacology*, vol. 157, no. 18, pp. 21–37, 2014.

[38] A. Ghorbani, "Studies on pharmaceutical ethnobotany in the region of Turkmen Sahra, north of Iran (part 1): general results," *Journal of Ethnopharmacology*, vol. 102, no. 1, pp. 58–68, 2005.

[39] S. K. Ghimire, O. Gimenez, R. Pradel, D. McKey, and Y. Aumeeruddy-Thomas, "Demographic variation and population viability in a threatened Himalayan medicinal and aromatic herb *Nardostachys grandiflora*: matrix modelling of harvesting effects in two contrasting habitats," *Journal of Applied Ecology*, vol. 45, no. 1, pp. 41–51, 2008.

[40] A. Cheikhyoussef, M. Shapi, K. Matengu, and H. M. Ashekele, "Ethnobotanical study of indigenous knowledge on medicinal plant use by traditional healers in Oshikoto region, Namibia," *Journal of Ethnobiology and Ethnomedicine*, vol. 7, no. 10, 2011.

[41] T. Flatie, T. Gedif, K. Asres, and T. Gebre-Mariam, "Ethnomedical survey of Berta ethnic group Assosa Zone, Benishangul-Gumuz regional state, mid-west Ethiopia," *Journal of Ethnobiology and Ethnomedicine*, vol. 5, article 14, 2009.

[42] R. Bajpai, N. Jain, and A. K. Pathak, "Standardization of ethanolic extract of *Cucurbita maxima* seed," *Journal of Applied Pharmaceutical Science*, vol. 2, no. 8, pp. 92–95, 2012.

[43] B. Malla, D. P. Gauchan, and R. B. Chhetri, "An ethnobotanical study of medicinal plants used by ethnic people in Parbat district of western Nepal," *Journal of Ethnopharmacology*, vol. 165, pp. 103–117, 2015.

[44] M. Y. Paksoy, S. Selvi, and A. Savran, "Ethnopharmacological survey of medicinal plants in Ulukişla (Niğde-Turkey)," *Journal of Herbal Medicine*, 2014.

[45] J.-L. Zhang, M. Cui, Y. He, H.-L. Yu, and D.-A. Guo, "Chemical fingerprint and metabolic fingerprint analysis of Danshen injection by HPLC-UV and HPLC-MS methods," *Journal of Pharmaceutical and Biomedical Analysis*, vol. 36, no. 5, pp. 1029–1035, 2005.

[46] M. S. Kpodar, P. Lawson-Evi, B. Bakoma et al., "Ethnopharmacological survey of plants used in the treatment of diabetes mellitus in south of Togo (Maritime Region)," *Journal of Herbal Medicine*, vol. 5, no. 3, pp. 147–152, 2015.

[47] K. Dhiman, A. Gupta, D. K. Sharma, N. S. Gill, and A. Goyal, "A review on the medicinally important plants of the family Cucurbitaceae," *Asian Journal of Clinical Nutrition*, vol. 4, no. 1, pp. 16–26, 2012.

[48] M. Katemo, P. T. Mpiana, B. M. Mbala et al., "Ethnopharmacological survey of plants used against diabetes in Kisangani city (DR Congo)," *Journal of Ethnopharmacology*, vol. 144, no. 1, pp. 39–43, 2012.

[49] E. Singh, S. Sharma, A. Pareek, J. Dwivedi, S. Yadav, and S. Sharma, "Phytochemistry, traditional uses and cancer chemopreventive activity of Amla (*Phyllanthus emblica*): the Sustainer," *Journal of Applied Pharmaceutical Science*, vol. 2, no. 1, pp. 176–183, 2012.

[50] H. J. Kim, T. Yokozawa, H. Y. Kim, C. Tohda, T. P. Rao, and L. R. Juneja, "Influence of amla (Emblica officinales Gaertn.) on hypercholesterolemia and lipid peroxidation in cholesterol-fed rats," *Journal of Nutritional Science and Vitaminology*, vol. 51, no. 6, pp. 413–418, 2005.

[51] S. Arora, K. Kaur, and S. Kaur, "Indian medicinal plants as a reservoir of protective phytochemicals," *Teratogenesis Carcinogenesis and Mutagenesis*, vol. 23, no. 1, pp. 295–300, 2003.

[52] K. Walia and R. Boolchandani, "Role of amla in type 2 diabetes mellitus—a review," *Research Journal of Recent Sciences*, vol. 4, pp. 31–35, 2015.

[53] S. Kumari, N. Sarmah, and K. Handique, "Antioxidant activities of the unripen and ripen *Citrus aurantifolia* of Assam," *International Journal of Innovative Research in Science, Engineering and Technology*, vol. 2, no. 9, pp. 4811–4816, 2013.

[54] N. K. Moorthy and G. S. Reddy, "Preliminary phytochemical and pharmacological study of *Morinda citrifolia*, Linn," *Antiseptic*, vol. 67, pp. 167–171, 1970.

[55] M. R. Alam, A. B. Rahman, M. Moniruzzaman et al., "Evaluation of antidiabetic phytochemicals in *Syzygium cumini* (L.) skeels (Family: Myrtaceae)," *Journal of Applied Pharmaceutical Science*, vol. 2, no. 10, pp. 94–98, 2012.

[56] X. Yang, B.-C. Wang, X. Zhang et al., "Evaluation of *Lysimachia christinae* Hance extracts as anticholecystitis and cholagogic agents in animals," *Journal of Ethnopharmacology*, vol. 137, no. 1, pp. 57–63, 2011.

[57] J. Tardío and M. Pardo-de-Santayana, "Cultural importance indices: a comparative analysis based on the useful wild plants of southern Cantabria (Northern Spain)," *Economic Botany*, vol. 62, no. 1, pp. 24–39, 2008.

[58] A. Jusu and A. C. Sanchez, "Economic Importance of the medicinal plant trade in Sierra Leone1," *Economic Botany*, vol. 67, no. 4, pp. 299–312, 2013.

[59] O. Hollup, "Islamic revivalism and political opposition among minority Muslims in Mauritius," 1996, http://sunnirazvi.net/society/mauritius.htm.

[60] S. Bisht and S. S. Sisodia, "Anti-hyperglycemic and antidyslipidemic potential of *Azadirachta indica* leaf extract in STZ-induced diabetes mellitus," *Journal of Pharmaceutical Sciences & Research*, vol. 2, no. 10, pp. 622–627, 2010.

[61] G. Saravanan and P. Leelavinothan, "Effects of *Syzygium cumini* bark on blood glucose, plasma insulin and C-peptide in streptozotocin -induced diabetic rats," *International Journal of Endocrinology and Metabolism*, vol. 4, pp. 96–105, 2006.

[62] S. O. Olagbende-Dada, S. O. Ogbonnia, H. A. B. Coker, and G. E. Ukpo, "Blood Glucose lowering effect of Aqueous extract of *Graptophyllum pictum* (Linn) Griff. on Alloxan-induced Diabetic Rats and its acute toxicity in Mice," *African Journal of Biotechnology*, vol. 10, no. 6, pp. 1039–1043, 2011.

[63] R. P. Ubillas, C. D. Mendez, S. D. Jolad et al., "Antihyperglycemic acetylenic glucosides from *Bidens pilosa*," *Planta Medica*, vol. 66, no. 1, pp. 82–83, 2000.

[64] J. Yousuf, R. K. Verma, and H. Dar, "Traditional plant based therapy among rural communities of some villages of Baramulla district (Jammu and Kashmir)," *Journal of Phytology*, vol. 4, no. 5, pp. 46–49, 2013.

[65] S. K. Gupta, O. P. Sharma, N. S. Raina, and S. Sehgal, "Ethnobotanical study of medicinal plants of Paddar Valley of Jammu and Kashmir, India," *African Journal of Traditional, Complementary and Alternative Medicine*, vol. 10, no. 4, pp. 59–65, 2013.

[66] N. A. Masevhe, L. J. McGaw, and J. N. Eloff, "The traditional use of plants to manage candidiasis and related infections in Venda, South Africa," *Journal of Ethnopharmacology*, vol. 168, pp. 364–372, 2015.

[67] R. T. Trotter II, "*Remedios caseros*: Mexican American home remedies and community health problems," *Social Science and Medicine B*, vol. 15, no. 2, pp. 107–114, 1981.

[68] R. Trotter and M. Logan, "Informant consensus: a new approach for identifying potentially effective medicinal plants," in *Plants in Indigenous Medicine and Diet: Bio-Behavioural Approaches*, N. L. Etkin, Ed., pp. 91–112, Redgrave Publishers, Bedford Hills, NY, USA, 1986.

[69] S. Vijayakumar, J. E. M. Yabesh, S. Prabhu, M. Ayyanar, and R. Damodaran, "Ethnozoological study of animals used by traditional healers in Silent Valley of Kerala, India," *Journal of Ethnopharmacology*, vol. 162, pp. 296–305, 2015.

[70] T. H. Malasanos and P. W. Stacpoole, "Biological effects of $\omega$-3 fatty acids in diabetes mellitus," *Diabetes Care*, vol. 14, no. 12, pp. 1160–1179, 1991.

[71] B. Mustafa, A. Hajdari, A. Pieroni, B. Pulaj, X. Koro, and C. L. Quave, "A cross-cultural comparison of folk plant uses among Albanians, Bosniaks, Gorani and Turks living in south Kosovo," *Journal of Ethnobiology and Ethnomedicine*, vol. 11, article 39, 2015.

# 7

# Inhibitory Effects of Angelica Polysaccharide on Activation of Mast Cells

Wei-An Mao,[1] Yuan-Yuan Sun,[2] Jing-Yi Mao,[3] Li Wang,[1] Jian Zhang,[1] Jie Zhou,[1] Khalid Rahman,[4] and Ying Ye[5]

[1]Department of Dermatology, Seventh People's Hospital, Shanghai University of Traditional Chinese Medicine, Shanghai 200137, China
[2]Department of Graduate, Bengbu Medical College, Bengbu 233000, China
[3]Yueyang Hospital, Shanghai University of Traditional Chinese Medicine, Shanghai 200437, China
[4]School of Pharmacy and Biomolecular Sciences, Faculty of Science, Liverpool John Moores University, Liverpool L3 3AF, UK
[5]Central Laboratory, Seventh People's Hospital, Shanghai University of Traditional Chinese Medicine, Shanghai 200137, China

Correspondence should be addressed to Jie Zhou; zjiegogo1199@163.com and Ying Ye; yy49453324@163.com

Academic Editor: Víctor López

This study was designed to investigate the inhibitory effects of Angelica polysaccharide (AP) on activation of mast cells and its possible molecular mechanism. In our study, we determined the proinflammatory cytokines and allergic mediators in anti-DNP IgE stimulated RBL-2H3 cells and found that AP (50, 100, and 200 $\mu$g/mL) significantly decreased the release of histamine, $\beta$-hexosaminidase, leukotrienes C4 (LTC4), IL-1, IL-4, TNF-$\alpha$, IL-6, and human monocyte chemotactic protein-1 (MCP-1/CCL2) ($p < 0.05$). In addition, $Ca^{2+}$ entry was inhibited by treatment with AP. AP also downregulated the protein expressions of p-Fyn, p-Akt, p-P38, IL-4, TNF-$\alpha$, and NF-$\kappa$B p65 in both Fyn gene upregulated and normal RBL-2H3 cells ($p < 0.05$). Collectively, our results showed that AP could inhibit the activation of mast cells via suppressing the releases of proinflammatory cytokines allergic mediators, Gab2/PI3-K/Akt and Fyn/Syk pathways.

## 1. Introduction

Allergic disorders, such as eczema, allergic rhinitis, and asthma, are generally considered as intractable diseases threatening people's health with an increasing prevalence in recent years [1, 2]. There is increasing evidence that mast cells play crucial roles in the development and pathogenesis of allergic diseases [3, 4]. In addition, allergic disorders are commonly caused by hypersensitive response to various allergens, such as proteins, pollen, chemicals, dust, and ultraviolet radiation [5]. Human's immune system would be sensitized after initial stimulation by an allergen. Thus, when rechallenged by the same allergen, the mast cells would be activated and degranulated; subsequently, various proinflammatory cytokines and allergic mediators would be released, leading to systemic allergic reactions [6, 7].

*Angelica sinensis* (Oliv.) Diels, belonging to the family of Apiaceae, is one of the well-known and commonly used traditional Chinese medicines. In traditional Chinese medicine theory, *A. sinensis* is a widely and commonly used drug for treating blood deficiency, inflammatory and gynecological diseases, and so forth. Current research indicates that *A. sinensis* is effective in the treatment of cardio- and cerebrovascular and immune nervous systems diseases, and so forth [8, 9]. In recent years, Angelica polysaccharide (AP) has been identified as one of the important and active components of *A. sinensis*. Increasing investigations have demonstrated that the AP possesses a wide range of pharmacological activities on the immune and circulatory system of humans including antitumor activity, immunoregulatory effect, radioprotective effect, and inhibition of platelet aggregation [10, 11].

As part of our continuing investigation on discovering candidate agents from TCMs, AP showed notable antiallergic effect *in vitro* in our preliminary experiment. Therefore, our present research was designed to systemically investigate the inhibitory effects of AP on activation of mast cells and its possible molecular mechanism, which would provide a scientific basis for the clinical use of AP to treat allergic disorders.

# 2. Materials and Methods

## 2.1. Chemicals and Reagents.

*2.1. Chemicals and Reagents.* Angelica polysaccharide (AP) was purchased from JRDUN Biotechnology Co. Ltd. (Shanghai, China); DMEM and fetal bovine serum (FBS) were purchased from Gibco. Co. (NY, USA); Cell Counting Kit-8 (CCK-8) was purchased from Dojindo Biochem (Shanghai, China); antidinitrophenol (DNP) IgE and DNP-HAS were purchased from Sigma-Aldrich (MO, USA); Fluo-3 AM reagents were purchased from Life Tech. Co. (CA, USA); rats histamine, IL-1, TNF-$\alpha$, IL-6, LTC4, $\beta$-hexosaminidase, and MCP-1/CCL2 ELISA kits were purchased from the Boster Co. (Wuhan, China); p-Fyn and Fyn primary antibodies were purchased from Abcam Co. (Cambridge, UK); p-Akt, Akt, p-P38, P38, and NF-$\kappa$B p65 primary antibodies were purchased from CST Co. (MA, USA); TNF-$\alpha$, IL-4, and GAPDH primary antibodies were purchased from Santa Cruz Biotech. (CA, USA); BCA protein kit and horseradish peroxidase- (HPR-) conjugated secondary antibodies were purchased from Beyotime Co. (Jiangsu, China); PVDF membrane was purchased from Millipore Biotech. (MA, USA).

*2.2. Cell Culture and Cell Viability Assay.* RBL-2H3 cells were purchased from the American Type Culture Collection (MD, USA) and were cultured in DMEM containing 10% (v/v) heat-inactivated FBS, 100 IU/mL penicillin, and 100 $\mu$g/mL streptomycin at 37°C in a humidified atmosphere with 5% $CO_2$.

Cell viability determination was carried out by using the CCK-8 assay [12]. Briefly, RBL-2H3 cells ($5 \times 10^4/100 \mu$L) were seeded in 96-well plates and cultured at 37°C for 24 h. Then, 100 $\mu$L serum-free DMEM containing 10% CCK-8 reagents (v/v) was added in each well, and cells were cultured for 1 h at 37°C. Subsequently, optical density (OD) values were determined at 450 nm by using a 96-well plate reader (DNM-9602, Pulang New technology, Beijing, China).

*2.3. Degranulation Assay in RBL-2H3 Cells.* RBL-2H3 cells ($2 \times 10^5$/well) were seeded in 24-well plates and stimulated with anti-DNPIgE (100 ng/mL) for 12 h. Then, the culture solution of RBL-2H3 cells was refreshed, and cells were treated with AP (50, 100, and 200 $\mu$g/mL) and azelastine (used as positive drugs, 30 $\mu$g/mL) for 1 h. The cells were then washed with Tyrode's buffer three times followed by incubation with DNP-HAS (20 ng/mL) for 30 and 120 min, respectively. (1) Then, for the cells incubated with DNP-HAS (20 ng/mL) for 30 min, the supernatant of the cell mixture was collected and the release of $\beta$-hexosaminidase, histamine, and LTC4 was determined by using commercial ELISA kits. In addition, the cells were also harvested for determining the releases of $\beta$-hexosaminidase and the inhibition of $\beta$-hexosaminidase release was calculated. (2) For the cells incubated with DNP-HAS (20 ng/mL) for 120 min, the supernatant of the cell mixture was collected, and IL-1, IL-4, TNF-$\alpha$, and CCL2 were

assayed by ELISA kits according to the instructions provided by the supplier [7].

*2.4. Determination of Intracellular $Ca^{2+}$ Concentrations.* The concentration of $Ca^{2+}$ was determined by using Fluo-3 AM Calcium Kits according to the manufacturer's instructions. Briefly, RBL-2H3 cells were seeded into the 6-well culture plate and treated with anti-DNP IgE. Subsequently, cells were incubated with 1 mL Fluo-3 AM for 1 h, and the fluorescent intensity was determined by using the flow cytometer (Accuri C6, BD, NJ, USA) [6].

*2.5. Western Blot Assay.* RBL-2H3 cells ($2 \times 10^5$/well) were seeded in 24-well plates and stimulated with anti-DNP IgE (100 ng/mL) for 12 h. Then, the culture solution of RBL-2H3 cells was refreshed, and cells were treated with AP (50, 100, and 200 $\mu$g/mL) for 1 h and the cells were washed with Tyrode's buffer three times. Following this, cells were incubated with DNP-HAS (20 ng/mL) for 10 min and the total proteins were extracted, and their concentration was determined by BCA protein kit and 30 $\mu$g total proteins were separated by sodium dodecyl sulfate- (SDS-) polyacrylamide gel electrophoresis (PAGE) and subsequently transferred to a PVDF membrane. The transferred protein PVDF membrane was probed with various primary antibodies, followed by incubation with HPR-conjugated secondary antibodies. Finally, chemiluminescence detection was used to visualize the target protein bands. To normalize protein loading, antibodies directed against GAPDH were used, and the proteins expression levels were expressed as a relative value to that of GAPDH.

*2.6. Plasmid Construction and Transient Transfection.* Fyn upregulated RBL-2H3 cells were constructed by the JRDUN Biotech. Co. (Shanghai, China). Briefly, the human Fyn gene was subcloned into a lentiviral vector [pCDNA3.1 (+)] to generate the lentiviral expression vector [pCDNA3.1 (+)-Fyn]. The recombinant lentiviruses were then produced by 293 T cells following the cotransfection of pCDNA3.1 (+)-Fyn. The resulting recombinant lentiviruses carrying Fyn were used to infect RBL-2H3 cells. The Fyn expression in untreated RBL-2H3 cells, cells treated with control vector (MOCK group), and Fyn gene overexpressed RBL-2H3 cells (Fyn-RBL-2H3) were detected by using real-time fluorogenic PCR (qRT-PCR) and western blotting assay.

*2.7. Real-Time Fluorogenic PCR Assays.* RBL-2H3 cells were harvested, and total RNA was extracted using Trizol reagent (Invitrogen, USA). Total RNA was used for cDNA synthesis of NF-$\kappa$B p65, TNF-$\alpha$, Fyn, IL-4, and GAPDH by reverse transcription using qRT-PCR (ABI-7300, USA). All mRNA primers were designed by Premier 5.0 and synthesized by JRDun Biotech. (Shanghai, China). Primers used for the real-time PCR are shown in Table 1. Reverse transcription was performed according to the manufacturer's recommendation of the quantitative RT-PCR reaction kits (SYBR Green, Thermo Fisher Scientific, Shanghai, China).

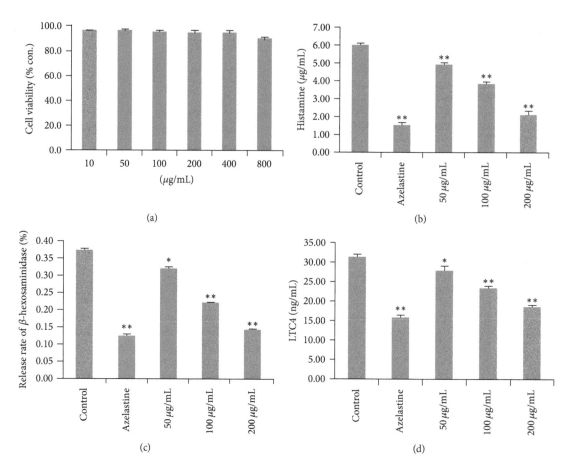

FIGURE 1: Effects of AP on degranulation in RBL-2H3 cells stimulated with anti-DNP IgE. (a) Cytotoxicity of AP on RBL-2H3 cells. (b) Effects of AP on histamine in RBL-2H3 cells. (c) Effects of AP on $\beta$-hexosaminidase in RBL-2H3 cells. (d) Effects of AP on LTC4 in RBL-2H3 cells. Azelastine was used as positive control. Data were represented as mean ± SD ($n$ = 6), $^{*}p$ < 0.05, and $^{**}p$ < 0.01, compared with control group.

TABLE 1: Primers used in our real-time PCR experiment.

| Genes | Sequences |
|---|---|
| NF-$\kappa$B p65 | F: 5′ AGACCTGGAGCAAGCCATTAG 3′ |
| | R: 5′ CGGACCGCATTCAAGTCATAG 3′ |
| TNF-$\alpha$ | F: 5′ TGGCGTGTTCATCCGTTC 3′ |
| | R: 5′ CTACTTCAGCGTCTCGTGTG 3′ |
| Fyn | F: 5′ ACCACCAAAGGTGCCTACTC 3′ |
| | R: 5′ ATGTAGTACCCGCCGTTGTC 3′ |
| IL-4 | F: 5′ CCTTGCTGTCACCCTGTTC 3′ |
| | R: 5′ CTCGTTCTCCGTGGTGTTC 3′ |
| GAPDH | F: 5′ GTCGGTGTGAACGGATTTG 3′ |
| | R: 5′ TCCCATTCTCAGCCTTGAC 3′ |

*2.8. Statistical Analyses.* Data are presented as means ± standard deviation. Statistically significant differences were analyzed using two-tailed Student's $t$-test; $p$ < 0.05 was considered to represent a statistically significant difference.

## 3. Results

*3.1. Effects of AP on Degranulation in RBL-2H3 Cells Stimulated with Anti-DNP IgE.* As can be seen from Figure 1(a), cell viability assay showed no obvious cytotoxic effect of AP on RBL-2H3 cells within the concentrations tested (0–800 $\mu$g/mL). Based on the results of cytotoxicity determination, the concentrations of 50, 100, and 200 $\mu$g/mL without cytotoxicity were selected following the experiments. Furthermore, our results showed that AP at concentrations of 50, 100, and 200 $\mu$g/mL possessed significant histamine suppressing activities compared to the control group, in a concentration-dependent manner ($p$ < 0.01) (Figure 1(b)). Additionally, AP (50, 100, and 200 $\mu$g/mL) also showed notable inhibitory effects on $\beta$-hexosaminidase and leukotrienes C4 (LTC4) in a concentration-dependent manner when compared to the control group ($p$ < 0.05, $p$ < 0.01, and $p$ < 0.01, resp.) (Figures 1(c) and 1(d)).

Furthermore, compared to the control group, IL-1, TNF-$\alpha$, IL-6, and human monocyte chemotactic protein-1 (MCP-1/CCL2) were also significantly inhibited by AP (50, 100, and 200 $\mu$g/mL) with a concentration-dependent manner ($p$ <

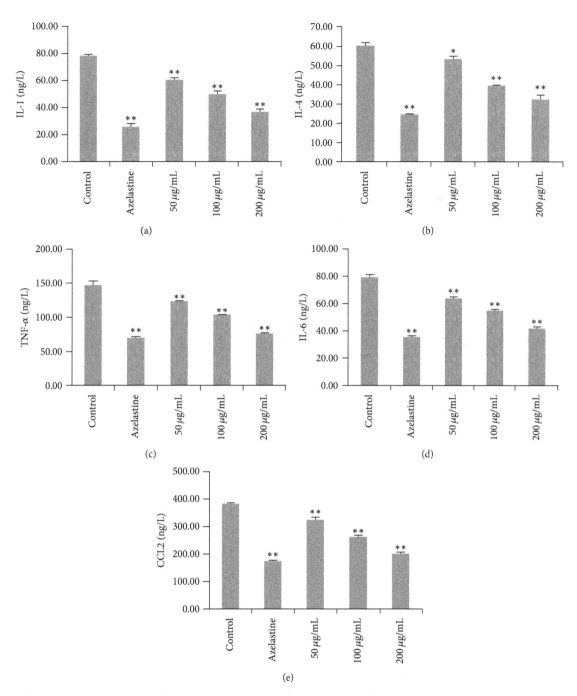

FIGURE 2: Effects of AP on the releases of IL-1 (a), IL-4 (b), TNF-$\alpha$ (c), IL-6 (d), and MCP-1/CCL2 (e) in RBL-2H3 cells stimulated with anti-DNP IgE. The azelastine was used as positive control. Data were represented as mean $\pm$ SD ($n = 6$), $^*p < 0.05$, and $^{**}p < 0.01$, compared to control group.

0.01) (Figure 2). Besides, AP (50, 100, and 200 $\mu$g/mL) also significantly decreased the release of IL-4 ($p < 0.05$, $p < 0.01$, and $p < 0.01$, resp.), in a concentration-dependent manner.

*3.2. Effects of AP on Ca²⁺ Entry in RBL-2H3 Cells Stimulated with Anti-DNP IgE.* In our present investigation, we also determined Ca²⁺ entry in RBL-2H3 cells induced by anti-DNP IgE by using Fluo-3-AM in conjunction with the FLIPR system. Our present results showed that AP could

significantly decrease the Ca²⁺ influx in RBL-2H3 cells stimulated with anti-DNP IgE at the concentrations of 50, 100, and 200 $\mu$g/mL ($p < 0.01$), compared to the control group (Figure 3). Besides, we can also find an obvious concentration-dependent manner for inhibiting Ca2+ influx in the present study.

*3.3. Effects of AP on Protein Expressions of p-Fyn, Fyn, p-Akt, Akt, p-P38, P38, IL-4, TNF-$\alpha$, and NF-$\kappa$B p65.* Furthermore,

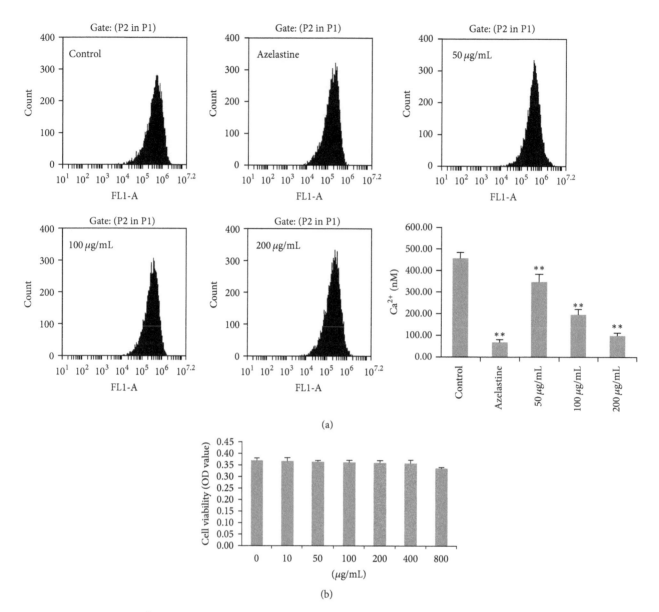

FIGURE 3: Effects of AP on $Ca^{2+}$ entry in RBL-2H3 cells stimulated with anti-DNP IgE. The azelastine was used as positive control. Data are represented as mean $\pm$ SD ($n = 6$), $^{**}p < 0.01$, compared to control group.

by using western bolt assay, our study also investigates the protein expressions of p-Fyn, Fyn, p-Akt, Akt, p-P38, P38, IL-4, TNF-$\alpha$, and NF-$\kappa$B in RBL-2H3 cells stimulated with anti-DNP IgE. The results indicate that the protein expressions of p-Akt, p-P38, IL-4, and TNF-$\alpha$ were significantly downregulated by treatment with AP (50, 100, and 200 $\mu$g/mL) in a concentration-dependent manner ($p < 0.01$), when compared to the control group. Similarly, treatment with AP also downregulated the protein expressions of p-Fyn and NF-$\kappa$B p65 (50, 100, and 200 $\mu$g/mL) ($p < 0.05$, $p < 0.01$, and $p < 0.01$, resp.), when compared to the control group. In contrast, no obvious difference was observed in the protein expressions of Fyn, Akt, and P38 ($p > 0.05$), compared to the control group (Figure 4).

### 3.4. Expression of Fyn in RBL-2H3 Cells after Transient Transfection.

In order to confirm the importance of Fyn gene in the activation of mast cells, the Fyn upregulated RBL-2H3 cells were constructed by transient transfection. As can be seen from Figure 5, after transient transfection, the Fyn gene was significantly upregulated in the RBL-2H3 cells ($p < 0.01$), compared to both untreated RBL-2H3 and MOCK groups (Figure 5(a)). Furthermore, the results of our western blotting assay also demonstrated that Fyn protein was upregulated after transient transfection (Figure 5(b)).

### 3.5. Effects of AP on mRNA Expressions of NF-$\kappa$B p65, IL-4, and TNF-$\alpha$ in Upregulated RBL-2H3 Cells Stimulated with Anti-DNP IgE.

After the Fyn upregulated RBL-2H3 cells were

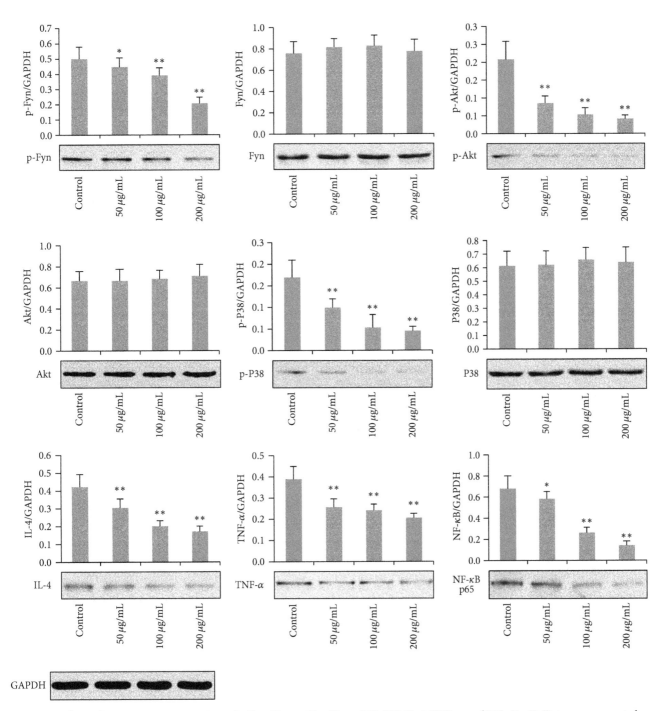

FIGURE 4: Effects of AP on protein expressions of p-Fyn, Fyn, p-Akt, Akt, p-P38, P38, IL-4, TNF-$\alpha$, and NF-$\kappa$B p65. Data are represented as mean ± SD ($n = 6$), $^*p < 0.05$, and $^{**}p < 0.01$, compared with control group.

established, we determined the mRNA expressions of NF-$\kappa$B p65, IL-4, and TNF-$\alpha$ in upregulated RBL-2H3 cells induced by anti-DNP IgE. Our results indicated that the mRNA expressions of NF-$\kappa$B p65, IL-4, and TNF-$\alpha$ genes in RBL-2H3 cells were significantly increased in both untreated RBL-2H3 cells ($p < 0.01$) and MOCK groups ($p < 0.01$). However, treatment with AP (50, 100, and 200 $\mu$g/mL) reversed these

increased mRNA expressions of NF-$\kappa$B p65 ($p < 0.01$), IL-4 ($p < 0.01$), and TNF-$\alpha$ ($p < 0.01$), in a concentration-dependent manner compared with the Fyn upregulated RBL-2H3 cells. In addition, our results also demonstrated that no obvious antiproliferation effect of AP (0–800 $\mu$g/mL) was found in the growth of Fyn upregulated RBL-2H3 cells (Figure 6).

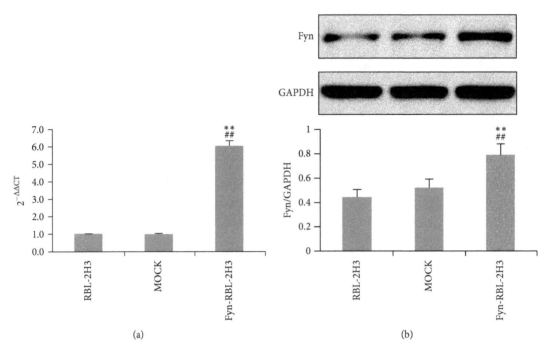

(a)                                                                 (b)

FIGURE 5: Expression of Fyn in RBL-2H3 cells after transient transfection. (a) mRNA expressions of Fyn determined by real-time PCR (qRT-PCR). (b) Protein expressions of Fyn determined by western blot assay. MOCK means the cells treated with control vector, and Fyn-RBL-2H3 means Fyn gene upregulated RBL-2H3 cells, $^{**}p < 0.01$, compared to untreated RBL-2H3 cells, and $^{##}p < 0.01$, compared to MOCK group.

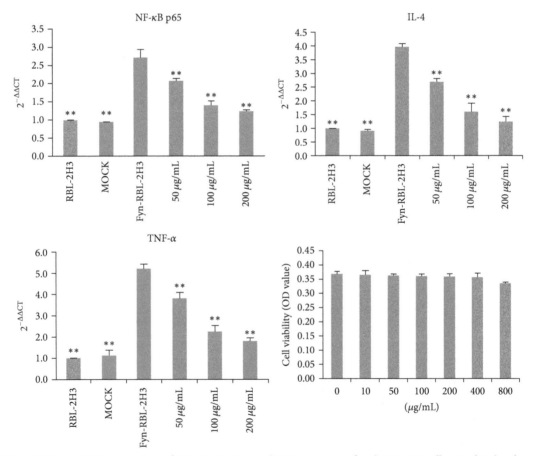

FIGURE 6: Effects of AP on mRNA expressions of NF-$\kappa$B p65, IL-4, and TNF-$\alpha$ in upregulated RBL-2H3 cells stimulated with anti-DNP IgE. MOCK means the cells treated with control vector, and Fyn-RBL-2H3 means Fyn gene upregulated RBL-2H3 cells, $^{**}p < 0.01$, compared to Fyn-RBL-2H3 cells.

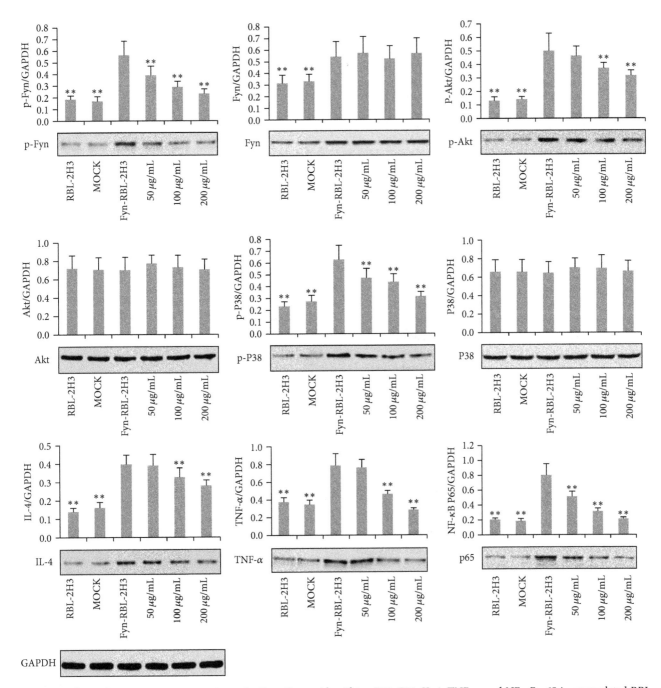

FIGURE 7: Effects of AP on protein expressions of p-Fyn, Fyn, p-Akt, Akt, p-P38, P38, IL-4, TNF-$\alpha$, and NF-$\kappa$B p65 in upregulated RBL-2H3 cells stimulated with anti-DNP IgE. MOCK means the cells treated with control vector, and Fyn-RBL-2H3 means Fyn gene upregulated RBL-2H3 cells, $^{**}p < 0.01$, compared to Fyn-RBL-2H3 cells.

*3.6. Effects of AP on Protein Expressions of p-Fyn, Fyn, p-Akt, Akt, p-P38, P38, IL-4, TNF-$\alpha$, and NF-$\kappa$B p65 in Upregulated RBL-2H3 Cells Stimulated with Anti-DNP IgE.* Furthermore, after treatment with AP (50, 100, and 200 $\mu$g/mL), we determined the protein expressions of p-Fyn, Fyn, p-Akt, Akt, p-P38, P38, IL-4, TNF-$\alpha$, and NF-$\kappa$B p65 in upregulated RBL-2H3 cells stimulated with anti-DNP IgE. As can be seen from Figure 7, the p-Fyn, Fyn, p-Akt, p-P38, IL-4, TNF-$\alpha$, and

NF-$\kappa$B p65 were upregulated ($p < 0.01$), compared with untreated RBL-2H3 cells. However, after treatment with AP (50, 100, and 200 $\mu$g/mL), the expressions of p-Fyn, p-P38, and NF-$\kappa$B p65 were downregulated significantly ($p < 0.01$) in a concentration-dependent manner, compared to the Fyn-RBL-2H3 cells. In addition, the AP (100 and 200 $\mu$g/mL) decreased the upregulated expressions of p-Akt, IL-4, and TNF-$\alpha$ ($p < 0.01$), when compared to the Fyn-RBL-2H3 cells.

## 4. Discussion

Eczema, one of the stubborn skin diseases with increasing prevalence, is closely correlated to the immune functions of human being. Currently, natural herbal medicines, such as TCMs, have aroused considerable interest due to their low toxicity and reliable therapeutic effects [12, 13]. Interestingly, *A. sinensis* is one of the most commonly used herbal medicines for treating eczema in China [14, 15]. However, no systemic investigation reporting the active substances and their therapeutic effect on eczema has been conducted. To the best of our knowledge, this is the first systemic investigation regarding inhibitory effect of Angelica polysaccharide (AP) on activation of mast cells and its possible molecular mechanism. In our present research, the AP showed significant inhibitory effect against the activation of RBL-2H3 cells. In addition, our present results also indicated that downregulating Fyn gene might be a possible molecular mechanism for responding to the activity of AP.

Previous researches reported that, after sensitization by various allergens, the mast cells would be activated and respond via degranulation [7, 16]. Subsequently, several of proinflammatory cytokines and allergic mediators are released, leading to immune response. Histamine and β-hexosaminidase are commonly considered as the notable markers in degranulation of mast cells [17]. Previous reports have demonstrated that they would be elevated in plasma or tissues in various allergic diseases. LTC4, IL-6, IL-1, MCP-1/CCL2, and TNF-$\alpha$ play important roles in the development of allergic diseases, and their release and synthesis could be increased in various allergic diseases [18, 19]. In our present study, we used the anti-DNP IgE, a commonly used allergen, to sensitize the RBL-2H3 cells. Then, we determined the releases of histamine, β-hexosaminidase, LTC4, and MCP-1/CCL2 in RBL-2H3 cells. Besides, mast cell degranulation and histamine production are $Ca^{2+}$ dependent, and $Ca^{2+}$ entry activates the degranulation of mast cells [7, 20]. Our present results showed that AP possessed significantly inhibitory effects on releases of proinflammatory cytokines, allergic mediators, and $Ca^{2+}$ entry in RBL-2H3 cells stimulated with anti-DNP IgE, indicating that AP could effectively inhibit the degranulation and activation of mast cells. Alleviating the inflammatory reactions would be beneficial for controlling the allergic symptoms. Our results also revealed that AP treatment could inhibit the expressions of some crucial inflammatory pathway cytokines including IL-1, IL-6, TNF-$\alpha$, and NF-$\kappa$B p65.

Fyn is a crucial signaling molecule for activation of mast cells stimulated by various antigens. Increasing reports have demonstrated that Gab2/PI3-K/Akt and Fyn/Syk pathway plays an essential role in the development of allergic diseases [21, 22]. Interestingly, in our present study, we also found that AP could downregulate phosphorylated Fyn in anti-DNP IgE stimulated RBL-2H3 cells. Furthermore, the phosphorylated downstream signaling molecules Gab2/PI3-K/Akt and Fyn/Syk pathway in anti-DNP IgE stimulated RBL-2H3 cells, including p-Akt and p-P38, were also downregulated. Thus, we proposed that the Fyn might be a potential molecular mechanism of AP for treating allergic diseases. To confirm

our hypothesis, the gene upregulated RBL-2H3 cells were constructed by transient transfection. Importantly, similar results were also obtained in the Fyn upregulated RBL-2H3 cells stimulated with anti-DNP IgE. Our results showed that the AP treatment could downregulate the related cytokines and proteins in inflammatory pathway and essential proteins in Gab2/PI3-K/Akt and Fyn/Syk pathways.

## 5. Conclusions

In conclusion, our present investigation demonstrated that AP could inhibit the releases of proinflammatory cytokines and allergic mediators. In addition, our results also demonstrated that AP downregulated the related cytokines and proteins in inflammatory pathway and essential proteins in Gab2/PI3-K/Akt and Fyn/Syk pathways. Collectively, our results suggested that AP could inhibit the activation of mast cells.

## Competing Interests

The authors declare that they have no competing interests.

## Acknowledgments

This work was funded by Key Disease Type (eczema) Construction Project of Shanghai (no. zxbz2012-04) and Key Discipline Construction Project of Pudong Health Bureau of Shanghai (no. PWZx2014-16).

## References

[1] W. Peng, Q.-L. Ming, P. Han et al., "Anti-allergic rhinitis effect of caffeoylxanthiazonoside isolated from fruits of *Xanthium strumarium* L. in rodent animals," *Phytomedicine*, vol. 21, no. 6, pp. 824–829, 2014.

[2] A. S. Kemp, "Allergic rhinitis," *Paediatric Respiratory Reviews*, vol. 10, no. 2, pp. 63–68, 2009.

[3] M. Kim, S. J. Lim, H.-J. Lee, and C. W. Nho, "Cassia tora seed extract and its active compound aurantio-obtusin inhibit allergic responses in ige-mediated mast cells and anaphylactic models," *Journal of Agricultural and Food Chemistry*, vol. 63, no. 41, pp. 9037–9046, 2015.

[4] J. B. Wechsler, C.-L. Hsu, and P. J. Bryce, "IgE-mediated mast cell responses are inhibited by thymol-mediated, activation-induced cell death in skin inflammation," *Journal of Allergy and Clinical Immunology*, vol. 133, no. 6, pp. 1735–1743, 2014.

[5] L. Zhu, L. Zhao, R. Qu et al., "Adrenergic stimulation sensitizes TRPV1 through upregulation of cystathionine β-synthetase in a rat model of visceral hypersensitivity," *Scientific Reports*, vol. 5, Article ID 16109, 2015.

[6] L. Huang, T. Li, H. Zhou, P. Qiu, J. Wu, and L. Liu, "Sinomenine potentiates degranulation of RBL-2H3 basophils via upregulation of phospholipase $A_2$ phosphorylation by Annexin A1 cleavage and ERK phosphorylation without influencing on calcium mobilization," *International Immunopharmacology*, vol. 28, no. 2, pp. 945–951, 2015.

[7] J. Huang, T. Zhang, S. Han, J. Cao, Q. Chen, and S. Wang, "The inhibitory effect of piperine from Fructus piperis extract on the

degranulation of RBL-2H3 cells," *Fitoterapia*, vol. 99, no. 1, pp. 218–226, 2014.

[8] L. Fang, X.-F. Xiao, C.-X. Liu, and X. He, "Recent advance in studies on *Angelica sinensis*," *Chinese Herbal Medicines*, vol. 4, no. 1, pp. 12–25, 2012.

[9] J.-P. Ma, Z.-B. Guo, L. Jin, and Y.-D. Li, "Phytochemical progress made in investigations of *Angelica sinensis* (Oliv.) Diels," *Chinese Journal of Natural Medicines*, vol. 13, no. 4, pp. 241–249, 2015.

[10] Q. Zeng, Y.-W. Jia, P.-L. Xu et al., "Quick and selective extraction of *Z*-ligustilide from *Angelica sinensis* using magnetic multi-walled carbon nanotubes," *Journal of Separation Science*, vol. 38, no. 24, pp. 4269–4275, 2015.

[11] W.-J. Zhou, S. Wang, Z. Hu, Z.-Y. Zhou, and C.-J. Song, "Angelica sinensis polysaccharides promotes apoptosis in human breast cancer cells via CREB-regulated caspase-3 activation," *Biochemical and Biophysical Research Communications*, vol. 467, no. 3, pp. 562–569, 2015.

[12] W. Peng, C. Hu, Z. Shu, T. Han, L. Qin, and C. Zheng, "Antitumor activity of tatariside F isolated from roots of *Fagopyrum tataricum* (L.) Gaertn against H22 hepatocellular carcinoma via up-regulation of p53," *Phytomedicine*, vol. 22, no. 7-8, pp. 730–736, 2015.

[13] B. Patwardhan, "Ethnopharmacology and drug discovery," *Journal of Ethnopharmacology*, vol. 100, no. 1-2, pp. 50–52, 2005.

[14] J. Lee, Y. Y. Choi, M. H. Kim et al., "Topical Application of *Angelica sinensis* improves pruritus and skin inflammation in mice with atopic dermatitis-like symptoms," *Journal of Medicinal Food*, vol. 19, no. 1, pp. 98–105, 2015.

[15] J. E. Wang, C. H. Zhu, and C. Ye, "Observation on 96 cases of chronic eczema scrotum treated with modified Chinese Angelica decoction and sanhuang oil," *Clinic Medicine and Engineering*, vol. 19, no. 7, pp. 71–72, 2012.

[16] N. A. El-Shitany and K. El-Desoky, "Cromoglycate, not ketotifen, ameliorated the injured effect of warm ischemia/reperfusion in rat liver: role of mast cell degranulation, oxidative stress, proinflammatory cytokine, and inducible nitric oxide synthase," *Drug Design, Development and Therapy*, vol. 9, pp. 5237–5246, 2015.

[17] F. Tang, F. Chen, X. Ling et al., "Inhibitory effect of methyleugenol on IgE-mediated allergic inflammation in RBL-2H3 cells," *Mediators of Inflammation*, vol. 2015, Article ID 463530, 9 pages, 2015.

[18] H.-H. Park, S. Lee, H.-Y. Son et al., "Flavonoids inhibit histamine release and expression of proinflammatory cytokines in mast cells," *Archives of Pharmacal Research*, vol. 31, no. 10, pp. 1303–1311, 2008.

[19] M. Matsubara, S. Masaki, K. Ohmori, A. Karasawa, and K. Hasegawa, "Differential regulation of IL-4 expression and degranulation by anti-allergic olopatadine in rat basophilic leukemia (RBL-2H3) cells," *Biochemical Pharmacology*, vol. 67, no. 7, pp. 1315–1326, 2004.

[20] S.-S. Hsu, K.-L. Lin, C.-T. Chou et al., "Effect of thymol on $Ca^{2+}$ homeostasis and viability in human glioblastoma cells," *European Journal of Pharmacology*, vol. 670, no. 1, pp. 85–91, 2011.

[21] J. H. Lee, T. H. Kim, H. S. Kim et al., "An indoxyl compound 5-bromo-4-chloro-3-indolyl 1,3-diacetate, CAC-0982, suppresses activation of Fyn kinase in mast cells and IgE-mediated allergic responses in mice," *Toxicology and Applied Pharmacology*, vol. 285, no. 3, pp. 179–186, 2015.

[22] J. H. Kim, A.-R. Kim, H. S. Kim et al., "*Rhamnus davurica* leaf extract inhibits Fyn activation by antigen in mast cells

for anti-allergic activity," *BMC Complementary and Alternative Medicine*, vol. 15, article 80, 2015.

# 8

# Acupoints Stimulation for Anxiety and Depression in Cancer Patients: A Quantitative Synthesis of Randomized Controlled Trials

**Tao Wang,**[1] **Renli Deng,**[1] **Jing-Yu Tan,**[2] **and Feng-Guang Guan**[3]

[1]*The Fifth Affiliated (Zhuhai) Hospital of Zunyi Medical University, No. 1439, Zhufeng Road, Zhuhai, Guangdong 519100, China*
[2]*School of Nursing, Fujian University of Traditional Chinese Medicine, No. 1, Qiuyang Road, Fuzhou, Fujian 350122, China*
[3]*The Second Affiliated People's Hospital, Fujian University of Traditional Chinese Medicine,*
 *No. 282, Wusi Road, Fuzhou, Fujian 350003, China*

Correspondence should be addressed to Renli Deng; renli.deng@gmail.com and Feng-Guang Guan; fg_guan@hotmail.com

Academic Editor: Mary K. Garcia

This study aims at concluding the current evidence on the therapeutic effects of acupoints stimulation for cancer patients with anxiety and depression. Randomized controlled trials using acupoints stimulation for relieving anxiety and/or depression in cancer patients were searched, and 11 studies were finally included, of which eight trials compared acupoints stimulation with standard methods of treatment/care, and acupoints stimulation showed significantly better effects in improving depression than using standard methods of treatment/care. Four studies compared true acupoints stimulation with sham methods, and no significant differences can be found between groups for either depression or anxiety, although the pooled effects still favored true intervention. For the five studies that evaluated sleep quality, the results were conflicting, with three supporting the superiority of acupoints stimulation in improving sleep quality and two demonstrating no differences across groups. Acupoints stimulation seems to be an effective approach in relieving depression and anxiety in cancer patients, and placebo effects may partially contribute to the benefits. However, the evidence is not conclusive due to the limited number of included studies and the clinical heterogeneity identified among trials. More rigorous designed randomized, sham-controlled studies are necessary in future research.

## 1. Introduction

Cancer is one of the major health problems in the world. The incidence of cancer and the related death have significantly increased during the past decades. According to the global corresponding data reported by the International Agency for Research on Cancer (IARC), 14.1 million cancer patients were identified around the world and 8.2 million patients died in 2012 [1]. Cancer-related death has gradually surpassed the relative figure of all types of heart disease and stroke and has become the leading cause of death at present [2].

With the advance of medical technologies, cancer treatments have changed reasonably, and comprehensive treatment strategies including optimized pharmacological intervention [3] and palliative care can ease most physical symptoms effectively and let cancer survivors live a relatively symptom-free life [4, 5]. Although the survival rate has been rising over the past decade, the negative cancer experiences and the side effects associated with cancer treatments (e.g., pain, fatigue, nausea, and vomiting) can result in a wide range of health problems, which contain not only physical issues but also psychological and emotional distresses including depression, anxiety, and posttraumatic stress disorder (PTSD) [5–9]. The incidence of depression in cancer survivors is three to four times as much as that in general population [10], ranging from 10% to 50% [11, 12]. The percentages of anxiety and PTSD following cancer were reported to be 6% to 23% [13] and 0% to 32% [14], respectively. The negative emotional feelings can contribute to significantly undesirable impacts on cancer patients, leading to sleep disturbance, loss of appetite, deterioration of quality of life, and so forth [15]. In turn, the psychological and emotional disorders can also increase the risk of recurrence and mortality of cancer as psychological distresses could impair patients' immune response [16].

Healthcare professionals have recognized that cancer treatment should aim at not only expanding patients' life span but also improving their psychosocial well-being [17]. In recent years, healthcare professionals and patients are increasingly interested in using complementary therapies to relieve cancer survivors' emotional problems such as anxiety and depression and make them as alternatives to the mainstream medicine [18]. Acupoints stimulation as one kind of complementary therapies originates from ancient China, and it is based on the theory of main and collateral channels. For the modalities of acupoints stimulation, both acupuncture and acupressure are used in practice. The World Health Organization (WHO) has viewed acupoints stimulation as a beneficial intervention to deal with a wide range of health problems [19], and its therapeutic effects for psychological distresses, particularly with regard to anxiety and depression, have been explored in noncancer populations, and corresponding systematic reviews and clinical trials have been conducted to identify its positive effects [20–23]. Cancer patients as the special population suffer more from anxiety and depression [10], and acupoints stimulation can be a promising therapy, but the evidence remains unknown.

Preclinical research has indicated that both the hypothalamic-pituitary-gonadal axis (HPA) and the sympathetic nervous system (SNS) can be significantly affected by acupoints stimulation, which presents a possible explanation that acupoints stimulation may have a positive impact on reducing psychological distresses from the biological perspectives [24, 25]. A large number of clinical trials have also been conducted to explore whether acupoints stimulation is effective in controlling anxiety and depression in cancer patients but their findings were conflicting [26–36]. Some demonstrated that acupoints stimulation can effectively relieve anxiety and/or depression while some did not. The clinical heterogeneity in patient characteristics, intervention protocols, and outcome variables and the various degrees of methodological quality among those trials may partially contribute to the contradictory study results. However, to our knowledge, currently there is no systematic summary in regard to the methodological quality assessment of the trials on acupoints stimulation for anxiety and depression in cancer patients, and the overall evidence on its clinical efficacy remains uncertain. Therefore, the objectives of this systematic review are to explore the current evidence on acupoints stimulation for anxiety and depression in cancer patients and to offer recommendations for future research and practice.

## 2. Methods

*2.1. Search Strategies.* We retrieved relevant references by searching electronic databases. Ten databases were searched (up to November 20, 2014) which include PubMed, Cochrane Central Register of Controlled Trials (CENTRAL), Cumulative Index to Nursing and Allied Health Literature (CINAHL), Allied and Complementary Medicine (AMED), PsycINFO, ISI Web of Science, Science Direct, WanFang Data, China National Knowledge Infrastructure (CNKI), and Chinese Scientific Journal Database (VIP). When conducting the electronic search, we did not set restrictions for the publications in terms of types of language and types of study. Mesh terms and key words used in the search strategies were "acupuncture", "acupressure", "acupuncture, ear", "electroacupuncture", "neoplasms", "anxiety", "depression", "mood disorders", and so forth; we also searched the references of the final included articles and other Chinese core journals on Traditional Chinese Medicine (TCM) to see whether we can locate any publications for possible inclusion. The literature search was conducted independently by two reviewers. In Table 4, we list two search strategies for this systematic review.

*2.2. Study Selection and Data Extraction.* After completing literature search, the same two reviewers independently screened the title and abstract of all searched articles, and the final eligible articles were obtained and read in full text. Inclusion criteria for eligible studies were (1) randomized controlled trials comparing acupoints stimulation (including manual acupuncture, electroacupuncture, or acupressure) to one or more of the following situations: sham acupoints stimulation, standard treatment/care (usual care, standard medication, and attention control group were all defined as standard treatment/care in this systematic review), or waitlist control; (2) participants who should be cancer patients with anxiety and/or depression regardless of being children or adults; and (3) trials published in English or Chinese.

The primary outcome measures were anxiety and depression as measured by Hospital Anxiety and Depression Scale (HADS), Center for Epidemiologic Studies Depression Scale (CESD), Hamilton Depression Scale (HAMD), Beck Depression Inventory-Primary Care (BDI-PC), and so forth, while the secondary outcome was the status of sleep quality as measured by Pittsburgh Sleep Quality Index (PSQI), sleep log, and so forth. Characteristics of the included studies were extracted through a data extraction form which was piloted prior to the commencement of the study.

*2.3. Methodological Quality Assessment for the Included Studies.* We evaluated the methodological quality of each included trial with the 2015 risk of bias criteria provided by the Cochrane Back and Neck (CBN) Group [37], which include 13 specific domains: random sequence generation, allocation concealment, blinding of participants, blinding of caregiver, blinding of outcome assessor, description and acceptance of dropout rate, intention-to-treat analysis, selective outcome reporting, baseline similarity, cointerventions, acceptable compliance, timing of outcome assessment, and other sources of bias (e.g., validity of the outcome assessments and the report of the conflict of interest). The risk of bias criteria used in this study are adapted from the Cochrane Handbook of Reviews of Interventions and are appropriate for studies using nonpharmacological intervention [37]. Two reviewers independently assessed the risk of bias of the included RCTs. Each of the 13 risk of bias items was rated as "low risk of bias," "unclear risk of bias," or "high risk of bias."

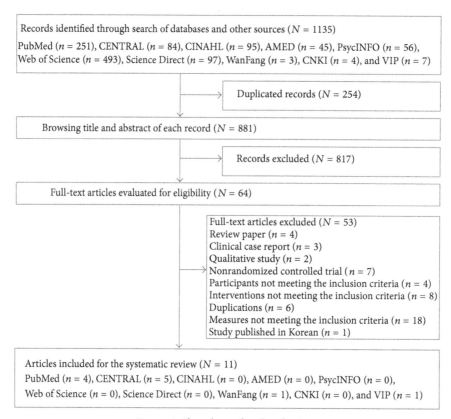

FIGURE 1: Flow chart of study selection.

Methodological quality assessment was further checked by a third review author and any disagreements on the risk of bias judgment were handled by discussion.

*2.4. Data Analysis.* We used the Review Manager 5.3 (Cochrane Collaboration) to conduct the data synthesis. Regarding the continuous outcome variables, we calculated the standardized mean difference (SMD) or the weighted mean difference (WMD) with 95% confidence intervals (CI). Fixed effect model was considered when the trials had a satisfactory statistical homogeneity which was evaluated by examining $I^2$ ($I^2 < 50\%$). Otherwise, a random effect model was applied. Both overall assessment and subgroup estimation were performed. The overall assessment on the effects of acupoints stimulation for mood problems and sleep quality was performed first regardless of the acupoints stimulation types. Subgroup analysis based on different acupoints stimulation modalities (manual acupuncture, electroacupuncture, and acupressure) was carried out afterwards. If the data synthesis could not be conducted owing to the absence of available data, different types of data, or a significant heterogeneity in the outcome effect, descriptive analysis was considered instead.

## 3. Results

*3.1. Characteristics of the Included Studies.* A total of 1135 potential records were yielded by searching the electronic databases, and 11 trials [26–36] were finally retrieved for

systematic review. The flow chart (Figure 1) presents the selection process of the qualified studies. The 11 included studies, with nine English and two Chinese articles, were all journal papers published between 2006 and 2014. The study sample ranged from 30 to 302 and the average sample size was 98. A total of 1073 participants (number of randomized participants) with various types of malignancies were involved. Six studies focused on breast cancer [26, 29, 31–34], one study was on lung cancer [30], one study was on gynecological cancer [36], and three studies [27, 28, 35] involved more than two types of malignancies. For the study design, eight [26–28, 31–33, 35, 36] were two-arm design and the other three [29, 30, 34] studies included three study arms.

Anxiety and/or depression were assessed in 11 studies. Seven of them assessed anxiety, out of which six studies [26, 27, 29, 30, 33, 34] used Hospital Anxiety and Depression Scale (HADS-A) which is commonly used in clinical research related to emotional problems in cancer [38] and the other one [32] adopted Psychological and General Well-Being Index (PGWB) which is a validated quality of life (QoL) instrument and "anxiety" is included as one of the subscales. Eleven studies assessed depression, out of which one study [26] employed CESD, one [36] applied HAMD only, two [28, 35] used both HAMD and Self-Rating Depression Scale (SDS) (only data from HAMD was used for data synthesis in order to ensure the homogeneity of outcome measures among trials), five [27, 29, 30, 33, 34] employed HADS subscale for depression (HADS-D) only, and two studies adopted BDI-PC [31] and Psychological and General Well-Being Index

(PGWB) [32], respectively. Sleep quality was assessed in five studies [26, 28–30, 32] and the PSQI was employed in four trials [26, 28–30], while in the other one study [32], sleep quality was measured by recording the times of wake-up and the hours of sleep on log book. Characteristics of the included studies are presented in Table 1.

*3.2. Description of the Intervention Protocol.* Intervention protocols used in the included studies are also summarized in Table 1. Three acupoints stimulation modalities were employed, of which seven [26–28, 31, 33, 34, 36] adopted manual acupuncture and three [29, 32, 35] used electroacupuncture while only one trial [30] chose acupressure. Of the seven studies that adopted manual acupuncture, two [26, 27] assessed its therapeutic effects by comparing true acupuncture with sham acupuncture (selected sham acupoints were located away from the true acupoints), four studies [28, 31, 33, 36] compared true acupuncture with standard treatment/care (two [28, 31] adopted standard medication, specifically antidepressant, as the standard treatment and the remaining two [33, 36] used attention control or usual care), and one trial [34] with three-arm design investigated the effects of acupuncture by comparing the true acupuncture which was conducted by acupuncture practitioners with two types of controls: the self-acupuncture control conducted by the participants and the standard treatment/care control without acupuncture. Of the three studies that used electroacupuncture, one compared true electroacupuncture with either sham electrostimulation or wait-list control [29] and the other two studies [32, 35] compared true electroacupuncture with standard treatment/care (standard medication in one study [32] and usual care in the other [35]). The only one study [30] employing acupressure was a three-arm design, with one group using acupressure plus oil and the other two adopting true acupressure and sham intervention, respectively. For this study, we only abstracted the data from the true and sham acupressure groups for analysis. Ten studies described the protocols of acupoints stimulation, which included the selection and identification of targeted acupoints, types of stimulation, and duration and frequency of treatment. Regarding the selected acupoints, *Sanyinjiao* (SP6), *Zusanli* (ST36), and *Hegu* (LI4), which can be identified in nearly half of the included studies, were the most frequently adopted acupoints for depression and/or anxiety.

*3.3. Methodological Quality and Risk of Bias of the Included Trials.* Table 2 shows the results of the risk of bias assessment for the included studies. Methodological quality of the trials was generally acceptable. All of the analyzed trials mentioned the method of randomization, and details of producing the random sequence were reported in nine studies by applying random number table, using computer software, or tossing coin. Treatment allocation was reported to be concealed in only five studies. Blinding of participants, care provider, or outcome assessor was performed in four studies. All studies reported the dropout of study subjects and in ten of them the dropout rates were deemed as acceptable (less than 20%) [37], whereas, in the other one study, the dropout rate exceeded 30% in the long-term observation (high risk of bias). In

eight trials, all subjects with randomization were included for data analysis based on missing data handling approach such as intention-to-treat analysis. Only one study [31] failed to specify whether it had selectively reported study outcomes or not. All studies were similar at baseline regarding the major demographic variables, and the timing of the outcome assessment was also reported to be similar in all the included trials.

*3.4. Therapeutic Effects of Acupoints Stimulation.* Results of the data synthesis for the systematic review are summarized in Table 3.

*3.4.1. Overall Assessment of Acupoints Stimulation for Anxiety and Depression*

*(i) Acupoints Stimulation versus Standard Methods of Treatment/Care.* Eight studies [28, 29, 31–36] compared the effects of acupoints stimulation with standard methods of treatment/care. All of the eight trials evaluated depression, four [29, 32–34] measured anxiety, and three [28, 29, 32] measured sleep quality. Meta-analysis indicated that acupoints stimulation can significantly relieve depression in cancer patients [random effect model, SMD = −1.08, 95% CI = −1.97 to −0.19, and $P$ = 0.02]. However, statistical heterogeneity ($P < 0.0001$, $I^2$ = 94%) was identified in the pooled effects, and removal of any suspicious trials did not change the heterogeneity significantly. For the eight studies that evaluated depression, two trials [28, 31] compared acupuncture with standard medication (antidepressant), and data synthesis was not conducted due to different kinds of outcome measures. According to the descriptive analysis of each single trial, acupoints stimulation (acupuncture) demonstrated a similar [31] or even better effect [28] in controlling depression than using antidepressant.

Data synthesis cannot be conducted for anxiety due to the insufficient number of studies and the inconsistent types of data. Descriptive analysis was adopted instead. Two trials [29, 33] showed significant improvements in anxiety. In the study conducted by Mao et al. [29], acupoints stimulation (electroacupuncture) was found to be effective in relieving anxiety in cancer survivors ($P$ = 0.044) after ten treatments over eight weeks. There are two articles [33, 34] reporting two different study phases from one large trial. In one paper published in 2012 [33], a 6-week acupuncture treatment led by the acupuncturists was compared with enhanced usual care (attention control) which was implemented by providing patients with an information booklet to maintain the consistency of the control group, and the results favored acupuncture in reducing anxiety ($P < 0.01$). Sample from the acupuncture group was rerandomized in a further trial [34] to compare the effects of 4-week acupuncturist-delivered acupuncture with either 4-week self-acupuncture or no maintenance group (usual care), and no marked differences in anxiety scores were detected across groups.

For sleep quality, conflicting study results were reported where one study [28] favored acupoints stimulation (acupuncture) in improving the quality of sleep ($P < 0.01$), while another one [29] reported that acupoints stimulation

TABLE 1: Characteristics of included trials.

| Study & setting | Types of cancer | Sample size | Acupoints stimulation intervention | | Control | Primary and/or secondary outcomes[*] |
| --- | --- | --- | --- | --- | --- | --- |
| | | | Types of acupoints stimulation | Selected acupoints | | |
| S[a]: Bao et al., 2014 [26] Two cancer centers, USA | Breast cancer | *Randomized* = 51 *Completed* = 47 *Intervention group*: 23, age (yr) = median 61 (45–85) *Control group*: 24, age (yr) = Median 61 (44–82) | *Intervention*: manual acupuncture *Practitioner*: acupuncturist *Frequency*: weekly treatment *Total duration*: 8 weeks | Guanyuan (CV4), Qihai (CV6), Zhongwan (CV12), Hegu (LI4) Master of Heart 6 (MH6), Yanglingquan (GB34), Zusanli (ST36), Taixi (KI3), and Shugu (BL65) | *Sham acupuncture*: nonpenetrating retractable needles at 14 sham acupoints located at the midpoint of the line connecting 2 real acupoints | (i) *Depression*: Center for Epidemiologic Studies Depression Scale (CESD) (ii) *Anxiety*: Hospital Anxiety and Depression Scale (HADS-A) (iii) *Sleep quality*: Pittsburgh Sleep Quality Index (PSQI) (iv) *Adverse events* |
| S2: Deng et al., 2013 [27] A cancer center, USA | Various types of cancer | *Randomized* = 101 *Completed* = 74 *Intervention group*: 47, age (yr) = median 54 (IRQ 46, 58) *Control group*: 50, age (yr) = median 53 (IRQ 45, 59) | *Intervention*: manual acupuncture *Practitioner*: acupuncturist *Frequency*: weekly treatment *Total duration*: 6 weeks | Qihai (CV6), Guanyuan (CV4), Taixi (KI3), Zusanli (ST36), Sanyinjiao (SP6), Quchi (LI11), Yinxi (HT6), and auricular point for antidepression | *Sham acupuncture*: Blunt-tipped needles used at a few millimeters off the meridians and away from the points used in true acupuncture | (i) *Anxiety and Depression*: Hospital Anxiety and Depression Scale (HADS) (ii) *Adverse events* |
| S3: Feng et al., 2011 [28] Department of TCM, General Hospital of PLA, China | Various types of cancer | *Randomized* = 80 *Completed* = 80 *Intervention group*: 40, age (yr) = 63.80 ± 5.47 *Control group*: 40, age (yr) = 63.60 ± 4.26 | *Intervention*: manual acupuncture *Practitioner*: acupuncturist *Frequency*: daily treatment *Total duration*: 30 days | Fenglong (ST40); Yinlingquan (SP9); Xuehai (SP10); Sanyinjiao (SP6); Yintang (EX-HN3); Baihui (DU20); Sishencong (EX-HN1); Neiguan (PC6); and Shenmen (TF4) | *Standard methods of treatment/care*: standard medication using antidepressant | (i) *Depression*: Self-Rating Depression Scale (SDS) and Hamilton Depression Scale (HAMD) (ii) *Sleep quality*: Pittsburgh Sleep Quality Index (PSQI) |
| S4: Mao et al., 2014 [29] A cancer center, USA | Breast cancer | *Randomized* = 67 *Completed* = 59 *Intervention group*: 22, age (yr) = 57.5 ± 10.1 *Control group 1*: 22 age (yr) = 60.9 ± 6.5 *Control group 2*: 23 age (yr) = 60.6 ± 8.2 | *Intervention*: electroacupuncture *Practitioner*: acupuncturist *Frequency*: twice per week for 2 weeks and weekly treatment for the following 6 weeks *Total duration*: 8 weeks | At least 4 local points around the joint with the most pain and at least 4 distant points to address nonpain symptoms commonly observed in conjunction with pain | *Sham electroacupuncture (control 1)*: nonpenetrating needles at nonacupuncture, nontrigger points at least 5 cm from the joint where pain was perceived to be maximal *Wait-list control (control 2)* | (i) *Anxiety and depression*: Hospital Anxiety and Depression Scale (HADS) (ii) *Sleep quality*: Pittsburgh Sleep Quality Index (PSQI) |
| S5: Tang et al., 2014 [30] A medical center, Taiwan | Lung cancer | *Randomized* = 57 *Completed* = 45 *Group 1*: 17, age (yr) = 53.9 ± 9.8 *Group 2*: 24, age (yr) = 54.8 ± 9.5 *Group 3*: 16, age (yr) = 66.1 ± 8.0 | *Intervention*: acupressure *Practitioner*: research assistant with acupressure training *Frequency*: daily treatment *Total duration*: 5 months | Hegu (LI4); Zusanli (ST36); Sanyinjiao (SP6) | *Sham acupressure*: sham acupressure at sham acupoints located at first metacarpal head, patella, and inner ankle | (i) *Anxiety and depression*: Hospital Anxiety and Depression Scale (HADS) (ii) *Sleep Quality*: Pittsburgh Sleep Quality Index (PSQI) |

TABLE 1: Continued.

| Study & setting | Types of cancer | Sample size | Acupoints stimulation intervention | | Control | Primary and/or secondary outcomes* |
|---|---|---|---|---|---|---|
| | | | Types of acupoints stimulation | Selected acupoints | | |
| S6: Walker et al., 2010 [31] Oncology clinics, USA | Breast cancer | Randomized = 50 Completed = 27, age (yr) = median 55 (35–77) Intervention group: 25 Control group: 25 | Intervention: manual acupuncture Practitioner: not reported Frequency: twice per week for the first 4 weeks and once per week for the following 8 weeks Total duration: 12 weeks for intervention and 1 year for follow-up | Kidney 3; Urinary bladder 23; Spleen 6; Gallbladder 20; Du 14; Du 20; Stomach 36; Liver 3; Heart 7; Pericardium 7; Ren 6; Lung 9 | Standard methods of treatment/care: standard medication using antidepressant | (i) Depression: Beck Depression Inventory-Primary Care (BDI-PC) (ii) Adverse events |
| S7: Frisk et al., 2012 [32] Three participating centers, Sweden | Breast cancer | Randomized = 45 Completed = 26 Intervention group: 26 age (yr) = mean 54.1 (47–69) Control group: 18 age (yr) = mean 53.4 (43–67) | Intervention: electroacupuncture Practitioner: physiotherapist Frequency: twice a week the first two weeks and then once a week for 10 weeks Total duration: 12 weeks | Xinshu (BL15); Shenshu (BL23); Ciliao (BL32); Baihui (GV20); Shenmen (HE7); Neiguan (PC6); Taichong (LR3); Sanyinjiao (SP6); Yinlingquan (SP9) | Standard methods of treatment/care: standard medication (sequential or continuous combined estrogen/progestagen therapy for hot flushes) | (i) Depression/anxiety: Psychological and General Well-Being Index (PGWB) and Women's Health Questionnaire (WHQ) (ii) Sleep data: the numbers of times wake-up/night and hours of sleep (iii) Adverse events |
| S8: Molassiotis et al., 2012 [33] Two cancer hospitals, four cancer centers, and three treatment centers of a national voluntary breast cancer organization, United Kingdom | Breast cancer | Randomized = 302 Completed = 246 Intervention group: 227, age (yr) = mean 52 (30–75) Control group: 75, age (yr) = mean 53 (25–80) | Intervention: manual acupuncture Practitioner: therapists with acupuncture training Frequency: 6 sessions with each session lasting 20 min Total duration: 6 weeks | Zusanli (ST36); Sanyinjiao (SP6); Hegu (LI4); and some alternative points [Yanglingquan (GB34) and Yinlingquan (SP9)] | Standard methods of treatment/care: enhanced usual care with information booklet on how to cope with fatigue | (i) Anxiety and depression: Hospital Anxiety and Depression Scale (HADS) (ii) Adverse events |

TABLE 1: Continued.

| Study & setting | Types of cancer | Sample size | Acupoints stimulation intervention | | Control | Primary and/or secondary outcomes* |
| --- | --- | --- | --- | --- | --- | --- |
| | | | Types of acupoints stimulation | Selected acupoints | | |
| S9: Molassiotis et al., 2013 [34] Two cancer hospitals, four cancer centers, and three treatment centers of a national voluntary breast cancer organization, United Kingdom | Breast cancer | Randomized = 198 Completed = 151, age (yr) = mean: 53 Intervention group: 65 Control group 1: 67 Control group 2: 65 | Intervention: manual acupuncture Practitioner: acupuncturist Frequency: weekly treatment Total duration: 4 weeks | Zusanli (ST36); Sanyinjiao (SP6); Hegu (LI4) | Self-acupuncture (control 1): self-acupuncture at Zusanli (ST36) and Sanyinjiao (SP6) No acupuncture (control 2) | (i) Anxiety and depression: Hospital Anxiety and Depression Scale (HADS) (ii) Adverse events |
| S10: Xiang et al., 2006 [35] A TCM hospital, Beijing, China | Various types of cancer (details not given) | Randomized = 92 Completed = 92 Intervention group: 46, age (yr) = 41–82 Control group: 46, age (yr) = 37–89 | Intervention: electroacupuncture + music therapy Practitioner: doctor Frequency: daily treatment Total duration: 4 weeks | Neiguan (PC6); Zusanli (ST36); Sanyinjiao (SP6); Baihui (DU20); Taixi (KI3); Yintang (EX-HN3); and so forth. | Music therapy + standard methods of treatment/care (usual care) | Depression: Hamilton Depression Scale (HAMD) and Self-Rating Depression Scale (SDS) |
| S11: Shi et al., 2013 [36] A hospital, Anhui, China | Gynecological cancer | Randomized = 30 Completed = 30 Intervention group: 15, age (yr) = 43.3 ± 1.94 Control group: 15, age (yr) = 45.0 ± 1.49 | Intervention: manual acupuncture Practitioner: not reported Frequency: twice per week Total duration: 3 months | Neiguan (PC6); Zusanli (ST36); Sanyinjiao (SP6); Taichong (LR3); Hegu (LI4); Guanyuan (RN4); Qihai (RN6); Taixi (KI3); Shenshu (BL23); Ganshu (BL18); Pishu (BL20) | Standard methods of treatment/care: usual care | Depression: Hamilton Depression Scale (HAMD) |

aS = study, * Primary and/or secondary outcomes which were determined by the systematic review.

TABLE 2: Methodological and quality assessment of included trials.

| Criteria | S[a]1 | S2 | S3 | S4 | S5 | S6 | S7 | S8 | S9 | S10 | S11 |
|---|---|---|---|---|---|---|---|---|---|---|---|
| (1) "Was the method of randomization adequate?" | ✓ | ✓ | ✓ | ✓ | ✓ | ? | ✓ | ✓ | ✓ | ✓ | ? |
| (2) "Was the treatment allocation concealed?" | X | ✓ | ? | ✓ | ? | ? | ✓ | ✓ | ✓ | ? | ? |
| (3) "Was the patient blinded to the intervention?" | ✓ | ✓ | ? | ✓ | ✓ | ? | ? | X | X | ? | ? |
| (4) "Was the care provider blinded to the intervention?" | X | X | ? | X | X | ? | ? | X | X | ? | ? |
| (5) "Was the outcome assessor blinded to the intervention?" | ✓ | ✓ | ? | ✓ | ✓ | ? | ? | X | X | ? | ? |
| (6) "Was the drop-out rate described and acceptable?" | ✓ | ✓ | ✓ | ✓ | ✓ | ✓ | X | ✓ | ✓ | ✓ | ✓ |
| (7) "Were all randomized participants analyzed in the group to which they were allocated?" | ✓ | ✓ | ✓ | ✓ | ✓ | ✓ | X | X | X | ✓ | ✓ |
| (8) "Are reports of the study free of suggestion of selective outcome reporting?" | ✓ | ✓ | ✓ | ✓ | ✓ | ? | ✓ | ✓ | ✓ | ✓ | ✓ |
| (9) "Were the groups similar at baseline regarding the most important prognostic indicators?" | ✓ | ✓ | ✓ | ✓ | ✓ | ✓ | ✓ | ✓ | ✓ | ✓ | ✓ |
| (10) "Were co-interventions avoided or similar?" | ✓ | ✓ | ? | ✓ | ? | ? | ✓ | ? | ? | ✓ | ? |
| (11) Was the compliance acceptable in all groups? | ? | ? | ? | ✓ | ✓ | ? | ✓ | ✓ | ✓ | ? | ? |
| (12) "Was the timing of the outcome assessment similar in all groups?" | ✓ | ✓ | ✓ | ✓ | ✓ | ✓ | ✓ | ✓ | ✓ | ✓ | ✓ |
| (13) "Are other sources of potential bias unlikely?" | ? | ? | ? | ? | ? | ? | ? | ? | ? | ? | ? |

Based on [37].
[a]S: study, ✓: low risk of bias; X: high risk of bias; ?: unclear risk of bias.

(electroacupuncture) failed to contribute to significant improvement in PSQI score ($P = 0.058$) when comparing with the wait-list control.

*(ii) Acupoints Stimulation versus Sham Acupoints Stimulation.* Acupoints stimulation was compared with sham intervention in four trials [26, 27, 29, 30]. All of them involved anxiety and depression and three [26, 29, 30] assessed sleep quality. For anxiety and depression, only two studies were eligible for synthesis. Although the differences between groups did not reach a statistical significance, the pooled effects still favored true acupoints stimulation in relieving either anxiety [random effect model, MD = −0.65, 95% CI = −2.84 to 1.53, and $P = 0.56$] or depression [random effect model, MD = −0.27, 95% CI = −2.66 to 2.12, and $P = 0.82$]. For sleep quality, descriptive analysis from one trial [30] indicated that acupoints stimulation (acupressure) could improve sleep quality ($P = 0.040$).

*3.4.2. Subgroup Analysis on Manual Acupuncture*

*(i) Manual Acupuncture versus Standard Methods of Treatment/Care.* Manual acupuncture on anxiety and/or depression was compared with standard methods of treatment/care in five studies [28, 31, 33, 34, 36], and manual acupuncture was found to be superior in depression relief [random effect model, MD = −2.55, 95% CI = −3.61 to −1.49, and $P < 0.00001$]. However, significantly statistical heterogeneity ($P = 0.002$, $I^2 = 80\%$) was identified in the pooled effect. This might be caused by Feng et al.'s study [28] as the $I^2$ decreased to 0% ($P = 0.89$) after removing the mentioned trial, and the pooled effect was relatively stable, which still favored manual acupuncture [random effect model, MD = −2.10, 95% CI = −2.56 to −1.64, and $P < 0.00001$]. Descriptive analysis also supported the superiority of acupuncture in managing anxiety ($P < 0.01$) [33] and improving sleep quality ($P < 0.01$) [28] in cancer patients.

TABLE 3: Summary of meta-analyses.

| Study outcomes | Number of trials | Number of participants | Statistical method | Effect estimate | Test for overall effect Z | Test for overall effect P | Heterogeneity ($I^2$) |
|---|---|---|---|---|---|---|---|
| Overall assessment of acupoints stimulation: acupoints stimulation versus different comparisons (for anxiety) | | | | | | | |
| Acupoints stimulation versus standard methods of treatment/care | 3 | 567 | NR | NR | NR | NR | NA |
| Acupoints stimulation versus sham acupoints stimulation | 2 | 137 | Mean difference (IV, random, 95% CI) | −0.65 [−2.84, 1.53] | 0.59 | 0.56 | >50% |
| Overall assessment of acupoints stimulation: acupoints stimulation versus different comparisons (for depression) | | | | | | | |
| Acupoints stimulation versus standard methods of treatment/care | 5 | 485 | Mean difference (IV, random, 95% CI) | −1.08 [−1.97, −0.19] | 2.39 | 0.02 | >50% |
| Acupoints stimulation versus sham acupoints stimulation | 2 | 137 | Mean difference (IV, random, 95% CI) | −0.27 [−2.66, 2.12] | 0.23 | 0.82 | 50% |
| Subgroup analysis: different types of acupoints stimulation versus standard methods of treatment/care (for anxiety) | | | | | | | |
| Electroacupuncture | 2 | 112 | NR | NR | NR | NR | NA |
| Acupuncture | 2 | 302* | NR | NR | NR | NR | NA |
| Subgroup analysis: different types of acupoints stimulation versus standard methods of treatment/care (for depression) | | | | | | | |
| Electroacupuncture | 2 | 159 | NR | NR | NR | NR | NA |
| Acupuncture | 4 | 393 | Mean difference (IV, random, 95% CI) | −2.55 [−3.61, −1.49] | 4.72 | <0.00001 | >50% |
| Subgroup analysis: different types of acupoints stimulation versus sham comparison (for anxiety) | | | | | | | |
| Acupuncture | 2 | 152 | NR | NR | NR | NR | NA |
| Acupressure | 1 | 57 | NR | NR | NR | NR | NA |
| Subgroup analysis: different types of acupoints stimulation versus sham comparison (for depression) | | | | | | | |
| Acupuncture | 2 | 152 | NR | NR | NR | NR | NA |
| Acupressure | 1 | 57 | NR | NR | NR | NR | NA |

IV: inverse variance, CI: confidence interval, NR: not reported because pooling was not conducted due to the insufficient number of studies, different models of data, or absence of data, NA: not applicable
* Sample was adopted from one study (as the sample of the other study was based on the study we adopted).

TABLE 4: Selected search strategies.

| ID | Searching strategies | Records |
|---|---|---|
| | PubMed | |
| #1 | Search "acupuncture"[MeSH Terms] | 17708 |
| #2 | Search "acupuncture therapy"[MeSH Terms] | 16944 |
| #3 | Search "acupressure"[MeSH Terms] | 465 |
| #4 | Search "acupuncture, ear"[MeSH Terms] | 267 |
| #5 | Search "acupuncture points"[MeSH Terms] | 4063 |
| #6 | Search "electroacupuncture"[MeSH Terms] | 2566 |
| #7 | Search "auriculotherapy"[MeSH Terms] | 277 |
| #8 | #1 OR #2 OR #3 OR #4 OR #5 OR #6 OR #7 | 17958 |
| #9 | Search ((((((((acupunctur*[Title/Abstract]) OR acupressure*[Title/Abstract]) OR auriculotherap*[Title/Abstract]) OR electroacupunctur*[Title/Abstract]) OR acupoint*[Title/Abstract]) OR needl*[Title/Abstract]) OR acupuncture therapy[Title/Abstract]) OR "ear acupuncture"[Title/Abstract]) OR acupuncture points[Title/Abstract] | 104918 |
| #10 | #8 or #9 | 108214 |
| #11 | Search "neoplasms"[MeSH Terms] | 2609885 |
| #12 | Search (((((((((cance*[Title/Abstract]) OR carcinom*[Title/Abstract]) OR neoplasm*[Title/Abstract]) OR tumo*[Title/Abstract]) OR tumou*[Title/Abstract]) OR neoplasia[Title/Abstract]) OR oncolog*[Title/Abstract]) OR malignan*[Title/Abstract]) OR neoplasms[Title/Abstract] | 2345516 |
| #13 | #11 OR #12 | 3231222 |
| #14 | Search "anxiety"[MeSH Terms] | 56178 |
| #15 | Search "anxiety disorders"[MeSH Terms] | 67844 |
| #16 | Search "depression"[MeSH Terms] | 153512 |
| #17 | Search "depressive disorder"[MeSH Terms] | 80897 |
| #18 | Search "mood disorders"[MeSH Terms] | 115156 |
| #19 | Search "affective disorders, psychotic"[MeSH Terms] | 33045 |
| #20 | Search "stress, psychological"[MeSH Terms] | 92744 |
| #21 | #14 OR #15 OR #16 OR #17 OR #18 OR #19 OR #20 | 346299 |
| #22 | Search (((((((anxiet*[Title/Abstract]) OR anxiou*nervousness[Title/Abstract]) OR hypervigilanc*[Title/Abstract]) OR depression*[Title/Abstract]) OR depressiv*[Title/Abstract]) OR emotion*[Title/Abstract]) OR psycholog*[Title/Abstract]) OR affective*[Title/Abstract] | 518732 |
| #23 | #21 OR #22 | 687179 |
| #24 | #10 AND #13 AND #23 | 251 |
| | Cochrane Central Register of Controlled Trials (CENTRAL) | |
| #1 | MeSH descriptor: [Acupuncture Therapy] explode all trees | 3132 |
| #2 | MeSH descriptor: [Acupuncture] explode all trees | 151 |
| #3 | MeSH descriptor: [Acupressure] explode all trees | 227 |
| #4 | MeSH descriptor: [Acupuncture Points] explode all trees | 1069 |
| #5 | MeSH descriptor: [Acupuncture, Ear] explode all trees | 123 |
| #6 | MeSH descriptor: [Auriculotherapy] explode all trees | 129 |
| #7 | MeSH descriptor: [Electroacupuncture] explode all trees | 473 |
| #8 | acupunctur* or acupressure* or auriculotherap* or electroacupunctur* or acupoint* or needl*:ti,ab,kw (Word variations have been searched) | 13648 |
| #9 | #1 or #2 or #3 or #4 or #5 or #6 or #7 or #8 | 13710 |
| #10 | MeSH descriptor: [Neoplasms] explode all trees | 52791 |
| #11 | neoplasm* or tumo* or tumou* or neoplasia or cance* or carcinom* or malignan* or oncolog*:ti,ab,kw (Word variations have been searched) | 94737 |
| #12 | #10 or #11 | 100138 |
| #13 | MeSH descriptor: [Anxiety] explode all trees | 5187 |

TABLE 4: Continued.

| ID | Searching strategies | Records |
|----|---------------------|---------|
| #14 | MeSH descriptor: [Anxiety Disorders] explode all trees | 4954 |
| #15 | MeSH descriptor: [Depression] explode all trees | 5472 |
| #16 | MeSH descriptor: [Affective Disorders, Psychotic] explode all trees | 1648 |
| #17 | MeSH descriptor: [Emotions] explode all trees | 11649 |
| #18 | anxiet* or anxiou* or nervousness or hypervigilanc* or depression* or depressiv* or emotion* or Psycholog* or affective*:ti,ab,kw (Word variations have been searched) | 102362 |
| #19 | #13 or #14 or #15 or #16 or #17 or #18 | 103970 |
| #20 | #9 and #12 and #19 | 108 |
| #21 | #20 in Tails | 84 |

*(ii) Acupuncture versus Sham Acupuncture.* Sham acupuncture was adopted in two studies [26, 27]. Due to different types of data, we used descriptive analysis here. One study [26] indicated that there were no significant differences for between-groups comparison in depression ($P = 0.442$), anxiety ($P = 0.526$), and sleep quality ($P = 0.557$). While for within-group comparisons, only true acupuncture group showed a noticeable difference in depression after intervention ($P = 0.022$). For another one [27], effects were similar for both depression and anxiety in within-group comparisons, and also, there were no statistically significant differences between the true acupuncture group and the sham acupuncture group.

*3.4.3. Subgroup Analysis on Electroacupuncture.* Descriptive analysis was adopted as data synthesis could not be conducted for subgroup analysis on electroacupuncture due to the insufficient number of studies and the inconsistent types of outcome data. Three studies [29, 32, 35] compared electroacupuncture with standard methods of treatment/care and the results were different. One trial [29] with a three-arm design indicated that both true electroacupuncture ($P = 0.015$) and sham electroacupuncture ($P = 0.0088$) presented a more effective improvement in HADS-D scores than waitlist control, while, for anxiety, only true intervention was found to be effective ($P = 0.044$). Meanwhile, this study [29] also found no significant improvement in sleep quality (as measured by PSQI) in both true and sham intervention groups, with the $P$ values 0.058 and 0.31, respectively. However, based on the reported data, we still cannot judge whether true electroacupuncture is superior to the sham approach as between-groups comparisons were not reported in this article [29].

In another study [35], apart from the standard treatment/care in both groups, the intervention group adopted electroacupuncture plus music therapy to compare with the control arm using music therapy only, and the within-group analysis showed that the HAMD-D scores significantly decreased in both groups after the intervention with the $P$ values, 0.013 and 0.022, respectively. However, between-groups comparisons revealed no statistical differences after the intervention ($P = 0.431$). In the study conducted by Frisk et al. [32], subscales of Women's Health Questionnaire (WHQ) and PGWB were employed to evaluate the status of depression and anxiety, and the subscale scores for anxiety (both WHQ and PGWB) were found to be improved significantly in the electroacupuncture group after the treatment, and all sleep parameters (including number of hours slept/night, times of wake-up/night, and WHQ sleep scores) also improved significantly in the electroacupuncture group (within-group comparison).

*3.4.4. Subgroup Analysis on Acupressure.* There was only one trial [30] adopting acupressure as the intervention approach, and it was found that the acupressure group had lower anxiety and depression scores than the sham acupressure group, but these differences did not reach a significant level.

*3.4.5. Subgroup Analysis on Sham Acupoints Stimulation versus Wait-List Control.* Comparison between sham acupoints stimulation and wait-list control was only mentioned in one study [29]. In this study, the true electroacupuncture group selected the acupoints located around the joint with the most pain and the acupoints were inserted with needles until receiving "*de qi*," while the sham comparison used nonpenetrating needles at nonacupuncture and nontrigger points located at least 5 cm from the joint without evoking the sensation of "*de qi*." This study indicated that sham electroacupuncture can produce some treatment effects to improve the HADS-D scores in cancer patients ($P = 0.0088$), while, for anxiety and sleep quality, there were no significant differences between groups.

*3.5. Adverse Events Associated with Acupoints Stimulation.* Six trials [26, 27, 31–34] mentioned the potential adverse events as the safety outcomes, of which three studies [26, 31, 32] reported that there were no adverse events associated with acupoints stimulation. In Deng et al.'s study [27], a total of 11 serious side effects occurred during the intervention such as low blood counts, renal failure, and nausea, but all these negative events were deemed to be not related to acupuncture. The other two studies conducted by Molassiotis et al. [33, 34] monitored adverse events, but the one published in 2012 [33] did not report the details of adverse events in the study results, while the latter one, which was published in 2013 [34], reported that a small number of cases suffered from mild side effects including spot bleeding and minor pain/discomfort.

None of the included trials assessed the causality between the intervention and the possible adverse events.

## 4. Discussion

In this systematic review, 11 trials with a total of 1073 participants were included. The study findings supported that acupoints stimulation can be a beneficial approach for managing anxiety and depression in cancer patients. However, some methodological flaws were still found in some studies. Considering the potential risks of bias identified in the analyzed trials and the limited number of included trials. The findings of this review should be interpreted prudently, and the current evidence on acupoints stimulation for anxiety and depression in cancer survivors can be rated as suggestive but still not fully conclusive.

Based on the overall analysis, acupoints stimulation as a complementary therapy could improve the mood of depression in patients with malignancy. The possible explanation for it might be that different levels of cortisol, epinephrine, and adrenocorticotropic hormone are associated with the negative moods in cancer patients, which are regulated by HPA and SNS, and acupoints stimulation could positively influence the HPA and SNS based on its potential immune-modulatory effect [24, 25]. It is noted that significant heterogeneity was identified in the overall assessment, and the possible explanations are as follows. Firstly, various types of acupoints stimulation were used among trials which more or less contribute to the heterogeneity in nature. Secondly, the measures for depression in the analyzed five studies were quite inconsistent, with three trials employing HAMD, and the other two applying HADS-D and BDI-PC, respectively, and the inconsistent outcome assessment tools could be another source for introducing the heterogeneity.

In the subgroup analyses, both manual acupuncture and electroacupuncture showed positive effects on depression when comparing with standard methods of treatment/care, among which two trials compared acupuncture with antide-pressant, and one study [28] even demonstrated a more significant effect of acupuncture in relieving depression than using antidepressant. However, conclusion on the superiority of acupuncture to antidepressant should be interpreted with caution because some methodological flaws were identified in the mentioned trial such as the absence of blinding and allocation concealment and unbalanced cointerventions, all of which could increase the risks of bias inevitably.

For anxiety, encouraging results on acupoints stimulation were also reported in corresponding studies. Based on the results of data syntheses as well as descriptive analyses, acupoints stimulation can be a beneficial approach for relieving psychological distresses among oncology patients. However, the evidence concluded from the included studies is not fully conclusive at the current stage as a number of methodological flaws, such as the unclear statement of randomization, blinding and allocation concealment, and unbalanced cointerventions across groups, were identified. It is noted that the studies' effect size would be more inclined to be overestimated when the methodological quality of those studies is unsatisfactory [39].

Our study findings did not reach a conclusion on the evidence of acupoints stimulation for improving sleep quality for the following reasons: conflicting results were reported in the analyzed studies, the number of studies reporting sleep quality was quite limited, and those trials reporting sleep quality only included it as a secondary outcome. Effects of acupoints stimulation on sleep quality in cancer patients should be explored in future studies.

It is noted that several kinds of assessment tools, including CESD, HAMD, SDS, BDI-PC, and HADS, were used in the included studies for measuring anxiety and depression. These tools are generic instruments which can be applied in different populations, and their psychometric properties have also been well documented as valid and reliable measures used in cancer patients. For instance, Cronbach's alpha was greater than 0.75 for CESD [40], HAMD [41], SDS [42], and BDI-PC [43] which indicated a satisfactory internal consistency, and the construct validity of HADS was also tested through the factor analysis [38], and Cronbach's alphas for the anxiety and depression subscales were 0.887 and 0.703, respectively [44].

Placebo effects of acupoints stimulation should be explored in studies incorporating a true, sham, and usual care group. Based on the study findings, both true and sham acupoints stimulation can relieve anxiety and/or depression more effectively than standard methods of treatment/care, and the true interventions were somewhat better than the sham comparisons although the differences did not reach the statistical significance. Based on these findings, it seems that the treatment effects of acupoints stimulation may be associated with large placebo effects. According to a series of recent randomized controlled trials, placebo effects might partially contribute to the overall therapeutic effects of acupoints stimulation [45–48]. However, specific therapeutic effects of acupoints stimulation still play a crucial role in improving patients' functional status, as a large number of rigorously designed randomized controlled trials and systematic reviews have proved the superiority of true acupuncture/acupressure to the sham comparisons [49–52].

Several reasons could be employed to explain the non-significant differences between the true and sham acupoints stimulation in our study findings. Firstly, the nonspecific placebo effects might be exaggerated in the analyzed trials as the outcome measures for anxiety and/or depression were all scales measured by patients themselves or caregivers which can be easily affected by their expectancy to treatment, especially when the blinding design is not well performed. Secondly, it is still uncertain whether the sham procedures used in the included studies are really inert or not. One of the preconditions for developing a sham intervention is that it is indistinguishable from the true treatment but it should be inert in nature, which means having no specific therapeutic effects for the targeted health problem but only producing nonspecific physiological and/or psychological effects (placebo effects) [53]. In the analyzed trials, the design of sham acupoints stimulation might not be very appropriate. For example, nonspecific acupoints (one type of sham modality) which were close to the true acupoints might also produce some treatment effects, because, based on the holistic concept of Traditional Chinese Medicine (TCM) theory, acupoints stimulation performs its effects by regulating the whole body functions. The "nonacupoints" described in some trials might be potential, active acupoints which have not been identified on current acupoints chart. All of these designs could generate some specific treatment effects for patients in the sham intervention group. Moreover, in our included trials, only four incorporated a sham intervention arm. The relative small sample size and the methodological flaws identified in those trials made the final data analysis on sham intervention only a preliminary finding and not fully convincing.

Adverse events associated with acupoints stimulation were measured in six studies [26, 27, 31–34] and no serious harm data related to acupoints stimulation were reported. Acupoints stimulation could be a safe intervention used in clinical practice. Other systematic reviews, as well as prospective or retrospective surveys with a large sample size, also supported the idea that acupoints stimulation can be a relatively safe approach [54, 55]. However, it is noted that some analyzed studies in this review failed to include the safety issue as the outcome measure, and none of the included trials incorporated standardized criteria to assess the causality between the intervention and the reported adverse events.

Our findings suggested that acupoints stimulation can be a promising approach to managing the psychological distresses in cancer patients, but definite evidence still cannot be concluded from this review and the study finding can only be interpreted as suggestive due to the following limitations. Firstly, although the quality of the included studies was generally acceptable, methodological flaws still existed in some trials which could affect the reliability of our findings. Secondly, language bias cannot be excluded as all of the analyzed studies were only English or Chinese publications. In addition, publication bias might exist because there were seldom negative findings reported in our included studies, and we did not perform funnel plot as the number of trials included for each comparison was quite limited (less than ten).

## 5. Implications for Future Research and Practice

This study concluded several implications for future research and practice. Firstly, future research should elaborate more details on the protocols of acupoints stimulation in both true and sham intervention groups including the practitioner, duration of intervention and number of sessions, the selection and location of the true and sham acupoints, and the styles of stimulation. Secondly, apart from the certain psychological measures, some biomarkers [56] such as Interleukin-6 (IL-6), Interleukin-1$\beta$ (IL-1$\beta$), and tumor necrosis factor-$\alpha$ (TNF-$\alpha$) could be adopted as the potential indicators for emotional problems in future studies, which might minimize the exaggeration of treatment effects to some extent. Moreover, design of sham acupoints stimulation should be more reasonable; sham acupoints should be prudently selected

to avoid choosing potentially effective true acupoints. An experienced TCM practitioner could be invited or consulted when developing the intervention protocol and some special-designed needles which cannot penetrate the acupoints could be adopted as the sham intervention. Furthermore, standard criteria should be applied to assess the causality between the adverse events and the acupoints stimulation. In addition, clinical researchers should take every effort to minimize the potential risks of bias. Although we understand it is difficult to reach blinding design among research personnel who conduct acupuncture or acupressure, some measures can still be considered to control the potential bias induced by study participants and outcome assessors in clinical settings; for example, researchers could use eye-patches to cover the participants' eyes when providing the intervention, and outcome assessors could be those people who are not involved in any other procedures of the study except for the data collection process [52, 57]. Finally, future studies should follow the CONSORT [58] and STRICTA [59] guidelines to enhance the report quality of the RCTs on acupoints stimulation.

## Conflict of Interests

The authors declare that there is no conflict of interests regarding the publication of this paper.

## Authors' Contribution

Tao Wang undertook the study design, literature searching, data extraction and analysis, and data interpretation and drafted and revised this paper. Renli Deng supported the study design and revised this paper. Jing-Yu Tan undertook the study design, literature searching, and data extraction and revised this paper. Feng-Guang Guan undertook the study design and revised this paper.

## References

[1] J. Ferlay, I. Soerjomataram, R. Dikshit et al., "Cancer incidence and mortality worldwide: sources, methods and major patterns in GLOBOCAN 2012," *International Journal of Cancer*, vol. 136, no. 5, pp. E359–E386, 2015.

[2] World Health Organization, "Global health observatory data repository. 2011. Number of deaths (World) by cause," February 2015, http://www.who.int/features/qa/15/en/.

[3] O. Minton, A. Richardson, M. Sharpe, M. Hotopf, and P. Stone, "A systematic review and meta-analysis of the pharmacological treatment of cancer-related fatigue," *Journal of the National Cancer Institute*, vol. 100, no. 16, pp. 1155–1166, 2008.

[4] E. Dean-Clower, A. M. Doherty-Gilman, A. Keshaviah et al., "Acupuncture as palliative therapy for physical symptoms and quality of life for advanced cancer patients," *Integrative Cancer Therapies*, vol. 9, no. 2, pp. 158–167, 2010.

[5] M. Hamer, Y. Chida, and G. Y. Molloy, "Psychological distress and cancer mortality," *Journal of Psychosomatic Research*, vol. 66, no. 3, pp. 255–258, 2009.

[6] K. D. Stein, K. L. Syrjala, and M. A. Andrykowski, "Physical and psychological long-term and late effects of cancer," *Cancer*, vol. 112, no. 11, supplement, pp. 2577–2592, 2008.

[7] A. Molassiotis, P. Fernandez-Ortega, D. Pud et al., "Complementary and alternative medicine use in colorectal cancer patients in seven European countries," *Complementary Therapies in Medicine*, vol. 13, no. 4, pp. 251–257, 2005.

[8] S.-M. Wang, D. Gaal, I. Maranets, A. Caldwell-Andrews, and Z. N. Kain, "Acupressure and preoperative parental anxiety: a pilot study," *Anesthesia & Analgesia*, vol. 101, no. 3, pp. 666–669, 2005.

[9] J.-Y. Tan, A. Molassiotis, T. Wang, and L. K. P. Suen, "Current evidence on auricular therapy for chemotherapy-induced nausea and vomiting in cancer patients: a systematic review of randomized controlled trials," *Evidence-Based Complementary and Alternative Medicine*, vol. 2014, Article ID 430796, 18 pages, 2014.

[10] D. Polsky, J. A. Doshi, S. Marcus et al., "Long-term risk for depressive symptoms after a medical diagnosis," *Archives of Internal Medicine*, vol. 165, no. 11, pp. 1260–1265, 2005.

[11] W. F. Pirl, "Evidence report on the occurrence, assessment, and treatment of depression in cancer patients," *JNCI Monographs*, no. 32, pp. 32–39, 2004.

[12] M. Pasquini and M. Biondi, "Depression in cancer patients: a critical review," *Clinical Practice & Epidemiology in Mental Health*, vol. 3, no. 3, article 2, 2007.

[13] D. P. H. Stark and A. House, "Anxiety in cancer patients," *British Journal of Cancer*, vol. 83, no. 10, pp. 1261–1267, 2000.

[14] M. Kangas, J. L. Henry, and R. A. Bryant, "Posttraumatic stress disorder following cancer: a conceptual and empirical review," *Clinical Psychology Review*, vol. 22, no. 4, pp. 499–524, 2002.

[15] G. P. Zhou, J. Y. Cai, Z. G. Huang, and F. Xu, "Effect of depression on adverse drug reactions from antineoplastics among cancer patients," *Chinese Remedies & Clinics*, vol. 9, pp. 916–917, 2009 (Chinese).

[16] E. M. V. Reiche, S. O. V. Nunes, and H. K. Morimoto, "Stress, depression, the immune system, and cancer," *The Lancet Oncology*, vol. 5, no. 10, pp. 617–625, 2004.

[17] P. B. Jacobsen and H. S. Jim, "Psychosocial interventions for anxiety and depression in adult cancer patients: achievements and challenges," *CA: A Cancer Journal for Clinicians*, vol. 58, no. 4, pp. 214–230, 2008.

[18] M. M. Lee, S. S. Lin, M. R. Wrensch, S. R. Adler, and D. Eisenberg, "Alternative therapies used by women with breast cancer in four ethnic populations," *Journal of the National Cancer Institute*, vol. 92, no. 1, pp. 42–47, 2000.

[19] World Health Organization, "Acupuncture: review and analysis of reports on controlled clinical trials," *Parkinsonism & Related Disorders*, supplement 2, p. S163, 2002.

[20] C. A. Smith, P. P. J. Hay, and H. MacPherson, "Acupuncture for depression," *The Cochrane Database of Systematic Reviews*, no. 1, Article ID CD004046, 2010.

[21] S. Horiuchi, A. Tsuda, Y. Honda, H. Kobayashi, M. Naruse, and A. Tsuchiyagaito, "Mood changes by self-administered acupressure in Japanese college students: a randomized controlled trial," *Global Journal of Health Science*, vol. 7, no. 4, pp. 40–44, 2014.

[22] D. W. H. Au, H. W. H. Tsang, P. P. M. Ling, C. H. T. Leung, P. K. Ip, and W. M. Cheung, "Effects of acupressure on anxiety: a systematic review and meta-analysis," *Acupuncture in Medicine*, vol. 33, no. 5, pp. 353–359, 2015.

[23] Y. Y. Chan, W. Y. Lo, S. N. Yang, Y. H. Chen, and J. G. Lin, "The benefit of combined acupuncture and antidepressant medication for depression: a systematic review and meta-analysis," *Journal of Affective Disorders*, vol. 176, pp. 106–117, 2015.

[24] H. J. Park, H. J. Park, Y. Chae, J. W. Kim, H. Lee, and J.-H. Chung, "Effect of acupuncture on hypothalamic-pituitary-adrenal system in maternal separation rats," *Cellular and Molecular Neurobiology*, vol. 31, no. 8, pp. 1123–1127, 2014.

[25] L. M. Thornton, B. L. Andersen, and W. P. Blakely, "The pain, depression, and fatigue symptom cluster in advanced breast cancer: covariation with the hypothalamic-pituitary-adrenal axis and the sympathetic nervous system," *Health Psychology*, vol. 29, no. 3, pp. 333–337, 2010.

[26] T. Bao, L. Cai, C. Snyder et al., "Patient-reported outcomes in women with breast cancer enrolled in a dual-center, double-blind, randomized controlled trial assessing the effect of acupuncture in reducing aromatase inhibitor-induced musculoskeletal symptoms," *Cancer*, vol. 120, no. 3, pp. 381–389, 2014.

[27] G. Deng, Y. Chan, D. Sjoberg et al., "Acupuncture for the treatment of post-chemotherapy chronic fatigue: a randomized, blinded, sham-controlled trial," *Supportive Care in Cancer*, vol. 21, no. 6, pp. 1735–1741, 2013.

[28] Y. Feng, X.-Y. Wang, S.-D. Li et al., "Clinical research of acupuncture on malignant tumor patients for improving depression and sleep quality," *Journal of Traditional Chinese Medicine*, vol. 31, no. 3, pp. 199–202, 2011.

[29] J. J. Mao, J. T. Farrar, D. Bruner et al., "Electroacupuncture for fatigue, sleep, and psychological distress in breast cancer patients with aromatase inhibitor-related arthralgia: a randomized trial," *Cancer*, vol. 120, no. 23, pp. 3744–3751, 2014.

[30] W.-R. Tang, W.-J. Chen, C.-T. Yu et al., "Effects of acupressure on fatigue of lung cancer patients undergoing chemotherapy: an experimental pilot study," *Complementary Therapies in Medicine*, vol. 22, no. 4, pp. 581–591, 2014.

[31] E. M. Walker, A. I. Rodriguez, B. Kohn et al., "Acupuncture versus venlafaxine for the management of vasomotor symptoms in patients with hormone receptor-positive breast cancer: a randomized controlled trial," *Journal of Clinical Oncology*, vol. 28, no. 4, pp. 634–640, 2010.

[32] J. Frisk, A.-C. Källström, N. Wall, M. Fredrikson, and M. Hammar, "Acupuncture improves health-related quality-of-life (HRQoL) and sleep in women with breast cancer and hot flushes," *Supportive Care in Cancer*, vol. 20, no. 4, pp. 715–724, 2012.

[33] A. Molassiotis, J. Bardy, J. Finnegan-John et al., "Acupuncture for cancer-related fatigue in patients with breast cancer: a pragmatic randomized controlled trial," *Journal of Clinical Oncology*, vol. 30, no. 36, pp. 4470–4476, 2012.

[34] A. Molassiotis, J. Bardy, J. Finnegan-John et al., "A randomized, controlled trial of acupuncture self-needling as maintenance therapy for cancer-related fatigue after therapist-delivered acupuncture," *Annals of Oncology*, vol. 24, no. 6, pp. 1645–1652, 2013.

[35] C. Y. Xiang, Q. Guo, J. Liao, S. G. Wang, Y. F. Yang, and Y. H. Feng, "Effect of therapy of traditional Chinese medicine five element music and electroacupuncture on the depression levels of cancer patients," *Chinese Journal of Nursing*, vol. 41, no. 11, pp. 969–972, 2006.

[36] M. Q. Shi, K. Han, and Y. L. Xia, "Study about soothing liver and reinforcing essence of kidney by acupuncture in adjusting depression of gynecological malignancies after surgery and chemotherapy," *Journal of Liaoning University of TCM*, vol. 15, no. 2, pp. 164–168, 2013.

[37] A. D. Furlan, A. Malmivaara, R. Chou et al., "2015 Updated method guideline for systematic reviews in the Cochrane back and neck group," *Spine*, vol. 40, no. 21, pp. 1660–1673, 2015.

[38] A. B. Smith, P. J. Selby, G. Velikova et al., "Factor analysis of the hospital anxiety and depression scale from a large cancer population," *Psychology and Psychotherapy: Theory, Research and Practice*, vol. 75, no. 2, pp. 165–176, 2002.

[39] R. Kunz, G. Vist, and A. D. Oxman, "Randomisation to protect against selection bias in healthcare trials," *The Cochrane Database of Systematic Reviews*, no. 2, Article ID MR000012, 2007.

[40] M. J. Schroevers, R. Sanderman, E. van Sonderen, and A. V. Ranchor, "The evaluation of the Center for Epidemiologic Studies Depression (CES-D) scale: depressed and positive affect in cancer patients and healthy reference subjects," *Quality of Life Research*, vol. 9, no. 9, pp. 1015–1029, 2000.

[41] M. Olden, B. Rosenfeld, H. Pessin, and W. Breitbart, "Measuring depression at the end of life: is the hamilton depression rating scale a Valid instrument?" *Assessment*, vol. 16, no. 1, pp. 43–54, 2009.

[42] W. Dugan, M. V. McDonald, S. D. Passik, B. D. Rosenfeld, D. Theobald, and S. Edgerton, "Use of the Zung self-rating depression scale in cancer patients: feasibility as a screening tool," *Psycho-Oncology*, vol. 7, no. 6, pp. 483–493, 1998.

[43] K. Mystakidou, E. Tsilika, E. Parpa, V. Smyrniotis, A. Galanos, and L. Vlahos, "Beck depression inventory: exploring its psychometric properties in a palliative care population of advanced cancer patients," *European Journal of Cancer Care*, vol. 16, no. 3, pp. 244–250, 2007.

[44] K. Mystakidou, E. Tsilika, E. Parpa, E. Katsouda, A. Galanos, and L. Vlahos, "The Hospital Anxiety and Depression Scale in Greek cancer patients: psychometric analyses and applicability," *Supportive Care in Cancer*, vol. 12, no. 12, pp. 821–825, 2004.

[45] K. Linde, K. Niemann, A. Schneider, and K. Meissner, "How large are the nonspecific effects of acupuncture? A meta-analysis of randomized controlled trials," *BMC Medicine*, vol. 8, article 75, 2010.

[46] Y. H. Koog, S. R. We, and B.-I. Min, "Three-armed trials including placebo and no-treatment groups may be subject to publication bias: systematic review," *PLoS ONE*, vol. 6, no. 5, Article ID e20679, 2011.

[47] S. R. We, Y. H. Koog, M. S. Park, and B.-I. Min, "Placebo effect was influenced by publication year in three-armed acupuncture trials," *Complementary Therapies in Medicine*, vol. 20, no. 1-2, pp. 83–92, 2012.

[48] Y. H. Koog and W. Y. Jung, "Time course of placebo effect of acupuncture on pain: a systematic review," *ISRN Pain*, vol. 2013, Article ID 204108, 7 pages, 2013.

[49] A. F. Molsberger, T. Schneider, H. Gotthardt, and A. Drabik, "German randomized acupuncture trial for chronic shoulder pain (GRASP)—a pragmatic, controlled, patient-blinded, multi-centre trial in an outpatient care environment," *Pain*, vol. 151, no. 1, pp. 146–154, 2010.

[50] K. Itoh, Y. Katsumi, S. Hirota, and H. Kitakoji, "Effects of trigger point acupuncture on chronic low back pain in elderly patients—a sham-controlled randomised trial," *Acupuncture in Medicine*, vol. 24, no. 1, pp. 5–12, 2006.

[51] Y. Sun and T. J. Gan, "Acupuncture for the management of chronic headache: a systematic review," *Anesthesia and Analgesia*, vol. 107, no. 6, pp. 2038–2047, 2008.

[52] J. Y. Tan, L. K. Suen, T. Wang, and A. Molassiotis, "Sham acupressure controls used in randomized controlled trials: a systematic review and critique," *PLoS ONE*, vol. 10, no. 7, Article ID e0132989, 2015.

[53] I. Lund, J. Näslund, and T. Lundeberg, "Minimal acupuncture is not a valid placebo control in randomised controlled trials of acupuncture: a physiologist's perspective," *Chinese Medicine*, vol. 4, article 1, 2009.

[54] S. Xu, L. Wang, E. Cooper et al., "Adverse events of acupuncture: a systematic review of case reports," *Evidence-Based Complementary and Alternative Medicine*, vol. 2013, Article ID 581203, 15 pages, 2013.

[55] J.-E. Park, M. S. Lee, J.-Y. Choi, B.-Y. Kim, and S.-M. Choi, "Adverse events associated with acupuncture: a prospective survey," *The Journal of Alternative and Complementary Medicine*, vol. 16, no. 9, pp. 959–963, 2010.

[56] C. X. Liu, L. L. Han, Z. Z. Yang, and Q. J. Yuan, "An analysis of serum levels of cytokines and relative factors in depression patients," *Chinese Journal of Behavioral Medicine & Brain Science*, vol. 23, no. 9, pp. 801–804, 2014.

[57] D. Kondziolka, T. Lemley, J. R. W. Kestle, L. D. Lunsford, G. H. Fromm, and P. J. Jannetta, "The effect of single-application topical ophthalmic anesthesia in patients with trigeminal neuralgia: a randomized double-blind placebo-controlled trial," *Journal of Neurosurgery*, vol. 80, no. 6, pp. 993–997, 1994.

[58] K. F. Schulz, D. G. Altman, and D. Moher, "CONSORT 2010 statement: updated guidelines for reporting parallel group randomised trials," *BMC Medicine*, vol. 8, no. 1, article 18, 2010.

[59] H. MacPherson, D. G. Altman, R. Hammerschlag et al., "Revised standards for reporting interventions in clinical trials of acupuncture (STRICTA): extending the CONSORT statement," *Journal of Evidence-Based Medicine*, vol. 3, no. 3, pp. 140–155, 2010.

# 9

# Bee Pollen as a Promising Agent in the Burn Wounds Treatment

**Paweł Olczyk,**[1] **Robert Koprowski,**[2] **Justyna Kaźmierczak,**[3] **Lukasz Mencner,**[3]
**Robert Wojtyczka,**[4] **Jerzy Stojko,**[5] **Krystyna Olczyk,**[3] **and Katarzyna Komosinska-Vassev**[3]

[1]*Department of Community Pharmacy, School of Pharmacy and Division of Laboratory Medicine in Sosnowiec,*
*Medical University of Silesia in Katowice, Kasztanowa 3, 41-200 Sosnowiec, Poland*
[2]*Department of Biomedical Computer Systems, Faculty of Computer Science and Materials Science, Institute of Computer Science,*
*University of Silesia, Bedzinska 39, 41-200 Sosnowiec, Poland*
[3]*Department of Clinical Chemistry and Laboratory Diagnostics, School of Pharmacy and Division of Laboratory Medicine in*
*Sosnowiec, Medical University of Silesia in Katowice, Jednosci 8, 41-200 Sosnowiec, Poland*
[4]*Department and Institute of Microbiology and Virology, School of Pharmacy and Division of Laboratory Medicine in Sosnowiec,*
*Medical University of Silesia in Katowice, Jagiellonska 4, 41-200 Sosnowiec, Poland*
[5]*Center of Experimental Medicine, Medics 4, Faculty of Medicine in Katowice, Medical University of Silesia in Katowice,*
*40-752 Katowice, Poland*

Correspondence should be addressed to Paweł Olczyk; polczyk@sum.edu.pl

Academic Editor: José Maurício Sforcin

The aim of the present study was to visualize the benefits and advantages derived from preparations based on extracts of bee pollen as compared to pharmaceuticals commonly used in the treatment of burns. The bee pollen ointment was applied for the first time in topical burn treatment. Experimental burn wounds were inflicted on two white, domestic pigs. Clinical, histopathological, and microbiological assessment of specimens from burn wounds, inflicted on polish domestic pigs, treated with silver sulfadiazine or bee pollen ointment, was done. The comparative material was constituted by either tissues obtained from wounds treated with physiological saline or tissues obtained from wounds which were untreated. Clinical and histopathological evaluation showed that applied apitherapeutic agent reduces the healing time of burn wounds and positively affects the general condition of the animals. Moreover the used natural preparation proved to be highly effective antimicrobial agent, which was reflected in a reduction of the number of microorganisms in quantitative research and bactericidal activity of isolated strains. On the basis of the obtained bacteriological analysis, it may be concluded that the applied bee pollen ointment may affect the wound healing process of burn wounds, preventing infection of the newly formed tissue.

## 1. Introduction

Wound healing, being the result of dynamic cooperation between many molecular factors, is a dynamic reaction whose undisturbed course enables restoring the continuity and functionality of damaged skin [1–3]. The process consists of 4 specific phases which smoothly proceed and change from one to the other even coexisting at times. The duration period of particular healing phases may vary depending on the type of the damage and possible coexistence of interfering additional factors, that is, the size and place of the damage, blood supply of the wound edges, cleanness of the wound, the degree of microbiological contamination, presence of necrotic tissue, and properly conducted healing management [1, 2, 4, 5].

The therapy of burn wounds may be properly conducted either by applying surgical methods or by topical application of therapeutic preparations. Besides contemporary, conventional treatment methods of thermal skin damage, apitherapy, which uses the therapeutic effect of standardized, pharmacologically active fractions obtained from bee products, is becoming more and more noticeable. Apitherapeutic agents have a beneficial effect on the skin condition, due to the reduction of water loss, and influence the reconstruction of the lipid barrier. One of the most frequently used apitherapeutic agents is bee pollen. This is a varied, natural product which is rich in such biologically active substances as amino acids, fatty acids, phytosterols, phospholipids, nucleic acids, carbohydrates, vitamins, mineral substances, enzymes, and coenzymes as well as phenolic compounds including phenolic acids and flavonoids [6–9]. The plethora of biologically active substances gives this natural raw material significant biotic properties such as antimicrobial, anti-inflammatory, immunomodulatory, or antioxidative activity [7, 10].

Such a high efficiency of this natural bee product with a significantly low risk of adverse reactions makes bee pollen a potentially optimal remedial factor in the therapy of local burn wounds [11, 12]. Therefore, the subject of this study was the assessment of efficiency and therapeutic usability of the bee pollen which has not been studied before.

Bee pollen, also flower pollen, is male reproductive organs produced by flowers of entomophilous plants. It is collected by worker bees, transported, and stored in beehives. It constitutes a basic ingredient in bee's nutrition used for current needs or stored for later period [13]. Bee pollen results from agglutination of flower pollen, nectar or honey, and bee's salivary substances [14].

Bee pollen treatment of topical, thermal damage of the skin was compared with the commonly applied pharmaceutical preparation such as silver sulfadiazine (SSD), which has many side effects.

AgSD not only may be responsible for the development of argyria and dysfunctions of liver, spleen, and kidney due to systemic accumulation of silver or determined by sulphadiazine presence, dermatitis, erythema multiforme rashes, and acute hemolytic anemia but also unfortunately could be responsible for cytotoxic effect on fibroblasts and keratinocytes [15, 16].

The clinical assessment of the treatment process of burn wounds was conducted. It concerned wound pathomorphology including the extent and depth of the burn, wound maceration, occurrence, and character of the exudate as well as the process of scar formation. The histopathological assessment of the burn wound epithelialization of the dynamics was done together with qualitative and quantitative assessment of particular microorganisms in tissue samples collected from beds of experimental burn wounds.

## 2. Material and Methods

*2.1. Therapeutic Agents.* The following therapeutic preparations were used: 1% silver sulfadiazine (SSD) (Lek, Poland), 0.9% NaCl (Polpharma), and bee pollen formulation. The analyzed bee pollen came from the apiary "Barć" in Kamienna. These are clean and ecological regions of Poland. In this apiary the European Dark Bee also known as Western Honey Bee is bred. The pollen was a composition of many pollens of various plants. Taking into account the location of the apiary, the dominating pollens came from such plants as oilseed rape (lemon-yellow color), shamrock (brown color), coltsfoot (bright yellow), common dandelion (bright orange), linden (bright green), or heather (red-yellow). Macroscopically, it

was a multicolor blend of granules which were ground. 50 g of the ground pollen was added to 500 mL of 70% ethanol. The extraction of the solution was conducted for 4 weeks at room temperature. After that period, the solution underwent microfiltration. Next, the ethanol was distilled with vacuum evaporator. The result was dry matter which was used to prepare the bee pollen formulation (ointment containing 5% bee pollen ethanolic extract and 95% of petroleum jelly (according to Polish norm PN-R-78893)). The procedure was performed under general anesthesia according to the dosage regimen: atropine sulfate, 0.05 mg/kg body weight (Polfa Warszawa); ketamine hydrochloride, 3 mg/kg body weight (Biovet, Puławy); xylazine hydrochloride, 1 mg/kg body weight (Sandoz GMBH). Silver sulfadiazine was used in order to prolong the analgesic effect, 5 mg/kg body weight (Polpharma).

*2.2. Tissue Material.* The study protocol was approved by the Ethics Committee of the Medical University of Silesia. Two, 16-week-old, domestic pigs have been chosen as the useful experimental animals for the evaluation of wound repair because of many similarities of pig skin to human one. The usage of the limited number of experimental animals was consistent with validated animal model developed by Hoekstra et al. [17] in modification of Brans et al. [18]. The last mentioned pig model is based on the application of one experimental animal [18]. Moreover, in accordance with the guidelines of good laboratory practice for animal testing, the established principle is to use the minimum number of animals necessary to arrive at scientifically robust data and to ensure reliable data. Thus, the animals used in our study were bred and selected for the highest degree of genetic purity. This form of breeding purpose prevents genetic contamination and allows minimizing the number of animals necessary for the experiment, with very reliable results to be obtained.

Pigs were housed according to G.L.P. standards of Polish Veterinary Law. Each animal was inflicted with 18 skin burn wounds with equal gaps (9 wounds on each side along the line of the backbone). The size of each wound was identical, 1.5 cm × 3 cm. Totally, the wounds took about 2% of the surface of each animal's body subject to the experiment.

Burns were classified as 2nd-degree deep partial thickness burns. Animals were divided into two groups: control (C) and experimental ones (E). 36 dermal burns were inflicted. The wounds of animals in the control group were either untreated (subgroup C1) or treated with physiologic saline (subgroup C2).

The postburn wounds of the experimental group were also treated with SSD (subgroup E1) and with the bee pollen containing ointment (subgroup E2). The wounds in question were treated with mentioned substances twice a day, starting on the first day of the experiment. Three replications of biopsies were taken from the same wound of each animal, using surgical knife. Occlusive dressings were applied every 12 hours in all animals of all subgroups.

*2.3. Clinical Study.* Clinical observation was to assess the extent and depth of the burn, its maceration, and presence of necrotic tissue in it. Macroscopic reading of pathomorphological picture of the wound considered occurrence and intensification of typical symptoms of burn wounds: erythema, swelling, exudate, bleeding, and eschar. The process of granulation tissue formation together with the course of scar formation, ongoing on the burn wound surface, was also assessed.

*2.4. Histopathological Study.* The process of granulation, the type of the granulation tissue, intensification of swelling around the burn angiogenesis, and possible scarring of the wound were assessed. The microscopic picture of skin preparations included degree of the damage in the area and near the wound as well as the repair processes in next stages of the observation. Histopathological studies concerned the samples which were collected from burn wounds and from the adjacent, unchanged tissue in general anesthesia on 0, 3rd, 5th, 10th, 15th, and 21st day from the moment of inflicting the burn. After consolidation, tissues samples were collected form skin specimen in order to make histopathological preparations. The basic slides with samples were stained to achieve optical differentiation and verification of the elements of cell structure. Two different kinds of dyes were used: hematoxylin and eosin. Two histopathological preparations, which resulted from that process, underwent the microscopic assessment.

*2.5. Microbiological Study.* Microbiological study was performed from the material collected from the burn wounds on 0, 3rd, 5th, 10th, 15th, and 21st day of the experiment. In the case of quantitative study, the material was collected with a sterile swab stick from the burn wound surface of $1 \, cm^2$ and was subsequently put into the $10 \, cm^3$ of a sterile solution of 0.9% NaCl. This suspension of microorganisms served as the basis for a series of dilutions. Then, a $1 \, cm^3$ of the suspension was collected and spilt on the slide and dissolved in both the Mueller Hinton agar (MH), in order to assess the amount of bacteria, and Sabouraud agar, in order to assess the amount of fungi and mould. The material to microbiological purity test of the skin was simultaneously collected from the places where the burns were not inflicted. In the case of quantitative studies, the material was collected with AMIES transport medium with active carbon (HAGAMED, Poland), which was stored at $5°C$ up to the moment of performing microbiological tests (max. up to 2 hours). Simultaneously, the samples for microbiological purity test were collected from the skin of animals not taking part in the experiment. Microbiological diagnosis was conducted in accordance with the standards of National Committee for Clinical and Laboratory Standards [19]. The cultures were conducted on the following enrichment and differential media such as liquid media (Carbohydrate broth, an enrichment medium for aerobic bacteria) and solid media (blood agar, to enrich aerobic microorganisms and characterize the type of hemolysis; Mannitol Salt Agar (Chapman), to differentiate *Staphylococcus* spp.; MacConkey Agar, to differentiate *Enterobacteriaceae* species; Sabouraud Agar, to identify fungi; Agar D-Coccosel, to identify *Enterococcus*

*faecalis*; Cetrimide Agar, to identify *Pseudomonas* spp.). The identification of isolated bacteria species was conducted by microscopic tests, culture tests, and commercial biochemical test API (bioMerieux, France). The growth promotion test was carried out with reference strains. The next stage of the test was to assess the amount of bacteria on $1 \, cm^2$ of the burn wound surface. Therefore, the material was collected from $1 \, cm^2$ of the wound which was then shaken in $10 \, cm^3$ of the sterile solution of physiological saline.

*2.6. Data Analysis.* In addition to the analytical methods mentioned above, the automatic measurement of the time constants was proposed. They concern the change rate analysis of the number of bacteria, fungi, or moulds in the wound. Therefore, the electrical-analog method, the inertial first-order object with delay, was suggested. For such a proposed model, the time constants for particular groups C1, C2, E1, and E2 were measured.

The microbiological data analysis was performed using Statistica 7.0 package (StatSoft, Cracov, Poland). The normality of distribution was verified with Kolmogorov-Smirnov test. Statistical differences between variables were verified by analysis of variance (ANOVA), followed by post hoc NIR test.

# 3. Results

*3.1. Clinical Test Results.* The clinical view of the wounds was compared on 3rd, 5th, 10th, 15th, and 21st day after burn infliction.

Differences in the clinical view of healing wounds were noticed on the 5th day of the observation. In the control subgroups, untreated wounds (C1), wounds treated with 0.9% NaCl solution (C2), and the study subgroup (E1) in which the wounds were treated with silver sulfadiazine, the erythema was observed to exceed the area of the burn wound. The skin surrounding the wound was very swollen with visible exudate. In the case of the wounds treated with the ointment with a 5% bee pollen, the subgroup (E2), the area of the wound was covered with a thin, flexible eschar accompanied by bleeding. On 10th and 15th day of the experiment, the untreated wound, in the control subgroup (C1), was covered with a hard, dry, and cracked eschar strongly adhering in the center. Under the eschar, there was a pink granulation tissue. During the same days, in the control subgroup, treated with 0.9% NaCl solution (C2), the burn wound was covered with a softened eschar with a small amount of serosanguineous exudate. In the experimental subgroup (E1) treated with silver sulfadiazine, the area of the wound was covered with a hard eschar and there was an erythema. The burn wounds of subgroup (E2), treated with the bee pollen ointment on the 10th day, were covered with a thin, flexible eschar with a visible granulation, while, on the 15th day, there was a clear epithelium being formed. The area of the wound decreased. The tissues surrounding the wound were characterized by a weak, atrophic inflammatory condition. On the 21st day of the observation, the clinical view was still significantly differentiated. In subgroup (C1) the untreated wounds were covered with a dry, cracked eschar. In subgroup (C2),

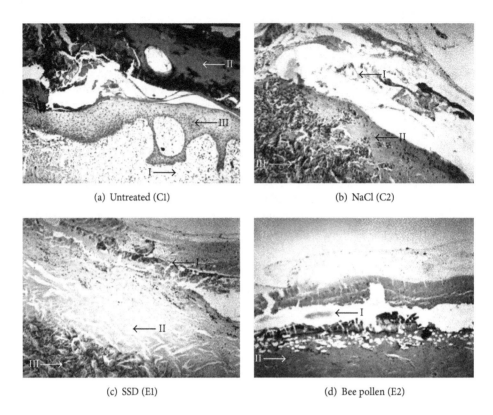

(a) Untreated (C1)

(b) NaCl (C2)

(c) SSD (E1)

(d) Bee pollen (E2)

FIGURE 1: The picture of microscopic changes of skin samples collected from burn wounds on the 10th day of the experiment: (a) untreated (I: swollen inflammatory granulation tissue in the area of dermis, II: eschar with a slight bleeding, and III: visible, pink, and swollen granulation tissue); (b) washed with NaCl (I: petechial hemorrhages, loss of stratified squamous epithelium, II: coagulative necrosis, and III: massive lymphocytic infiltration); (c) treated with SSD (I: petechial hemorrhages, II: area of aseptic necrosis with many inflammatory infiltrations, and III: inflammatory infiltrations on the verge of necrosis); (d) treated with bee pollen (I: petechial hemorrhages, II: area of necrosis with many inflammatory infiltrations).

the wounds, being constantly washed with 0.9% NaCl, were covered with an irregular eschar tightly adhering to the wound in its central part. After the eschar was removed mechanically, a pink granulation tissue without the features of epithelialization could be seen. The wound, treated with silver sulfadiazine (subgroup E1), was covered with a pink epithelium. The tissues surrounding the wound had no significant inflammatory features. The wound area did not decrease. The wounds, treated with the bee pollen ointment, in subgroup E2, were covered with a thick epithelium. The features of the healing process were strongly visible. Within the surrounding tissue there were not any signs of erythema or the ongoing inflammatory process.

*3.2. Histopathological Test Results.* The histological view of wound healing of animals from all groups until the 5th day of the experiment were identical. Figure 1 shows differentiated dynamics of repairing processes which occurred on the 10th day of the experimental healing process for all analyzed groups. Application of the bee pollen (E2) achieved its therapeutic effect on the 10th day of the experiment. The whole wound surface was filled with collagen fibers, which affected

scar formation, and the stratified squamous epithelium was being created.

On the 15th day of the observation, other changes in the histopathological view were observed. In the control subgroups C1 and C2 and in the E1 subgroup, a slow wound healing process in the phase of fibroplasia with the sustaining inflammation could be observed. In subgroup (E2), in which the wounds were treated with the ointment with 5% bee pollen extract, fibroplasia was significantly proceeding, while the present granulation tissue was covered with a regenerated epithelium. In the wound area there were no clear signs of inflammatory reaction. The regenerated stratified squamous epithelium was appearing on the wound edges together with existing inflammatory infiltrations in the histopathological view on the 21st day of the experiment in the case of the untreated wounds (subgroup C1). In case of wounds washed with 0.9% of NaCl (subgroup C2) as well as in subgroup (E1), in which the wounds were treated with silver sulfadiazine, the developed stratified squamous epithelium was covered with an eschar, under which there was a visible mature granulation tissue with a lot of fibers. In subgroup (E2), in which the wounds were treated with the bee pollen ointment, the whole wound surface was filled with a scar together with a thick

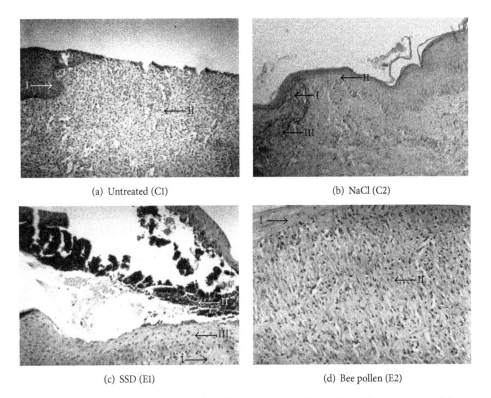

(a) Untreated (C1)

(b) NaCl (C2)

(c) SSD (E1)

(d) Bee pollen (E2)

FIGURE 2: The microscopic changes of skin samples collected from burn wounds on the 21st day of the experiment: (a) untreated (I: regenerated stratified squamous epithelium on the sample edge, II: vessel-rich and cell-rich granulation tissue); (b) washed with NaCl (I: eschar, II: regenerated stratified squamous epithelium, and III: vessel-rich and cell-rich inflammatory granulation tissue); (c) treated with SSD (I: a slightly swollen dermis, II: eschar with petechial hemorrhages, and III: regenerated stratified squamous epithelium); (d) treated with bee pollen (I: connective tissue scar covered with epithelium and II: inflammatory granulation tissue with predominating collagen fibers).

stratified squamous epithelium. There was no granulation tissue. The E2 subgroup showed a correctly healed burn wound. The description of histopathological observations on 21st day of the experiment is shown in Figure 2.

### 3.3. Microbiological Test Results

*3.3.1. Quantitative Study.* The Logarithmic CFU (colony forming unit) values of bacteria cultured on particular days of the burn wound healing are summarized in Table 1.

The result of the quantitative study conducted on the 0 day, immediately after burning, showed no microorganisms from none of the experimental groups. The effect of thermal feature made the skin sterilized. On the 3rd day of the study, the bacteria were isolated only from the tissue specimens collected from the untreated wounds. On the 5th day, the microorganisms were present in the tissue material of all studied groups. Further growth of the average number of bacteria in $1\,cm^2$ of the wound was found on the 10th day of the experiment. However, the number of bacteria decreased in wounds washed with 0.9% of NaCl (C2) and in wound treated with the bee pollen ointment (E2). A further decrease of the number of bacteria in most analyzed groups was observed on the 15th day after burning. However, the wounds treated with the bee pollen ointment were characterized by

the smallest number of bacteria in relation to the previous measurement. A systematic decrease of the number of bacteria in the wounds classifying to control and experimental groups was confirmed on the 21st day of the experiment and; what is more, the beds of thermal damage treated with silver sulfadiazine and with the bee pollen ointment were characterized by the biggest decrease of the bacteria number (Figures 3 and 4).

Logarithmic CFU (colony forming unit) values of fungi and mould cultured on particular days of the burn wound healing are summarized in Table 2.

The growth of fungi and mould in the wound area of animals, evaluated on 0 and 3rd day of the C1, C2, E1, and E2 subgroups, resulted in finding no such microorganisms. The experimental studies conducted on 5th and 10th day showed that the number of fungi and moulds increased particularly in the case of untreated wounds as well as those treated with silver sulfadiazine. Next days showed a decreased general number of fungi and mould in untreated wounds and those treated with SSD. The wounds washed with NaCl and those exposed to bee pollen ointment were characterized by the lowest number of fungi and mould on the 21st day of the experiment (Figures 5 and 6).

Variable number of fungi and moulds in time was analytically analyzed. This analysis is to approximate the

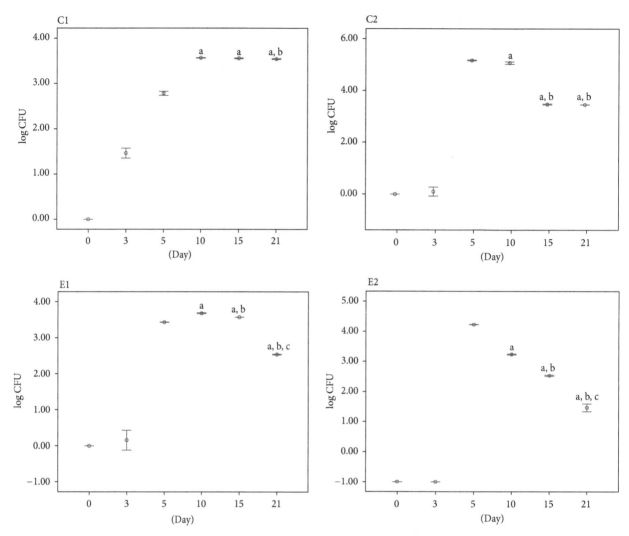

FIGURE 3: Quantitative study: log CFU value of bacteria cultured on particular days of the burn wound healing: C1: tissue material from untreated wounds; C2: tissue material collected from wounds washed with NaCl; E1: tissue material from wounds treated with silver sulfadiazine; E2: tissue material from wounds treated with bee pollen ointment. Results are expressed as mean ± standard error of the mean (SEM) of the assays performed in triplicate. [a]$p < 0.05$ compared with value determined on 5th day, [b]$p < 0.05$ compared with value determined on 10th day, and [c]$p < 0.05$ compared with value determined on 15th day.

TABLE 1: log CFU values of bacteria on the following days of the experiment.

|                  | 0 day | 3rd day | 5th day | 10th day | 15th day | 21st day |
|------------------|-------|---------|---------|----------|----------|----------|
| C1 (untreated)   | —     | 1.47    | 2.78    | 3.57     | 3.56     | 3.54     |
| C2 (NaCl)        | —     | —       | 5.18    | 5.08     | 3.48     | 3.46     |
| E1 (SSD)         | —     | —       | 3.43    | 3.68     | 3.57     | 2.53     |
| E2 (bee pollen)  | —     | —       | 5.23    | 4.24     | 3.53     | 2.48     |

TABLE 2: log CFU values of fungi and mould on the following days of the experiment.

|                  | 0 day | 3rd day | 5th day | 10th day | 15th day | 21st day |
|------------------|-------|---------|---------|----------|----------|----------|
| C1 (untreated)   | —     | —       | 1.59    | 1.47     | 1.19     | 0.99     |
| C2 (NaCl)        | —     | —       | 1.01    | 1.01     | 1.19     | 0.18     |
| E1 (SSD)         | —     | —       | 1.68    | 1.60     | 1.07     | 1.00     |
| E2 (bee pollen)  | —     | —       | 0.99    | 0.88     | 1.16     | 0.75     |

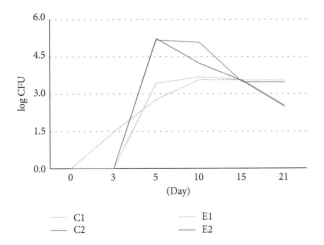

C1 ——    E1 ——
C2 ——    E2 ——

FIGURE 4: Dynamics of $\log$ CFU value of bacteria cultured on particular days of the burn wounds treated with NaCl (C2), silver sulfadiazine (E1), bee pollen ointment (E2), and untreated wounds (C1).

TABLE 3: The error value of matching the inertial first-order object model with the experimental data (bacteria, fungi, and mould) for given time constants $T_1$.

|  | C1 | C2 | E1 | E2 |
|---|---|---|---|---|
| $\delta^{(B)}$ [%] | 3 | 44 | 5 | 58 |
| $T_1$ [day] | 20 | 1 | 18 | 1 |
| $\delta^{(R)}$ [%] | 25 | 17 | 18 | 17 |
| $T_1$ [day] | 7 | 20 | 6 | 20 |

of the response relationship for the multi-inertial object is as follows:

$$G(s) = \frac{k}{(1 + sT_1)(1 + sT_2)\cdots(1 + sT_n)},\qquad(1)$$

where $k$ is amplification and $T_1, T_2, \ldots, T_n$ is time constant.

This was the basis for formulating the error of matching the model with the source data, for example, for the bacteria (superscript) and tissue material from untreated wounds (subscript) done as follows:

$$\delta_{C1}^{(B)} = \frac{100}{I \cdot \max_i y_{C1}^{(B)}(i)} \sum_{i=1}^{I} \left| y_{C1}^{(B)}(i) - y_{SC1}^{(B)}(i) \right| \ [\%],\qquad(2)$$

where $y_{C1}^{(B)}(i)$ is change in the number of bacteria (superscript $B$) in the next $i$-measurements, $y_{SC1}^{(B)}(i)$ is simulation of change in the number of bacteria (superscript $B$) in the next $i$-measurements for the model (unit response) described by transmittance, and $I$ is total number of measurements.

Similarly, the error of experimental data match with the standard for fungi and mould (superscript $R$) and different materials is calculated. For such a formulated error the method of a tuned model was applied in order to match the multi-inertial object with the data and to specify the order of the model. The smallest values of errors, shown in Table 3, were obtained for multi-inertial first-order object.

In Table 3 the calculated error values of the match $\delta^{(B)}$ and $\delta^{(R)}$ for the materials C1, C2, E1, and E2 were shown. The calculations were done for the inertial first-order object (with the time constant $T_1$) with delay (5 days) for which the value of particular errors is smaller. In the graph in Figure 7 the exemplary obtained results are shown, the behaviors of $y_{C1}^{(R)}(i)$ and $y_{SC1}^{(R)}(i)$ for $T_1 = 8$.

As it can be concluded from Figure 7, the biggest error values (>44%) occur for materials C2 and E2, which results from the specification of changes in the number of bacteria in the wound. Due to individual variation of pigs, this specification depends on many factors. The smallest error values and, simultaneously, the best match of the model with experimental data occur for materials C1 and E1. The time constants for them are 20 and 18 days. Similar error values were obtained for fungi and mould which fluctuate around the value of 18%. The time constants are also different (as in the case of bacteria) for materials C1 and E1 amounting to 6 and 7 days, while for materials C2 and E2 they are equal to 20 days. Summing up the obtained results, the time constant average value of the growth of bacteria, mould, and fungi in the wound is at the level of 18 up to 20 days.

mode of changes in time with a model. A model, being the inertial first-order object with delay, has been chosen. The very choice of the model results from earlier authors' experiences concerning the analysis of dynamic changes (e.g., linked to temperature) occurring in humans and animals. The model enables parameterization of characteristics linked to the change rate of the number of fungi and moulds. These parameters are time constant $T_1$ and delay. The time constant enables the determination of the change rate of the number of fungi and moulds in time. According to the theory of automatic control (the processes occurring in living organisms) the steady state takes place after third up to fifth time constants (95% and 99% of the steady state). For the cases in question it means that if the obtained results are approximated with this model (the inertial first-order object with delay) it will become possible to determine the time after which the decrease in the number of fungi and moulds to the values close to 0 (zero) will appear. It will be, for example, $3 * T_1$ for which only 5% of fungi and mould will remain when related to the maximum value. Similarly for $5 * T_1$ only 1% of fungi and mould will remain in relation to the maximum value. The approximation of changes of the number of fungi and mould in time with the inertial first-order object with delay enables obtaining one more error parameter of matching $\delta$, which gives the information about the matching compliance of the model with the obtained experimental data.

The time change of the average number of bacteria, fungi, and moulds is a nonlinear relationship. Due to the analogy to the control systems, the response of the system (in this case it is the number of bacteria, moulds, and fungi) may be approximated by the inertial first-order object with delay. It results from the biological and medical rationale concerning the growth rate (development) of the bacteria, fungi, and moulds on the healing wound surface (regardless of the fact if it was C1, C2 or E1, E2). The general transmittance form

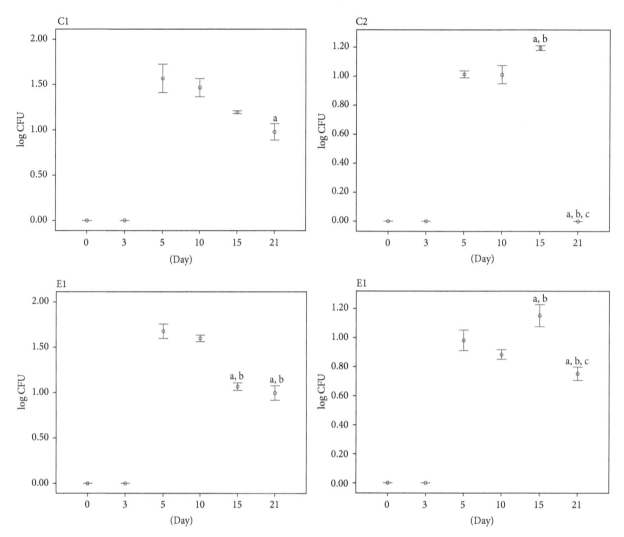

FIGURE 5: Quantitative study: log CFU value of fungi and mould cultured on particular days of the burn wound healing: C1: tissue material from untreated wounds; C2: tissue material collected from wounds washed with NaCl; E1: tissue material from wounds treated with silver sulfadiazine; E2: tissue material from wounds treated with bee pollen ointment. Results are expressed as mean ± standard error of the mean (SEM) of the assays performed in triplicate. [a]$p < 0.05$ compared with value determined on 5th day, [b]$p < 0.05$ compared with value determined on 10th day, and [c]$p < 0.05$ compared with value determined on 15th day.

*3.3.2. Qualitative Study.* In the qualitative study, changes of microbial species from the swabs of burn wounds treated with appropriate experimental agents and of the healthy skin surface were evaluated during next days of the experiment. On 0 day, the number of microorganisms, which constitute the physiological flora of the skin and the environment, increased in healthy skin (Table 4). However, no bacteria were cultured from none of the samples collected from the burn wounds immediately after burning.

On the 3rd day of the study, the wounds were colonized with microorganisms from *Micrococcus* species only in the subgroup in which the wounds were untreated (C1). On the 5th day of the study, the number of isolated microorganisms species significantly increased in the animals of all subgroups. Besides typical physiological flora of the skin and the environment (*Micrococcus* spp., *Bacillus* spp.) there were also microorganisms which are characteristic for wound

inflammation. In the subsequent days of the experiment, all burn wounds were characterized by a lower number of strains. On the 21st day of the study, in subgroups C2, E1, and E2, the bacterial flora was reduced to only one environmental species, such as *Bacillus* spp., while in the group of untreated wounds (C1), only *Staphylococcus hyicus* was found.

# 4. Discussion

Wound healing is a dynamic and time-synchronized reaction of the organism connected both with the actions of many cells, such as inflammatory cells, vascular cells, connective tissue cells, and epithelial cells, and with accumulating extracellular matrix (ECM) components, which leads to creation of a new tissue [20]. A significant role in the healing process is played by ECM components: glycosaminoglycans (GAGs), fibronectin, proteoglycans, vitronectin, and collagens [21, 22].

TABLE 4: Changing of species of microflora in burn wounds in the following days of the experiment; N: tissue material from healthy skin not inflicted with a burn; C1: tissue material from untreated wounds; C2: tissue material from places washed with 0.9% NaCl; E1: tissue material from places treated with silver sulfadiazine salt; E2: tissue material from places treated with the with bee pollen ointment.

| | 0 day | 3rd day | 5th day | 10th day | 15th day | 21st day |
|---|---|---|---|---|---|---|
| N | Micrococcus spp. Bacillus spp. Staphylococcus lentus | Micrococcus spp. Bacillus spp. Staphylococcus lentus | Micrococcus spp. Bacillus spp. Gemella spp. Aerococcus viridans | Micrococcus spp. Bacillus spp. Aerococcus viridans | Micrococcus spp. Bacillus spp. Aerococcus viridans Enterococcus faecalis | Micrococcus spp. Bacillus spp. Aerococcus viridans |
| C1 | — | Micrococcus spp. | Micrococcus spp. | Micrococcus spp. Staphylococcus hyicus Candida spp. | Candida spp. | Staphylococcus hyicus |
| C2 | — | — | Micrococcus spp. | Micrococcus spp. | Bacillus spp. | Bacillus spp. |
| E1 | — | — | Bacillus spp. Staphylococcus hyicus Enterococcus faecalis | Bacillus spp. Micrococcus spp. | Bacillus spp. | Bacillus spp. |
| E2 | — | — | Bacillus spp. Staphylococcus hyicus Pseudomonas aeruginosa | Bacillus spp. Pseudomonas aeruginosa | Bacillus spp. | Bacillus spp. |

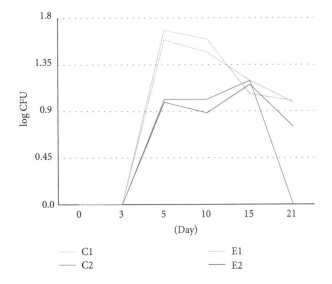

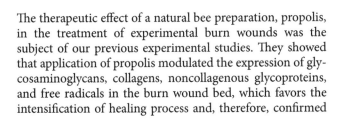

FIGURE 6: Dynamics of log CFU value of fungi and mould cultured on particular days of the burn wounds treated NaCl (C2), silver sulfadiazine (E1), bee pollen ointment (E2), and untreatedwounds (C1).

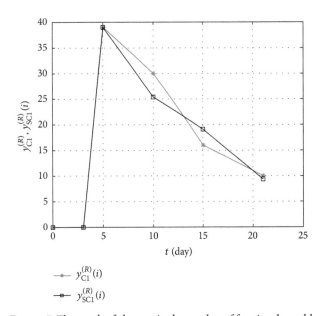

FIGURE 7: The graph of changes in the number of fungi and moulds in time for experimental and simulation data of the material C1.

The therapeutic effect of a natural bee preparation, propolis, in the treatment of experimental burn wounds was the subject of our previous experimental studies. They showed that application of propolis modulated the expression of glycosaminoglycans, collagens, noncollagenous glycoproteins, and free radicals in the burn wound bed, which favors the intensification of healing process and, therefore, confirmed a positive influence of the mentioned apitherapeutic agent on the metabolism of ECM components [21–24].

The aim of the present study was to compare the therapeutic efficiency of another natural agent based on bee pollen extract with a commonly used pharmaceutical silver sulfadiazine in treatment of thermal burns.

Although silver sulfadiazine is considered as a gold standard in the topical treatment of burn wounds, this therapeutic agent is characterized by many side effects such as the risk of crystalluria, methaemoglobinaemia, neutropenia, erythema multiforme, and prolonged reepithelialization and the impairment of the mechanical strength of newly created tissue [25, 26]. Such side effect cannot be found in the case of bee pollen. This apitherapeutic agent demonstrates strong immune-modulating properties, which accelerate epithelialization and has bacteriostatic, bactericidal, and anesthetic properties [9, 27]. Moreover, bee pollen has a strong anti-inflammatory activity, decreases the healing period, and reduces the duration and intensity of ailments [9, 28].

The experimental model implemented in the present study was based on the tissue material collected from the domestic pig skin. The choice of the animal was made mainly due to the similarity between pig skin and human one [29].

Clinical and histopathological observation comprising the assessment of the extent and depth of the burn wounds, wound maceration, presence of necrotic tissue, granulation tissue type, and swelling around the burn wound indicated that, on the first days of the experiment, the pathomorphological view of the wounds for every group was the same. It became significantly differentiated on the 5th day of the observation. In the case of the wounds treated with the ointment with bee pollen ointment (E2), the wound area was covered with a thin, flexible eschar with a slight bleeding. In the wound area there were signs of swelling and reddening.

On the next days of the observation of the wounds treated with the apitherapeutic agent, a strong granulation and, subsequently, epithelium formation with clearly visible fully healed characteristics were noted. The wound surface decreased and was the size of $1\,cm \times 1\,cm$. In the area of the tissues surrounding the healing wound there were no signs of swelling or the ongoing inflammatory process. The clinical and histopathological assessment led to a conclusion that the applied apitherapeutic agent ointment reduces the time of burn wound treatment. Similar results were obtained in our previous studies where the therapeutic usability of another apitherapeutic agent, propolis, was assessed in the course of regeneration of experimental thermal skin damage. Propolis ointments in comparison with SSD preparation significantly accelerated the regenerative-reparative process of tissue damage not demonstrating any undesirable effects at the same time [30]. The beneficial effect of standardized propolis formulation on the healing process was also proved in Jastrzębska-Stojko et al. experimental studies [31]. The healing process of burn wounds treated with Sepropol was faster as compared to the standard SSD therapy. Moreover, histopathological tests showed that the process of scar formation in wounds treated with propolis formulation started considerably earlier as compared to the control group [31]. The other part of our studies concerning microbiological examinations during experimental burn wound healing proved that bee pollen ointment had an effective antimicrobial activity, reducing both the number of microorganisms and presenting bactericidal activity in isolated strains. The antibacterial properties of another apitherapeutic agent, propolis, were already assessed in the study with animal model of burn wounds. The mentioned study indicated a higher antimicrobial effectiveness of propolis ointment as compared to SSD in

the course of burn wounds healing. A more beneficial action of the first from the mentioned preparations was manifested by a significant reduction of microorganisms as well as a more effective bactericidal action of the applied apitherapeutic agent. A similar trend in the effects of SSD action and a bee product in the range of antibacterial action were described by Kabała-Dzik et al. [32].

The therapeutic mechanism of bee natural products is based, among others, on antimicrobial activity and on inducing processes of damaged tissues regeneration. These characteristics proved their usability in wound healing and ulcerations of different etiology [31, 33].

The results in this study confirmed the beneficial effect of the bee pollen ointment on the burn wound healing process which could be seen in the decreased number of bacteria in the burn wounds during subsequent days of the experiment.

Different mechanisms could be responsible for the observed antibacterial effects of bee pollen. The first one results from the presence of active compounds, such as flavonoids and phenolic acids, whose forming complexes with bacterial cell walls lead to the disruption of cell wall integrity, blocking ion channels, and inhibiting electron flow in the electron transport chain [34].

The second mechanism by which bee pollen exerts antibacterial activity might be based on the inhibition of bacterial RNA-polymerase by phenolic compounds such as flavanone pinocembrin, flavonol galangin, and caffeic acid phenethyl ester [35].

Besides high antimicrobial activity, bee pollen ointment was also characterized by a bactericidal effect for isolated strains.

Moreover, the study also proved that thermal damage and bacterial infection of the wound favor yeast multiplication including *Candida albicans*. The yeast of the *Candida* species in proper conditions is saprophytes which live in the natural environment and colonize mucosa and human skin. However, they may induce life-threatening candidiases. Burns and necrotic lesions, which are the gates for fungal infection, may contribute to sepsis. *Bacillus cereus* and *Bacillus subtilis*, which are usually harmless, may induce infections in the condition of decreased immunity.

The clinical and histopathological observations performed in our study led to a conclusion that the bee pollen exerts a beneficial effect on wound healing cellular events providing reepithelization and wound closure. The microbiological studies proved that bee pollen ointment had an effective antimicrobial activity. The benefits and advantages of the bee pollen ointment in burn wound treatment imply the usability of the applied apitherapeutic agent preparation in topical burns therapy.

## Competing Interests

The authors declare that they have no conflict of interests.

## Acknowledgments

This work was supported by a grant from the Medical University of Silesia, Poland (KNW-1-018/K/4/0).

# References

[1] T. Velnar, T. Bailey, and V. Smrkolj, "The wound healing process: an overview of the cellular and molecular mechanisms," *Journal of International Medical Research*, vol. 37, no. 5, pp. 1528–1542, 2009.

[2] D. D. S. Tavares Pereira, M. H. M. Lima-Ribeiro, N. T. De Pontes-Filho, A. M. D. A. Carneiro-Leão, and M. T. D. S. Correia, "Development of animal model for studying deep second-degree thermal burns," *Journal of Biomedicine and Biotechnology*, vol. 2012, Article ID 460841, 7 pages, 2012.

[3] H. Sinno and S. Prakash, "Complements and the wound healing cascade: an updated review," *Plastic Surgery International*, vol. 2013, Article ID 146764, 7 pages, 2013.

[4] G. Gethin, "Understanding the inflammatory process in wound healing," *British Journal of Community Nursing*, vol. 17, no. 3, pp. S17–S22, 2012.

[5] J. M. Reinke and H. Sorg, "Wound repair and regeneration," *European Surgical Research*, vol. 49, no. 1, pp. 35–43, 2012.

[6] A. K. Kuropatnicki, E. Szliszka, and W. Krol, "Historical aspects of propolis research in modern times," *Evidence-Based Complementary and Alternative Medicine*, vol. 2013, Article ID 964149, 11 pages, 2013.

[7] M. R. Campos, S. Bogdanov, L. M. de Almeida-Muradian, T. Szczesna, Y. Mancebo, and C. Frigerio, "Pollen composition and standardisation of analytical methods," *Journal of Apicultural Research and Bee World*, vol. 47, no. 2, pp. 156–163, 2008.

[8] E. Szliszka and W. Krol, "Polyphenols isolated from propolis augment TRAIL-induced apoptosis in cancer cells," *Evidence-Based Complementary and Alternative Medicine*, vol. 2013, Article ID 731940, 10 pages, 2013.

[9] B. Kedzia, "Chemical composition of Polish propolis. Part I. The initial period of investigations," *Postepy Fitoterapii*, vol. 10, no. 1, pp. 39–44, 2009.

[10] A. Rzepecka-Stojko, B. Pilawa, P. Ramos, and J. Stojko, "Antioxidative properties of bee pollen extracts examined by EPR spectroscopy," *Journal of Apicultural Science*, vol. 56, no. 1, pp. 23–31, 2012.

[11] B. Kedzia and E. Holderna-Kedzia, "Właściwości biologiczne i działanie lecznicze pyłku kwiatowego zbieranego przez pszczoły," *Postepy Fitoterapii*, vol. 3, pp. 103–108, 2005.

[12] M. Hellner, D. Winter, R. Von Georgi, and K. Münstedt, "Apitherapy: usage and experience in German beekeepers," *Evidence-Based Complementary and Alternative Medicine*, vol. 5, no. 4, pp. 475–479, 2008.

[13] A. Pietrusa and K. Derbisz, "Produkty pszczele część II: pyłek pszczeli," *Przeglad Urologiczny*, vol. 6, no. 94, pp. 48–50, 2015.

[14] C. Nogueira, A. Iglesias, X. Feás, and L. M. Estevinho, "Commercial bee pollen with different geographical origins: a comprehensive approach," *International Journal of Molecular Sciences*, vol. 13, no. 9, pp. 11173–11187, 2012.

[15] O. Brandt, M. Mildner, A. E. Egger et al., "Nanoscalic silver possesses broad-spectrum antimicrobial activities and exhibits fewer toxicological side effects than silver sulfadiazine," *Nanomedicine: Nanotechnology, Biology, and Medicine*, vol. 8, no. 4, pp. 478–488, 2012.

[16] G. Sandri, M. C. Bonferoni, F. D'Autilia et al., "Wound dressings based on silver sulfadiazine solid lipid nanoparticles for tissue repairing," *European Journal of Pharmaceutics and Biopharmaceutics*, vol. 84, no. 1, pp. 84–90, 2013.

[17] M. J. Hoekstra, P. Hupkens, R. P. Dutrieux, M. M. C. Bosch, T. A. Brans, and R. W. Kreis, "A comparative burn wound model in the New Yorkshire pig for the histopathological evaluation of local therapeutic regimens: silver sulfadiazine cream as a standard," *British Journal of Plastic Surgery*, vol. 46, no. 7, pp. 585–589, 1993.

[18] T. A. Brans, R. P. Dutrieux, M. J. Hoekstra, R. W. Kreis, and J. S. du Pont, "Histopathological evaluation of scalds and contact burns in the pig model," *Burns*, vol. 20, no. 1, pp. S48–S51, 1994.

[19] M. K. York, "Aerobic Bacteriology. Quantitative cultures of wound tissues," in *Clinical Microbiology Procedures Handbook*, H. D. Isenberg, Ed., section 3.13.2, ASM Press, Washington, DC, USA, 2nd edition, 2004.

[20] I. I. A. Darby, B. Laverdet, F. Bonté, and A. Desmoulière, "Fibroblasts and myofibroblasts in wound healing," *Clinical, Cosmetic and Investigational Dermatology*, vol. 7, pp. 301–311, 2014.

[21] P. Olczyk, K. Komosinska-Vassev, K. Winsz-Szczotka, J. Stojko, K. Klimek, and E. M. Kozma, "Propolis induces chondroitin/dermatan sulphate and hyaluronic acid accumulation in the skin of burned wound," *Evidence-Based Complementary and Alternative Medicine*, vol. 2013, Article ID 290675, 8 pages, 2013.

[22] P. Olczyk, K. Komosinska-Vassev, K. Winsz-Szczotka et al., "Propolis modulates vitronectin, laminin, and heparan sulfate/heparin expression during experimental burn healing," *Journal of Zhejiang University: Science B*, vol. 13, no. 11, pp. 932–941, 2012.

[23] P. Olczyk, G. Wisowski, K. Komosinska-Vassev et al., "Propolis modifies collagen types I and III accumulation in the matrix of burnt tissue," *Evidence-Based Complementary and Alternative Medicine*, vol. 2013, Article ID 423809, 10 pages, 2013.

[24] P. Olczyk, P. Ramos, K. Komosińska-Vassev, J. Stojko, and B. Pilawa, "Positive effect of propolis on free radicals in burn wounds," *Evidence-Based Complementary and Alternative Medicine*, vol. 2013, Article ID 356737, pp. 1–12, 2013.

[25] T. Dai, Y.-Y. Huang, S. K. Sharma, J. T. Hashmi, D. B. Kurup, and M. R. Hamblin, "Topical antimicrobials for burn wound infections," *Recent Patents on Anti-Infective Drug Discovery*, vol. 5, no. 2, pp. 124–151, 2010.

[26] F. W. Fuller, "The side effects of silver sulfadiazine," *Journal of Burn Care and Research*, vol. 30, no. 3, pp. 464–470, 2009.

[27] U. Czyewska, J. Konończuk, J. Teul et al., "Verification of chemical composition of commercially available propolis extracts by gas chromatography-mass spectrometry analysis," *Journal of Medicinal Food*, vol. 18, no. 5, pp. 584–591, 2015.

[28] Y. Nakajima, K. Tsuruma, M. Shimazawa, S. Mishima, and H. Hara, "Comparison of bee products based on assays of antioxidant capacities," *BMC Complementary and Alternative Medicine*, vol. 9, article 4, 2009.

[29] V. Jayarama Reddy, S. Radhakrishnan, R. Ravichandran et al., "Nanofibrous structured biomimetic strategies for skin tissue regeneration," *Wound Repair and Regeneration*, vol. 21, no. 1, pp. 1–16, 2013.

[30] P. Olczyk, I. Wróblewska-Adamek, J. Stojko, K. Komosińska-Vassev, and K. Olczyk, "Histopathological evaluation of Propol-T and silver sulfadiazine therapeutic efficacy in burn healing," *Farmacja Polska*, vol. 63, no. 24, pp. 1108–1116, 2007.

[31] Ż. Jastrzębska-Stojko, R. Stojko, A. Rzepecka-Stojko, A. Kabała-Dzik, and J. Stojko, "Biological activity of propolis-honey balm in the treatment of experimentally-evoked burn wounds," *Molecules*, vol. 18, no. 11, pp. 14397–14413, 2013.

[32] A. Kabała-Dzik, E. Szaflarska-Stojko, R. D. Wojtyczka et al., "Efficiency assessment of antimicrobial activity of honey-balm

on experimental burn wounds," *Bulletin of the Veterinary Institute in Pulawy*, vol. 48, no. 2, pp. 109–112, 2004.

[33] M. Morais, L. Moreira, X. Feás, and L. M. Estevinho, "Honey-bee-collected pollen from five Portuguese Natural Parks: Palynological origin, phenolic content, antioxidant properties and antimicrobial activity," *Food and Chemical Toxicology*, vol. 49, no. 5, pp. 1096–1101, 2011.

[34] A. Rzepecka-Stojko, J. Stojko, A. Kurek-Górecka et al., "Polyphenols from bee pollen: structure, absorption, metabolism and biological activity," *Molecules*, vol. 20, no. 12, pp. 21732–21749, 2015.

[35] N. B. Takaisi-Kikuni and H. Schilcher, "Electron microscopic and microcalorimetric investigations of the possible mechanism of the antibacterial action of a defined propolis provenance," *Planta Medica*, vol. 60, no. 3, pp. 222–227, 1994.

# 10

# A Herbal Formula, CGXII, Exerts Antihepatofibrotic Effect in Dimethylnitrosamine-Induced SD Rat Model

**Hyo-Seon Kim,[1] Hyeong-Geug Kim,[1] Hye-Won Lee,[2] Sung-Bae Lee,[1] Jin-Seok Lee,[1] Hwi-Jin Im,[1] Won-Yong Kim,[1] Dong-Soo Lee,[3] and Chang-Gue Son[1]**

[1]Liver and Immunology Research Center, Daejeon Oriental Hospital, Oriental Medical College, Daejeon University, 176-9 Daeheung-ro, Jung-gu, Daejeon 34929, Republic of Korea
[2]TKM-Based Herbal Drug Research Group, Korea Institute of Oriental Medicine, Daejeon 34054, Republic of Korea
[3]Department of Internal Medicine, Daejeon St. Mary's Hospital, The Catholic University of Korea, 64 Daeheung-ro, Jung-gu, Daejeon 34943, Republic of Korea

Correspondence should be addressed to Chang-Gue Son; ckson@dju.ac.kr

Academic Editor: Xiao-Yan Wen

We aimed to evaluate the antihepatofibrotic effects of CGXII, an aqueous extract which is composed of *A. iwayomogi*, *A. xanthioides*, and *S. miltiorrhiza*, against dimethylnitrosamine- (DMN-) induced hepatofibrosis. Male Sprague Dawley rats were intraperitoneally injected with 10 mg/kg of DMN for 4 weeks (three consecutive days weekly). Rats were orally given distilled water, CGXII (50 or 100 mg/kg), or dimethyl dimethoxy biphenyl dicarboxylate (50 mg/kg) daily. DMN injection caused substantial alteration of total body weight and liver and spleen mass, whereas they were notably normalized by CGXII. CGXII treatment also markedly attenuated the elevation of serum aspartate aminotransferase and alanine aminotransferase levels, hepatic lipid peroxidation, and protein carbonyl contents. Collagen accumulation in hepatic tissue evidenced by histopathological analysis and quantitative assessment of hepatic hydroxyproline was ameliorated by CGXII. Immunohistochemistry analysis revealed decreased $\alpha$-smooth muscle actin supporting the antihepatofibrotic effect of CGXII. The profibrogenic cytokines transforming growth factor-$\beta$, platelet-derived growth factor-$\beta$, and connective tissue growth factor were increased by DMN injection. Administration of CGXII normalized the protein and gene expression levels of these cytokines. Our findings suggest that CGXII lowers the levels of profibrogenic cytokines and thereby exerts antifibrotic effects.

## 1. Introduction

Hepatic fibrosis is the critical step in the progression of chronic liver disease because it determines the clinical outcome to recovery or progression to liver cirrhosis or hepatocellular carcinoma [1]. Hepatic fibrosis is a common wound healing response to chronic liver injuries, including hepatitis viral infections, toxic agent invasions, and alcohol abuse [2–4]. In hepatic fibrosis, hepatic stellate cells (HSCs) can form excessive extracellular matrix (ECM) that includes collagen and $\alpha$-SMA [5]. Additionally, continuous HSC activation leads to myofibroblast transition via the release of profibrogenic cytokines including transforming growth factor (TGF)-$\beta$, platelet-derived growth factor (PDGF)-$\beta$, and

connective tissue growth factor (CTGF) [6, 7]. Thus, the HSC activations mainly affect the therapeutics response to liver fibrosis.

Despite many efforts to elucidate the pathophysiology of hepatofibrosis, hitherto no effective treatment or therapeutic drug has been established [8, 9]. Thus, a realistic strategy would be to prevent the underlying disease and inhibit fibrotic progression [10]. Additionally, herbal medicine has been expected to play a role in antihepatofibrosis treatment to improve quality of life (QOL) of patients with chronic liver disorders [11, 12].

To treat hepatofibrosis, various herbal medicines have been prescribed for thousands of years in clinical practice. The *Artemisia iwayomogi* Kitamura, *Amomum xanthioides*

Wallich, and *Salvia miltiorrhiza* Bunge have been most frequently used to treat especially the chronic liver diseases, due to their efficacies. According to the Traditional Oriental Medicine (TOM) theory, hepatofibrosis is generally attributed to impairment of two critical liver functions: metabolic activities and blood homeostasis [13, 14]. The abovementioned three herbal plants have demonstrated pharmacological efficacies using the animal-based pathophysiological conditions of "*dampness and Phlegm*" [15], "*stagnation of vital energy*" [16], and "*blood stasis*" [17], respectively. Based on data from clinical practice and animal-based studies, the CGXII mixture used in these experiments was a water extract mixture of *A. iwayomogi, A. xanthioides,* and *S. miltiorrhiza* prepared at an equal ratio [18, 19].

In order to support the clinical relevance of CGXII, we adapted a DMN-induced hepatofibrosis rat model and used dimethyl biphenyl dicarboxylate (DDB) as a reference compound, which is well known to be potent antihepatotherapeutics [20, 21]. We herein evaluated the antihepatofibrotic properties of CGXII and explored its underlying mechanisms responsible for the action of CGXII.

## 2. Materials and Methods

*2.1. Reagents and Chemicals.* Dimethylnitrosamine (N-nitrosodimethylamine or DMN), 1,1,3,3-tetraethoxypropane (TEP), chloramine-T, *p*-dimethylaminobenzaldehyde, hydroxyproline, potassium chloride (KCl), and trichloroacetic acid (TCA) were purchased from Sigma (St. Louis, MO, United States); Thiobarbituric acid (TBA) was purchased from Lancaster Co. (Lancashire, United Kingdom). Hydrochloric acid and phosphoric acid were from Kanto Chemical Co., Inc. (Tokyo, Japan); *n*-butanol was purchased from J. T. Baker (Center Valley, PA, United States); Mayer's haematoxylin and isopropanol were obtained from Wako Pure Chemical Industries (Osaka, Japan); Goat anti-human connective tissue growth factor (CTGF) antibody, CTFG standard solution, rabbit anti-human CTGF antibody, and anti-rabbit immunoglobulin G horseradish peroxidase conjugate were purchased from Santa Cruz Biotechnology (Santa Cruz, CA, United States), and DDB was purchased from Pharma King Co., Ltd. (Gyeonggi-do, Republic of Korea).

*2.2. Preparation of CGXII and Its Fingerprinting Analysis.* A. *iwayomogi, A. xanthioides,* and *S. miltiorrhiza* were obtained from the Jeong-Seong Oriental Medicine Company (Daejeon, Republic of Korea). Briefly, 100 g of each of the three fully dried herbs was mixed and boiled separately in distilled water for 90 minutes and concentrated nonstop for 120 minutes. After filtration and lyophilization, the extracts were stored at −70°C until use. The final yield of water extraction was 9.58%.

The reference standard stock solutions of quercitrin, quercetin-dehydrate, rosmarinic acid, salvianolic acid B, scopoletin, and tanshinone IIA (each component was dissolved at 250 μg/mL in 90% methanol) were prepared in methanol and stored at −4°C. The standard solutions were prepared using six concentrations of diluted solutions. All calibration curves were made by assessing the peak areas in

the range of 2.5–500 μg/mL. The linearity of the peak area ($y$) versus concentration ($x$, μg/mL) curve for each component was used to calculate the contents of the main components in CGXII.

A quantitative analysis was performed under the simultaneous conditions using an 1100 series high-performance liquid chromatography (HPLC, Agilent Technologies, Santa Clara, CA) equipped with an autosampler (G11313A), column oven (GA1316A), binary pump (G1312), diode-array-detector (G1315B), and degasser (G1379A). The analytical column with a Kinetex C18 (4.6 × 250 nm, particle size 5 μm, Phenomenex, Torrance, CA) was kept at 30°C during the experiment. The data were acquired and processed by ChemStation software (Agilent Technologies, USA). The mobile phase conditions contained 10% acetonitrile in distilled water (DW) with 0.05% formic acid (A) and 90% acetonitrile in water (B). The gradient flow was as follows: 0–30 min, 0%–20% B; 30–50 min, 20%–75% B; 50–60 min, 75%–100% B. The analysis was operated at a flow rate of 1.0 mL/min and detected at 280 nm. The injection volume was 10 μL.

*2.3. Animals and Experimental Schedule.* The design and performance of the experiments were approved by the Institutional Animal Care and Use Committee of Daejeon University (DJUARB2015-006) and conducted in accordance with the Policy on the Humane Care and Use of Laboratory Animals, as adopted and promulgated by the US National Institute of Health (NIH).

A total of 30 heads of specific pathogen-free SD rats (6-week-old, 190–210 g) were purchased from Daehan-Biolink (Chungbuk, Republic of Korea) and housed in a controlled temperature room at 22 ± 2°C, 55% ± 10% relative humidity, 12-hour light/dark cycles, and freely fed commercial pellets (Daehan-Biolink, Chungbuk, Republic of Korea) and tap water *ad libitum* for 7 days. After acclimation, rats were randomly divided into the following 5 groups ($n = 6$ for each group): normal (DW without DMN injection), DMN (DW with DMN injection), CGXII 50 or 100 (CGXII 50 or 100 mg/kg with DMN injection), and DDB 50 (DDB 50 mg/kg with DMN injection) groups. All animals were orally given DW, CGXII (50, or 100 mg/kg), or DDB (50 mg/kg) by gastric gavage once daily for 4 weeks. The DMN was intraperitoneally injected on three consecutive days per week for 4 weeks (10 mg/kg, dissolved in neutral saline), except for the normal group. The normal group was intraperitoneally injected with neutral saline. The body weights were recorded twice weekly during the experiment. On the final experimental day after 12 hours of fasting, all of the rats were weighed and sacrificed under ether anesthesia. Whole blood was isolated from the abdominal aorta using syringes for biochemical analyses. The livers and spleens were removed, immediately weighed, and photographed. Liver tissues were either fixed in 10% formalin solution for histopathological examination or RNA later solution or stored at −70°C for gene expression analysis and biochemical analysis, respectively.

*2.4. Complete Blood Count and Serum Biochemical Analysis.* Blood was collected from the abdominal aorta on the final day of experiment. After centrifuging at 3000 ×g for 15 min, the serum was separated and stored at $-70°C$. The serum levels of total bilirubin, aspartate transaminase (AST), and alanine transaminase (ALT) were determined using an Auto Chemistry Analyzer (AU400, Olympus, Tokyo, Japan).

### 2.5. Histomorphological Analysis and Immunohistochemical Staining.
For the histomorphological evaluations, a portion of liver tissue was fixed in 10% formalin solution and embedded in paraffin. The paraffin-embedded liver was sectioned (5 $\mu$m thickness), deparaffinized, hydrated, and stained for hematoxylin & eosin (H&E) staining. Masson's trichrome staining was performed to distinguish cells from surrounding connective tissue.

For immunohistochemical staining of $\alpha$-smooth muscle actin ($\alpha$-SMA), liver tissue sections were deparaffinized, hydrated, and heated in antibody specific retrieval buffer (1 mM EDTA in 0.05% Tween 20) at $100°C$ for 5 min and then treated with goat serum for 30 min. The slides were then incubated overnight with an anti-$\alpha$-SMA mouse monoclonal antibody (1:250, Abcam, Cambridge, UK) and incubated overnight. After washing with tap water, Histofine (Nichirei Biosciences, Tokyo, Japan) was added using TMB as a substrate. The slides were examined under an optical microscope (100x magnifications, Leica Microsystems, Wetzlar, Germany).

These histopathologic changes for inflammation were scored on a scale of 0 to 3, specifically 0 for normal state (<5% pathological changes), 1 for mild (<10%), 2 for moderate (15%–20%), and 3 for severe (>20%) [22]. A METAVIR fibrosis score from 0 to 4 was used to differentiate the levels of liver fibrosis. Briefly, stage 0 refers to no scarring, stage 1 to minimal scarring, stage 2 to scarring in other areas containing blood vessels than the liver, stage 3 to bridging fibrosis spread to other fibrotic areas, and stage 4 to advanced scarring of the liver or cirrhosis [23]. The percentage areas of positive $\alpha$-SMA staining cells were analyzed by the image analysis program, ImageJ 1.46 software (Rasband, Bethesda, MD, USA).

### 2.6. Determination of Hydroxyproline, Lipid Peroxidation, and Protein Carbonyl in Liver Tissues.
Hydroxyproline assays were performed as previously described with a slight modification [24]. Briefly, liver tissue (0.2 g) stored at $-70°C$ was homogenized in 2 mL of 6 N HCl and incubated overnight at $110°C$. After filtering the acid hydrolysates using filtering paper (Toyo Roshi Kaisha, Tokyo, Japan), 50 $\mu$L of samples and standards was incubated to completely evaporate the HCl. Then 50 $\mu$L of methanol and 1.2 mL of 50% of isopropanol were added after incubation, and 200 $\mu$L of chloramine-T solution was sequentially added to the samples. After further incubation at room temperature for 10 min, 1.3 mL of Ehrlich's solution was added to the mixture which was incubated at $50°C$ for 90 min. At the end of the incubation, the absorbance of the reaction mixtures was determined at 558 nm. A standard curve was constructed using 0–1.0 mg/50 $\mu$L of hydroxyproline solution.

Lipid peroxidation levels were evaluated by the thiobarbituric acid reactive substances (TBARS) method, as described previously [25]. Briefly, liver tissue (200 mg) was homogenized in ice-cold KCl (1.15%), and the homogenate

was mixed with 1% $H_3PO_4$ and 0.67% TBA solution. The mixture was heated for 45 min at $100°C$, $n$-butanol was added, and the solution was then mixed and centrifuged at 3000 $\times$g for 15 min. The absorbance of the supernatant was measured at 535 and 520 nm and compared to a standard value (freshly prepared TEP solution).

Hepatic protein carbonyl content was determined by detecting protein oxidation using the DNPH reaction, according to the previously described method [26]. Briefly, the liver tissue homogenate was prepared with cold phosphate buffer (50 mM, pH 6.7, containing 1 mM EDTA), and 200 $\mu$L of the homogenate was mixed with 800 $\mu$L of DNPH (10 mM dissolved in 2.5 M HCl). After incubation in the dark at room temperature for 1 h with vortexing every 15 min followed by the sequential addition of 1 mL of 20% TCA and 10% TCA and incubation for 5 min at $4°C$, a pellet was obtained by centrifugation at 10,000 $\times$g for 10 min at $4°C$. After resuspension in 1 mL of an ethanol/ethyl acetate mixture (1:1, v/v) and centrifugation, the protein pellets were re-suspended in 500 $\mu$L of guanidine hydrochloride by vortexing and centrifugation at 10,000 $\times$g for 10 min at $4°C$. Then, 220 $\mu$L of the supernatants were transferred to a 96-well plate. The absorbance was measured at 370 nm with a spectrophotometer (Molecular Device Corp).

### 2.7. Determination of Profibrogenic Cytokines and Tissue Inhibitor of Metalloproteinase-1 (TIMP-1).
Transforming growth factor-beta1 (TGF-$\beta$1), platelet-derived growth factor-BB (PDGF-BB), and TIMP-1 levels in the liver tissues were measured using commercial ELISA kits (R&D Systems, Minneapolis, MN). We also manually measured the level of CTGF in hepatic tissues. Briefly, after coating 96-well plates with goat anti-human CTGF antibody, the plates were incubated with blocking buffer (10 mM PBS with sodium azide and 1% bovine albumin) for 1 h at room temperature. Then, 100 $\mu$L of diluted homogenate samples and CTFG standard solution were added to the plates, followed by incubation for 1 h at room temperature. After binding of rabbit anti-human CTGF (100 $\mu$L, 2 $\mu$g/mL), 50 $\mu$L of anti-rabbit IgG-HRP was added to each well, and incubation was continued for 1 h. To each well, 100 $\mu$L of substrate solution was added and incubated for 20 min, followed by the addition of 50 $\mu$L stop solution. The absorbance at 405 nm was read within 15 min. All antibodies used for the measurement of CTGF were purchased from Santa Cruz Biotechnology.

### 2.8. Real-Time PCR for Analyzing Gene Expression in Liver Tissues.
Total RNA was extracted from liver tissue samples using the reagent Trizol (Molecular Research Center, Cincinnati, OH, USA). cDNA was synthesized from total RNA (2 $\mu$g) in a 20 $\mu$L reaction using the High-Capacity cDNA reverse transcription kit (Ambion, Austin, TX, USA). Real-time PCR was performed using SYBR Green PCR Master Mix (Applied Biosystems, Foster City, CA, USA) with PCR amplification performed in accordance with a standard protocol using the IQ5 PCR Thermal Cycler (Bio-Rad, Hercules, CA, USA). The primer sequences used were the following (shown $5' \rightarrow 3'$): for $\beta$-actin, AGG CCA ACC GTG AAA AGA TG and CCA GAG GCA TAC AGG GAC AAC; for

TGF-$\beta$1, AGC AGG AAG GGT CGG TTC AT and AGG AGA CGG AAT ACA GGG CTT T; for PDGF-BB, TGT GCT CGG GTC ATG TTC AA and ACC ACT CCA TCC GCT CCT TT; for CTGF, CAG TTG GCT CGC ATC ATA GTT G and GTG TGT GAT GAG CCC AAG GA; for collagen type 1 alpha (Col 1a1), GAT CCT GCC GAT GTC GCT AT and TGT AGG CTA CGC TGT TCT TGC A; for tissue inhibitor of metalloproteinase-1 (TIMP-1), ATG GAG AGC CTC TGT GGA TAT GTC and AGG CAG TGA TGT GCA AAT TTC C; for matrix metalloproteinase-2 (MMP-2), TGT GGC AGC CCA TGA GTT C and TCG GAA GTT CTT GGT GTA GGT GTA; for bone morphogenetic proteins and activating membrane-bound inhibitor (BAMBI), TTA TGT TGG CCT TGC GAA TG and TGG TGT CCA TGG AAG CTG TAG T; for Smad 7, TGC AAC CCC CAT CAC CTT AG and GAC AGT CTG CAG TTG GTT TGA GA. The final results are expressed as normalized fold values relative to the normal group.

*2.9. Statistical Analysis.* All data are expressed as the mean ± standard deviation (SD). Statistically significant differences between the groups were analyzed by one-way analysis of variance (ANOVA) followed by *post hoc* multiple comparison Fisher's least-significant difference (LSD) test using IBM SPSS version 20.0 (SPSS Inc. Chicago, IL, USA). Differences with $p < 0.05$, $p < 0.01$, or $p < 0.001$ were considered statistically significant.

# 3. Results

*3.1. Fingerprinting Analysis of CGXII.* The chemical constitutions of each individual herbal plant from the CGXII were evaluated using HPLC analysis. A total of six components, including scopoletin (in *A. iwayomogi*); quercitrin and quercetin dehydrate (in *A. xanthioides*); rosmarinic acid, salvianolic acid B, and tanshinone IIA (in *S. miltiorrhiza*), were observed in CGXII (Figures 1(a) and 1(b)). According to the results from the quantitative analysis, salvianolic acid, which is the most well-known reference compound, was most abundant in GGXII at 14.8 minutes of retention time (Figure 1(a)). The other compounds were detected at the following retention times: 12.7 min (scopoletin), 8.8 min (quercitrin), 16.8 min (quercetin dehydrate), 13.6 min (rosmarinic acid), and 37.2 min (tanshinone IIA) (Figure 1(b)). These chemical components ranged from 0.46 to 12.80 $\mu g/g$ (Table 1).

*3.2. Effects on the Total Body and Organ Weights.* DMN injection markedly lowered total body weights by 0.8-fold compared to that of the control group, and administration of CGXII did not normalize body weight. Absolute liver weight was not altered by DMN alone or DMN with CGXII treatment, but relative liver weight was notably increased in the DMN group compared with that of the normal group (approximately by 1.3-fold). Treatment with CGXII, particularly 50 mg/kg, significantly attenuated the elevation of relative liver weight ($p < 0.05$, Table 2). The DMN group also demonstrated considerable increases in absolute and relative spleen weights, compared with those of the normal group.

TABLE 1: The quantitative analysis of each component in CGXII.

| Compounds | RT (min) | Mean ± SD ($\mu g/mg$) |
|---|---|---|
| Quercitrin | 8.8 | 16.16 ± 0.11 |
| Scopoletin | 12.7 | 10.97 ± 0.04 |
| Rosmarinic acid | 13.6 | 5.63 ± 0.04 |
| Salvianolic acid B | 14.8 | 12.8 ± 0.09 |
| Quercetin dihydrate | 16.8 | 0.71 ± 0.02 |
| Tanshinone II A | 37.2 | 0.46 ± 0.01 |

Treatment with CGXII did not affect the weight changes produced by DMN. DDB (50 mg/kg) efficiently recovered the total body weights but not others.

*3.3. Effects on the Liver Enzymes and Platelet Counts.* DMN injection strikingly increased serum AST and ALT by approximately 9.6- and 18.3-fold compared with those of the normal group. Treatment with CGXII significantly attenuated the elevations of serum AST and ALT levels compared with those of the DMN group ($p < 0.05$ for 100 mg/kg in AST and ALT, Table 2). The platelet counts were markedly depleted by approximately 0.2-fold by DMN injection compared with those of the normal group, and CGXII did not affect them. DDB demonstrated a similar effect as CGXII platelet counts but showed the superior efficacy on both serum AST and ALT level.

*3.4. Effects on Histopathological Findings.* The effects of CGXII on DMN injection-induced chronic hepatic injury were evaluated by histopathological examination of hepatic tissue using H&E staining. DMN injection resulted in a striking formation of bridging necrosis, inflammation, and wide infiltration of inflammatory cells around central veins, whereas CGXII significantly ameliorated this response ($p < 0.05$ for 50 and $p < 0.001$ for 100 mg/kg, Figures 2(a) and 2(d)). Masson's trichrome staining was performed to visualize collagen deposition in hepatic tissue. In the DMN group, substantial fibrotic change (blue staining) was shown, whereas both CGXII treatments significantly inhibited collagen accumulation in hepatic tissues ($p < 0.05$ for 50 and $p < 0.001$ for 100 mg/kg, Figures 2(b) and 2(e)). To investigate HSC activation, $\alpha$-SMA level was analyzed by immunohistochemistry. The $\alpha$-SMA signal (brown staining) was strongly enhanced by DMN injection; this effect was reduced by CGXII administration ($p < 0.001$ for 50 and 100 mg/kg, Figures 2(c) and 2(f)). DDB treatment also moderately attenuated these morphological alterations.

*3.5. Effects on Hydroxyproline, Lipid Peroxidation, and Protein Carbonyl Content in Liver Tissues.* DMN injection dramatically increased the hepatic level of hydroxyproline (2.1-fold), MDA (2.4-fold), and protein carbonyl (1.9-fold) compared to those in the normal group. Administration of CGXII significantly reduced the hepatic level of hydroxyproline ($p < 0.05$ for 100 mg/kg), MDA ($p < 0.001$ for 50 and 100 mg/kg), and protein carbonyl ($p < 0.05$ for 50 and 100 mg/kg) compared with those of the DMN group (Figure 3). DDB showed

TABLE 2: Body and organ weights, serum biochemistries, and platelet counts.

| Parameter | Normal | DMN | CGXII 50 | CGXII 100 | DDB 50 |
|---|---|---|---|---|---|
| Body weight (g) | 334.8 ± 18.0 | 259.8 ± 23.7[###] | 270.3 ± 9.0 | 271.3 ± 19.4 | 286.2 ± 7.7[*] |
| Liver weight (g) | 10.2 ± 1.0 | 9.6 ± 1.7 | 9.1 ± 1.1 | 10.3 ± 0.9 | 11.1 ± 1.1 |
| Relative liver weight (%) | 3.0 ± 0.3 | 4.0 ± 0.3[##] | 3.3 ± 0.4[*] | 3.3 ± 1.0 | 3.5 ± 0.4 |
| Spleen weight (g) | 0.8 ± 0.1 | 1.5 ± 0.2[###] | 1.7 ± 0.1 | 1.7 ± 0.3 | 1.7 ± 0.2 |
| Relative spleen weight (%) | 0.2 ± 0.01 | 0.6 ± 0.09[###] | 0.6 ± 0.05 | 0.7 ± 0.11 | 0.6 ± 0.07 |
| AST (IU/dL) | 173.3 ± 24.2 | 2180 ± 1983.2[##] | 1061.6 ± 741.6 | 853.3 ± 359.5[*] | 481.6 ± 53.1[**] |
| ALT (IU/dL) | 38.3 ± 21.4 | 885 ± 515.9[###] | 543.3 ± 212.2 | 478 ± 186.4[*] | 235 ± 51.3[***] |
| Total bilirubin (mg/dL) | 0.1 ± 0.0 | 2.2 ± 1.3[###] | 1.1 ± 0.4[**] | 0.8 ± 0.1[**] | 0.6 ± 0.1[***] |
| Platelet (k/$\mu$L) | 933.8 ± 41.2 | 222.8 ± 29.7[###] | 251 ± 82.6 | 260.6 ± 143.2 | 290.3 ± 50.4 |

Following DMN injection, rats were orally given distilled water, CGXII (50 mg and 100 mg/kg), or DDB (50 mg/kg) daily for four weeks. Data are expressed as mean ± SD ($n = 6$). [##]$p < 0.01$ and [###]$p < 0.001$, compared with normal group; [*]$p < 0.05$, [**]$p < 0.01$, and [***]$p < 0.001$, compared with DMN group.

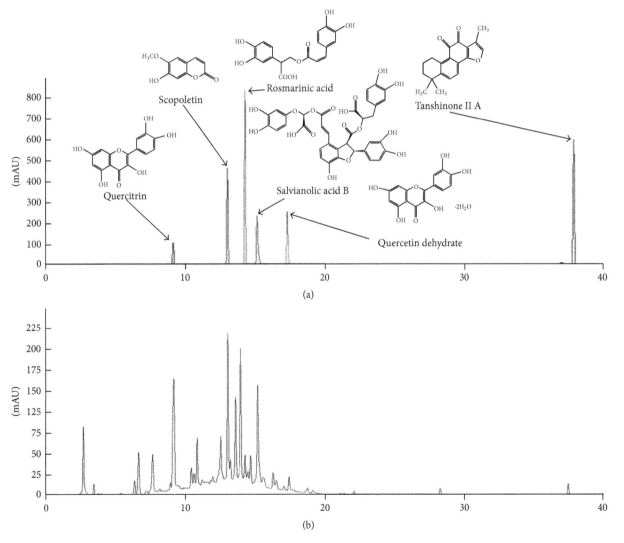

FIGURE 1: Chemical composition analysis based on high-performance liquid chromatography (HPLC). The water extract of CGXII and their standard compounds were subjected to HPLC. Chromatogram of reference compound mixtures (a) and CGXII (b). See Table 1.

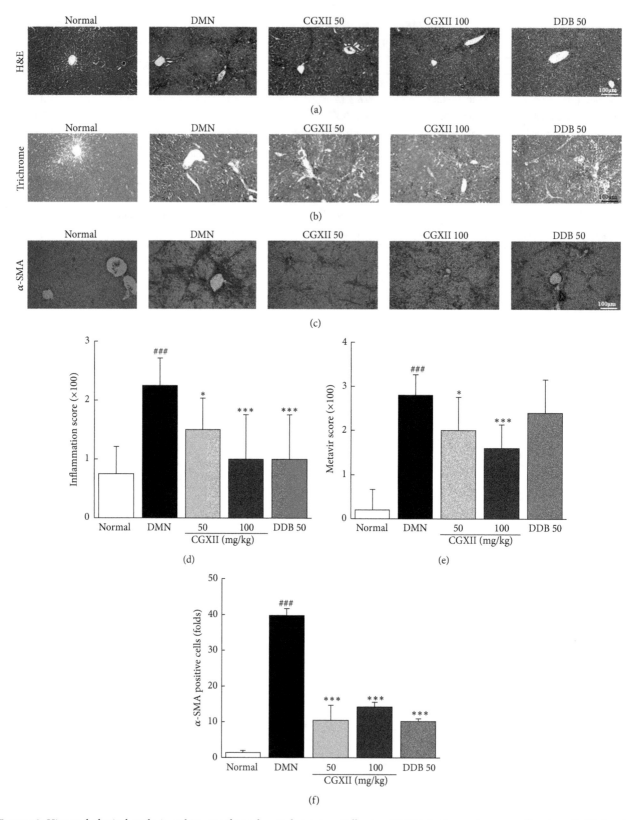

FIGURE 2: Histopathological analysis and immunohistochemical staining. Following DMN injection, rats were orally given distilled water, CGXII (50 mg and 100 mg/kg), or DDB (50 mg/kg) daily for 4 weeks. The liver tissues were examined using hematoxylin and eosin (a), Masson's trichrome (b), and immunohistochemistry for $\alpha$-SMA (c); pathophysiologic examinations were performed under light microscopy (100x magnification). The inflammation scores (d), METAVIR scores (e), and the $\alpha$-SMA positive cells (f) were analyzed. Data are expressed as the mean ± SD ($n = 6$). ### $p < 0.001$, compared with the normal group; * $p < 0.05$ and *** $p < 0.001$, compared with the DMN group.

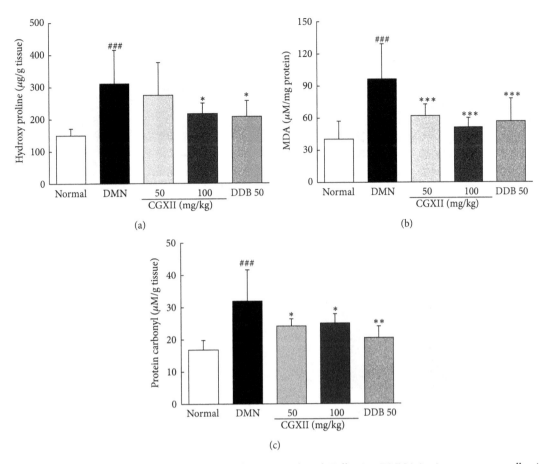

FIGURE 3: Contents of hydroxyproline, malondialdehyde, and protein carbonyl. Following DMN injection, rats were orally given distilled water, CGXII (50 mg and 100 mg/kg), or DDB (50 mg/kg) daily for 4 weeks. Hydroxyproline (a), malondialdehyde (MDA) (b), and protein carbonyl (c) content in the liver tissues. Data are expressed as the mean ± SD ($n = 6$). $^{###}p < 0.001$, compared with the normal group; $^{*}p < 0.05$, $^{**}p < 0.01$, and $^{***}p < 0.001$, compared with the DMN group.

an analogous effect on the levels of hydroxyproline, MDA, and protein carbonyl content (Figure 3).

### 3.6. Effects on the Protein Levels of Profibrogenic Cytokines and TIMP-1 in the Liver Tissues.
DMN injection substantially increased TGF-$\beta$1 by 10.0-fold compared with that of the normal group, whereas this abnormal elevation was significantly ameliorated by administration of CGXII ($p < 0.001$ for 50 and 100 mg/kg, Figure 4(a)). The DMN group showed remarkable increases in PDGF-BB of approximately 3.4-fold compared with that of the normal group, whereas CGXII significantly decreased the levels of PDGF-BB ($p < 0.01$ for 50 and 100 mg/kg, Figure 4(b)). Following the DMN injection both CTGF and TIMP-1 increased by approximately 1.7- and 13.6-fold, respectively, compared to the control group. Administration of CGXII did not significantly affect the levels of CTGF and TIMP-1. Administration with DDB also effectively improved the protein levels of TGF-$\beta$1, CTGF, and TIMP-1, but not PDGF-BB.

### 3.7. Effects on Fibrosis and Antifibrosis Related Gene Expression Analysis.
The gene expression levels of fibrogenic molecules including TGF-$\beta$1, PDGF-BB, CTGF, Col 1a1, and TIMP-1

were, respectively, higher in DMN group by 1.8-, 2.1-, 4.1-, and 1.8-fold compared with the levels of the normal group. The ECM turnover related molecules such as TIMP-1 and MMP-2 were markedly altered by DMN injection (6.0-fold higher in TIMP-1 and 2.5-fold higher in MMP-2 than that of the normal group). The antihepatofibrosis related molecules such as BAMBI and Smad7 showed remarkable downregulation by approximately 0.5- and 0.3-fold compared with those of the normal group. Administration of CGXII, however, significantly normalized TGF-$\beta$1, PDGF-BB, and BAMBI compared with those of the DMN group ($p < 0.001$ for 100 mg/kg in TGF-$\beta$1 and PDGF-BB, $p < 0.01$ for 50 mg/kg, and $p < 0.05$ for 100 mg/kg in BAMBI, Figures 5(a) and 5(b)). Administration with DDB also normalized the abnormal gene expression levels of TGF-$\beta$1, PDGF-BB, and BAMBI.

## 4. Discussion

Hepatofibrosis is a medical issue of great concern [27]. The social costs of treating hepatic fibrosis or cirrhosis have also steadily increased each year. The pathological mechanisms of hepatic fibrosis are unclear. Previously, many groups have made efforts to develop antihepatofibrosis agents, such as

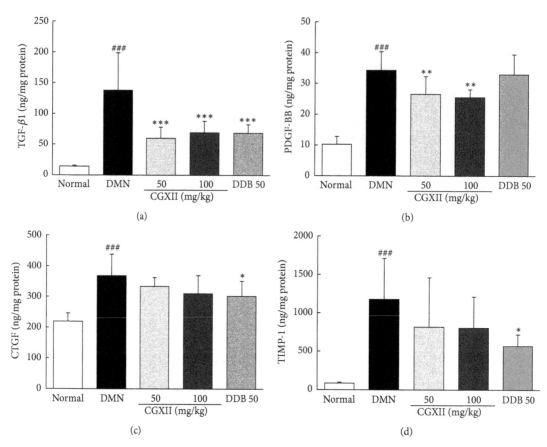

FIGURE 4: Determination of profibrogenic cytokines and TIMP-1. Following DMN injection, rats were orally given distilled water, CGXII (50 mg and 100 mg/kg), or DDB (50 mg/kg) daily for 4 weeks. Quantitative analysis of TGF-$\beta$1 (a), PDGF-BB (b), CTGF (c), and TIMP-1 (d) was performed in the liver tissues using ELISA kits. Data are expressed as the mean ± SD ($n = 6$). $^{\#\#\#}p < 0.001$, compared with the normal group; $^{*}p < 0.05$, $^{**}p < 0.01$, and $^{***}p < 0.001$, compared with the DMN group.

anti-TNF-$\alpha$ and UDCA [28, 29]; however no therapies have been approved. As a potential resource for therapies for hepatofibrosis, various herbal medicines have recently been suggested [30, 31].

Here, we aimed to determine the antifibrotic properties of CGXII in a chronic DMN-induced hepatofibrosis rat model. DMN has been widely used as an experimental model to study liver fibrosis [32, 33]. In our study, the DMN injection led to striking total body weight loss and increased the relative liver mass and spleen mass. The CGXII treatment resulted in a pattern of improvement with regard to these alterations, but no statistical significance was found except for relative liver mass (Table 2). One case of severe ascites (grade of 3) was observed in the DMN group but not in other groups (data not shown). The repeated DMN injection led to considerable hepatocyte destruction and inflammation, as evidenced by abnormal elevation of serum AST and ALT levels. These results were consistent with the histology findings, including inflamed cell infiltrations and necrotic cell bodies (Table 2 and Figures 2(a) and 2(d)). Additionally, total bilirubin in the serum level was elevated by 22-fold, and blood platelet counts were drastically depleted in the DMN group. The above alterations were significantly attenuated by CGXII (no statistically significant result in platelet count) in

both histopathological findings and serum levels of hepatic enzymes analysis.

As we predicted, four-week DMN injections induced a moderate degree of hepatic fibrosis, with an average 2.8 METAVIR fibrosis scores as evidenced by Masson's trichrome staining (Figures 2(b) and 2(e)). This result is consistent with approximately 2-fold elevation in hydroxyproline content observed in the study (Figure 3(a)). Administration of CGXII significantly attenuated the changes in histopathology and the level of hepatic hydroxyproline induced by DMN. The CGXII treatment also improved the oxidative end product of lipid peroxidation determined by MDA, as well as the protein carbonyl content in hepatic tissues (Figures 3(b) and 3(c)). Oxidative stress is thought to participate in the pathological changes of hepatic fibrosis via continuous damage of hepatocytes [34, 35].

In the progression of hepatic fibrosis, HSCs play critical roles in producing ECM. TGF-$\beta$, PDGF-$\beta$, and CTGF, as profibrogenic cytokines, are known to be humoral factors that activate and stimulate the proliferation of HSCs, leading to excessive accumulation of ECM [36]. Accordingly, these cytokines are critical indicators of the pathogenesis of hepatic fibrosis [37]. DMN markedly activated HSCs as shown by immunohistochemistry staining of $\alpha$-SMA, which is a potent

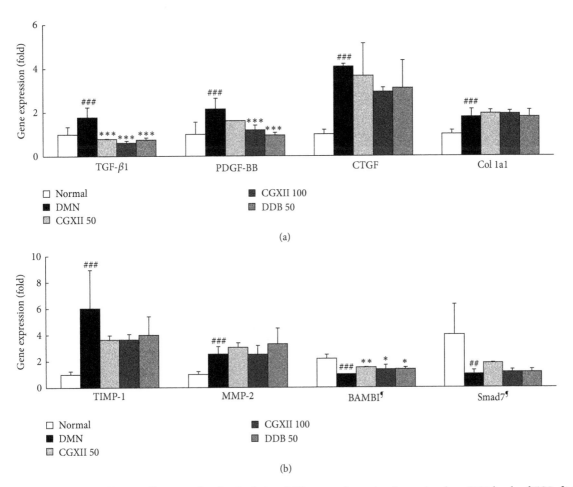

FIGURE 5: mRNA expression of hepatic fibrosis molecules. Real-time PCR was performed to determine the mRNA levels of TGB-$\beta$1, PDGF-BB, CTGF, Col 1a1 and TIMP-1, MMP-2 and BAMBI, and Smad7 in hepatic tissues. Expression was normalized as a ratio to $\beta$-actin. Data are expressed as the mean $\pm$ SD ($n = 6$). [##] $p < 0.01$ and [###] $p < 0.001$, compared with the normal group. [*] $p < 0.05$, [**] $p < 0.01$, and [***] $p < 0.001$, compared with the DMN group. [§] Both BAMBI and Smad7 were normalized in the DMN group, and the others were expressed as fold changes, which were normalized in the normal group.

marker of ECM, whereas CGXII opposed this action (Figures 2(c) and 2(f)). In our study, these three profibrogenic cytokines substantially increased both their protein and their mRNA expression levels in hepatic tissues in the DMN group; however these changes were significantly normalized, especially for TGF-$\beta$, in response to CGXII treatment (Figures 4(a)–4(c) and 5(a)). TGF-$\beta$, which leads to direct or indirect activation of HSCs, mainly induces the expression of PDGF-$\beta$ and CTGF receptors [38]. Our results well demonstrated strikingly elevated protein levels of hepatic TGF-$\beta$, which plays a central role in hepatic fibrosis. PDGF-$\beta$ is known to be a potent mitogen or activator of HSCs [39] and CTGF acts as a mediator of TGF-$\beta$-induced ECM formation in hepatic tissues in the progression of hepatic fibrosis [40]. TGF-$\beta$ levels were greatly modulated by CGXII treatment, as compared with the response of the other two cytokines.

Additionally, activation of HSCs resulted in upregulation of collagen 1a1 mRNA in hepatic tissue. This event was not reversed by administration of CGXII (Figure 5(a)). BAMBI and Smad7 are well-known TGF-$\beta$ inhibitors associated with a negative feedback response to TGF-$\beta$ signals [41]. The gene expressions of BAMBI and Smad7 were notably downregulated in the DMN group, but this alteration was attenuated by BAMBI (Figure 5(b)). The accumulation of hepatic collagen is the consequence of an unbalance between excessive production and reduced degradation of ECM [42]. The ECMs are principally degraded by MMPs, while TIMPs are potent inhibitors of MMPs [43]. In the present study, we therefore explored the protein or mRNA expression level of MMP-2 and TIMP-1. DMN strikingly activated TIMP-1 (protein and gene expression) and upregulated the gene expression of MMP-2, whereas these changes were slightly attenuated by CGXII treatment, although not in a statistically significance manner (Figures 4(d) and 5(b)). The upregulated gene expression of MMP-2 was thought to be a compensatory response to excessive accumulation of ECM.

CGXII is originated from an antihepatofibrotic herbal formula, CGX, which was developed by the TOM theory for treating patients with chronic liver diseases. Additionally, CGX has been widely prescribed at the Oriental Hospital in republic of Korea since 2001, based on the clinical experience and many experimental data [18, 19, 44]. The CGX is composed of thirteen herbs including *A. iwayomogi*, *A. xanthioides*, and *S. miltiorrhiza*. We previously compared the antihepatofibrotic activities of thirteen herbs of CGX with respect to TGF-$\beta$ inhibition using the HSC T-6 cell line [45, 46]. From those experimental data and practical theory of the traditional Korean pharmacology, we finally selected the abovementioned three herbal plants. The synergistic actions of three herbs of CGXII were proved comparing their individual abilities (data not shown). We have showed the six chemical compounds in CGXII; however we still lack knowledge regarding the active ingredient responsible

We have also reported the individual pharmaceutical activities of *A. iwayomogi* and *A. xanthioides* on hepatic injuries including hepatic fibrosis [47, 48]. *S. miltiorrhiza* also affected hepatic fibrosis in an animal study [49]. This study, however, is the first to evaluate their antihepatofibrotic activity as a combination formula of *A. iwayomogi*, *A. xanthioides*, and *S. miltiorrhiza*. Generally, the traditional practices of herbal medicine include mixing multiple medicinal plants. The mixing of herbs has been believed to have higher activity and lower toxicity than individual herb administration, and this effect has been partially proved by a few experimental studies [50–52].

In this study, we used DDB as a positive control. The previous studies reported the antifibrotic effects and antioxidant effects of DDB animal models [20, 21]. The antihepatofibrotic properties of DDB were observed in our study, in which the activity of DDB (50 mg/kg) was roughly similar to CGXII (100 mg/kg).

## 5. Conclusions

Taken together, our findings demonstrated the antihepatofibrotic properties of CGXII in a DMN injection rat model. The underlying mechanisms responsible for the effects may involve the inactivation of HSCs through the regulation of fibrogenic cytokines, especially TGF-$\beta$.

## Competing Interests

The authors declare that there is no conflict of interests.

## Acknowledgments

This study was supported by the Oriental Medicine Research and Development Project, Ministry of Health and Welfare, Republic of Korea no. HI12C-1920-010014.

## References

[1] A. Mallat, J. Lodder, F. Teixeira-Clerc, R. Moreau, P. Codogno, and S. Lotersztajn, "Autophagy: a multifaceted partner in liver fibrosis," *BioMed Research International*, vol. 2014, Article ID 869390, 7 pages, 2014.

[2] M. Friedrich-Rust, K. Wunder, S. Kriener et al., "Liver fibrosis in viral hepatitis: noninvasive assessment with acoustic radiation force impulse imaging versus transient elastography," *Radiology*, vol. 252, no. 2, pp. 595–604, 2009.

[3] B. Raynard, A. Balian, D. Fallik et al., "Risk factors of fibrosis in alcohol-induced liver disease," *Hepatology*, vol. 35, no. 3, pp. 635–638, 2002.

[4] J. B. Dixon, P. S. Bhathal, and P. E. O'Brien, "Nonalcoholic fatty liver disease: predictors of nonalcoholic steatohepatitis and liver fibrosis in the severely obese," *Gastroenterology*, vol. 121, no. 1, pp. 91–100, 2001.

[5] J.-H. Kim, S. Lee, M.-Y. Lee, and H.-K. Shin, "Therapeutic effect of Soshiho-tang, a traditional herbal formula, on liver fibrosis or cirrhosis in animal models: a systematic review and meta-analysis," *Journal of Ethnopharmacology*, vol. 154, no. 1, pp. 1–16, 2014.

[6] S. Tsukada, C. J. Parsons, and R. A. Rippe, "Mechanisms of liver fibrosis," *Clinica Chimica Acta*, vol. 364, no. 1-2, pp. 33–60, 2006.

[7] J.-H. Wang, J.-W. Shin, J.-Y. Son, J.-H. Cho, and C.-G. Son, "Antifibrotic effects of CGX, a traditional herbal formula, and its mechanisms in rats," *Journal of Ethnopharmacology*, vol. 127, no. 2, pp. 534–542, 2010.

[8] F. Li and J.-Y. Wang, "Targeted delivery of drugs for liver fibrosis," *Expert Opinion on Drug Delivery*, vol. 6, no. 5, pp. 531–541, 2009.

[9] J. A. Talwalkar, "Antifibrotic therapies—emerging biomarkers as treatment end points," *Nature Reviews Gastroenterology & Hepatology*, vol. 7, no. 1, pp. 59–61, 2010.

[10] P. Ginès and A. Cárdenas, "The management of ascites and hyponatremia in cirrhosis," *Seminars in Liver Disease*, vol. 28, no. 1, pp. 43–58, 2008.

[11] C. Levy, L. D. Seeff, and K. D. Lindor, "Use of herbal supplements for chronic liver disease," *Clinical Gastroenterology and Hepatology*, vol. 2, no. 11, pp. 947–956, 2004.

[12] J.-Y. Liu, C.-C. Chen, W.-H. Wang, J.-D. Hsu, M.-Y. Yang, and C.-J. Wang, "The protective effects of Hibiscus sabdariffa extract on CCl4-induced liver fibrosis in rats," *Food and Chemical Toxicology*, vol. 44, no. 3, pp. 336–343, 2006.

[13] Donguibogam: Principles and Practice of Eastern Medicine/ United Nations Educational, Scientific and Cultural Organization, http://www.unesco.org/new/en/communication-and-information/flagship-project-activities/memory-of-the-world/register/full-list-of-registered-heritage/registered-heritage-page-2/donguibogam-principles-and-practice-of-eastern-medicine/.

[14] F. Lozano, "Basic theories of traditional chinese medicine," in *Acupuncture for Pain Management*, Y.-C. Lin and E. S.-Z. Hsu, Eds., pp. 13–43, Springer, New York, NY, USA, 2014.

[15] H.-S. Shin, J.-M. Han, H.-G. Kim et al., "Anti-Atherosclerosis and hyperlipidemia effects of herbal mixture, Artemisia iwayomogi Kitamura and Curcuma longa Linne, in apolipoprotein E-deficient mice," *Journal of Ethnopharmacology*, vol. 153, no. 1, pp. 145–150, 2014.

[16] J.-H. Wang, J.-W. Shin, M.-K. Choi, H.-G. Kim, and C.-G. Son, "An herbal fruit, Amomum xanthoides, ameliorates thioacetamide-induced hepatic fibrosis in rat via antioxidative system," *Journal of Ethnopharmacology*, vol. 135, no. 2, pp. 344–350, 2011.

[17] Y. Zhang, Y. Zhang, Y. Xie et al., "Multitargeted inhibition of hepatic fibrosis in chronic iron-overloaded mice by Salvia miltiorrhiza," *Journal of Ethnopharmacology*, vol. 148, no. 2, pp. 671–681, 2013.

[18] H.-G. Kim, J.-M. Han, H.-W. Lee et al., "CGX, a multiple herbal drug, improves cholestatic liver fibrosis in a bile duct ligation-induced rat model," *Journal of Ethnopharmacology*, vol. 145, no. 2, pp. 653–662, 2013.

[19] J.-H. Wang, M.-K. Choi, J.-W. Shin, S.-Y. Hwang, and C.-G. Son, "Antifibrotic effects of *Artemisia capillaris* and *Artemisia iwayomogi* in a carbon tetrachloride-induced chronic hepatic fibrosis animal model," *Journal of Ethnopharmacology*, vol. 140, no. 1, pp. 179–185, 2012.

[20] O. M. E. Abdel-Salam, A. A. Sleem, and F. A. Morsy, "Effects of biphenyldimethyl-dicarboxylate administration alone or combined with silymarin in the $CCL_4$ model of liver fibrosis in rats," *TheScientificWorldJOURNAL*, vol. 7, pp. 1242–1255, 2007.

[21] H. A. El-Beshbishy, "The effect of dimethyl dimethoxy biphenyl dicarboxylate (DDB) against tamoxifen-induced liver injury in rats: DDB use is curative or protective," *Journal of Biochemistry and Molecular Biology*, vol. 38, no. 3, pp. 300–306, 2005.

[22] E. M. Brunt, C. G. Janney, A. M. Di Bisceglie, B. A. Neuschwander-Tetri, and B. R. Bacon, "Nonalcoholic steatohepatitis: a proposal for grading and staging the histological lesions," *American Journal of Gastroenterology*, vol. 94, no. 9, pp. 2467–2474, 1999.

[23] T. Şahin, Z. Begeç, H. İ. Toprak et al., "The effects of dexmedetomidine on liver ischemia-reperfusion injury in rats," *Journal of Surgical Research*, vol. 183, no. 1, pp. 385–390, 2013.

[24] M. Fujita, J. M. Shannon, O. Morikawa, J. Gauldie, N. Hara, and R. J. Mason, "Overexpression of tumor necrosis factor-$\alpha$ diminishes pulmonary fibrosis induced by bleomycin or transforming growth factor-$\beta$," *American Journal of Respiratory Cell and Molecular Biology*, vol. 29, no. 6, pp. 669–676, 2003.

[25] M. Uchiyama and M. Mihara, "Determination of malonaldehyde precursor in tissues by thiobarbituric acid test," *Analytical Biochemistry*, vol. 86, no. 1, pp. 271–278, 1978.

[26] R. L. Levine, J. A. Williams, E. R. Stadtman, and E. Shacter, "Carbonyl assays for determination of oxidatively modified proteins," *Methods in Enzymology*, vol. 233, pp. 346–357, 1994.

[27] R. Lozano, M. Naghavi, K. Foreman et al., "Global and regional mortality from 235 causes of death for 20 age groups in 1990 and 2010: a systematic analysis for the Global Burden of Disease Study 2010," *The Lancet*, vol. 380, no. 9859, pp. 2095–2128, 2012.

[28] I. H. Bahcecioglu, S. S. Koca, O. K. Poyrazoglu et al., "Hepatoprotective effect of infliximab, an anti-TNF-$\alpha$ agent, on carbon tetrachloride-induced hepatic fibrosis," *Inflammation*, vol. 31, no. 4, pp. 215–221, 2008.

[29] N. Mas, I. Tasci, B. Comert, R. Ocal, and M. R. Mas, "Ursodeoxycholic acid treatment improves hepatocyte ultrastructure in rat liver fibrosis," *World Journal of Gastroenterology*, vol. 14, no. 7, pp. 1108–1111, 2008.

[30] G.-Y. Li, H.-Y. Gao, J. Huang, J. Lu, J.-K. Gu, and J.-H. Wang, "Hepatoprotective effect of *Cichorium intybus* L., a traditional Uighur medicine, against carbon tetrachloride-induced hepatic fibrosis in rats," *World Journal of Gastroenterology*, vol. 20, no. 16, pp. 4753–4760, 2014.

[31] S.-C. Chien, W.-C. Chang, P.-H. Lin et al., "A Chinese herbal medicine, Jia-Wei-Xiao-Yao-San, prevents dimethylnitrosamine-induced hepatic fibrosis in rats," *The Scientific World Journal*, vol. 2014, Article ID 217525, 7 pages, 2014.

[32] H. Yasuda, E. Imai, A. Shiota, N. Fujise, T. Morinaga, and K. Higashio, "Antifibrogenic effect of a deletion variant of hepatocyte growth factor on liver fibrosis in rats," *Hepatology*, vol. 24, no. 3, pp. 636–642, 1996.

[33] M. Weerawatanakorn, Y.-L. Lee, C.-Y. Tsai et al., "Protective effect of theaflavin-enriched black tea extracts against dimethylnitrosamine-induced liver fibrosis in rats," *Food and Function*, vol. 6, no. 6, pp. 1832–1840, 2015.

[34] G. Poli, "Pathogenesis of liver fibrosis: role of oxidative stress," *Molecular Aspects of Medicine*, vol. 21, no. 3, pp. 49–98, 2000.

[35] Y. Yamamoto, S. Yamashita, A. Fujisawa, S. Kokura, and T. Yoshikawa, "Oxidative stress in patients with hepatitis, cirrhosis, and hepatoma evaluated by plasma antioxidants," *Biochemical and Biophysical Research Communications*, vol. 247, no. 1, pp. 166–170, 1998.

[36] S. L. Friedman, "Molecular regulation of hepatic fibrosis, an integrated cellular response to tissue injury," *Journal of Biological Chemistry*, vol. 275, no. 4, pp. 2247–2250, 2000.

[37] S. L. Friedman, "Liver fibrosis—from bench to bedside," *Journal of Hepatology*, vol. 38, supplement 1, pp. 38–53, 2003.

[38] D. Black, S. Lyman, T. Qian et al., "Transforming growth factor beta mediates hepatocyte apoptosis through Smad3 generation of reactive oxygen species," *Biochimie*, vol. 89, no. 12, pp. 1464–1473, 2007.

[39] M. Pinzani, "PDGF and signal transduction in hepatic stellate cells," *Frontiers in Bioscience*, vol. 7, pp. d1720–d1726, 2002.

[40] A. Leask and D. J. Abraham, "TGF-$\beta$ signaling and the fibrotic response," *The FASEB Journal*, vol. 18, no. 7, pp. 816–827, 2004.

[41] X. Yan, Z. Lin, F. Chen et al., "Human BAMBI cooperates with Smad7 to inhibit transforming growth factor-$\beta$ signaling," *Journal of Biological Chemistry*, vol. 284, no. 44, pp. 30097–30104, 2009.

[42] T. N. Wight and S. Potter-Perigo, "The extracellular matrix: an active or passive player in fibrosis?" *American Journal of Physiology—Gastrointestinal and Liver Physiology*, vol. 301, no. 6, pp. G950–G955, 2011.

[43] M. Consolo, A. Amoroso, D. A. Spandidos, and M. C. Mazzarino, "Matrix metalloproteinases and their inhibitors as markers of inflammation and fibrosis in chronic liver disease (review)," *International Journal of Molecular Medicine*, vol. 24, no. 2, pp. 143–152, 2009.

[44] J. W. Shin, J. H. Wang, H. G. Kim, H. J. Park, H. S. Bok, and C. G. Son, "CGX, a traditional Korean medicine ameliorates concanavalin A-induced acute liver injury," *Food and Chemical Toxicology*, vol. 48, no. 12, pp. 3308–3315, 2010.

[45] H. G. Kim, J. H. Wang, J. M. Han, S. Y. Hwang, D. S. Lee, and C. G. Son, "Chunggan extract (CGX), a traditional Korean herbal medicine, exerts hepatoprotective effects in a rat model of chronic alcohol consumption," *Phytotherapy Research*, vol. 27, no. 12, pp. 1854–1862, 2013.

[46] H.-G. Kim, J.-M. Kim, J.-M. Han et al., "Chunggan extract, a traditional herbal formula, ameliorated alcohol-induced hepatic injury in rat model," *World Journal of Gastroenterology*, vol. 20, no. 42, pp. 15703–15714, 2014.

[47] J.-M. Han, H.-G. Kim, M.-K. Choi et al., "Aqueous extract of *Artemisia iwayomogi* Kitamura attenuates cholestatic liver fibrosis in a rat model of bile duct ligation," *Food and Chemical Toxicology*, vol. 50, no. 10, pp. 3505–3513, 2012.

[48] J.-H. Wang, J. Wang, M.-K. Choi et al., "Hepatoprotective effect of *Amomum xanthoides* against dimethylnitrosamine-induced sub-chronic liver injury in a rat model," *Pharmaceutical Biology*, vol. 51, no. 7, pp. 930–935, 2013.

[49] T.-Y. Lee, G.-J. Wang, J.-H. Chiu, and H.-C. Lin, "Long-term administration of *Salvia miltiorrhiza* ameliorates carbon tetrachloride-induced hepatic fibrosis in rats," *Journal of Pharmacy and Pharmacology*, vol. 55, no. 11, pp. 1561–1568, 2003.

[50] C.-T. Che, Z. J. Wang, M. S. S. Chow, and C. W. K. Lam, "Herb-herb combination for therapeutic enhancement and advancement: theory, practice and future perspectives," *Molecules*, vol. 18, no. 5, pp. 5125–5141, 2013.

[51] H. Kiyohara, T. Matsumoto, and H. Yamada, "Combination effects of herbs in a multi-herbal formula: expression of Juzen-taiho-to's immuno-modulatory activity on the intestinal immune system," *Evidence-Based Complementary and Alternative Medicine*, vol. 1, no. 1, pp. 83–91, 2004.

[52] T. Efferth and B. Kaina, "Toxicities by herbal medicines with emphasis to traditional Chinese medicine," *Current Drug Metabolism*, vol. 12, no. 10, pp. 989–996, 2011.

# 11

# Chongcao-Shencha Attenuates Liver and Kidney Injury through Attenuating Oxidative Stress and Inflammatory Response in D-Galactose-Treated Mice

Cailan Li,[1] Zhizhun Mo,[1] Jianhui Xie,[2] Lieqiang Xu,[1] Lihua Tan,[1] Dandan Luo,[1] Hanbin Chen,[1] Hongmei Yang,[1] Yucui Li,[1] Ziren Su,[1] and Zuqing Su[3]

[1]*School of Chinese Materia Medica, Guangzhou University of Chinese Medicine, Guangzhou 510006, China*
[2]*Guangdong Provincial Key Laboratory of Clinical Research on Traditional Chinese Medicine Syndrome, The Second Affiliated Hospital, Guangzhou University of Chinese Medicine, Guangzhou 510120, China*
[3]*The Second Affiliated Hospital, Guangzhou University of Chinese Medicine, Guangzhou 510120, China*

Correspondence should be addressed to Ziren Su; suziren@126.com and Zuqing Su; 895075750@163.com

Academic Editor: Yoshiji Ohta

The Chongcao-Shencha (CCSC), a Chinese herbal compound formula, has been widely used as food material and medicine for enhancing physical strength. The present study investigated the possible effect of CCSC in alleviating the liver and kidney injury in D-galactose- (D-gal-) treated mice and the underlying mechanism. Mice were given a subcutaneous injection of D-gal (200 mg/kg) and orally administered CCSC (200, 400, and 800 mg/kg) daily for 8 weeks. Results indicated that CCSC increased the depressed body weight and organ index induced by D-gal, ameliorated the histological deterioration, and decreased the levels of ALT, AST, BUN, and CRE as compared with D-gal group. Furthermore, CCSC not only elevated the activities of antioxidant enzymes SOD, CAT, and GPx but also upregulated the mRNA expression of SOD1, CAT, and GPx1, while decreasing the MDA level in D-gal-treated mice. Results of western blotting analysis showed that CCSC significantly inhibited the upregulation of expression of nuclear factor kappa B (NF-$\kappa$B) p65, p-p65, p-I$\kappa$B$\alpha$, COX2, and iNOS and inhibited the downregulation of I$\kappa$B$\alpha$ protein expression caused by D-gal. This study demonstrated that CCSC could attenuate the liver and kidney injury in D-gal-treated mice, and the mechanism might be associated with attenuating oxidative stress and inflammatory response.

## 1. Introduction

Researches have demonstrated that chronic administration of D-gal induced changes resembling natural aging in rodents [1–3]. In animals, D-gal is normally metabolized by D-galactokinase and galactose-1-phosphate uridyltransferase, but oversupply of D-gal results in its abnormal metabolism and induces oxidative stress, inflammation response, and tissue damage, including the brain, liver, and kidney [4, 5]. It is observed that there is high production of reactive oxygen species (ROS) and low activities of antioxidant enzymes in the body fluids and tissues in D-gal-treated rats [6–8]. Since then, D-gal injection has been gradually used to establish an aging model for antiaging or organ injury research.

Oxidative damage caused by ROS is expected to play a role in D-gal-induced age-related changes in tissues [9]. The excess ROS formation can damage cellular macromolecules such as lipids, proteins, and DNA and cause cell damage [10, 11]. However, the endogenous antioxidant system, including superoxide dismutases (SOD), catalase (CAT), and glutathione peroxidase (GPx), is especially necessary to scavenge the excess ROS and meanwhile may cause the changes of some biomarkers [12]. In addition, it has been well demonstrated that inflammation is one of a variety of biological phenomena caused by oxidative stress [13]. Nuclear factor kappa B (NF-$\kappa$B) is a ubiquitous transcription factor critically involved in the proinflammatory response. And active NF-$\kappa$B is also one of the most important regulators of transcription of response genes encoding inflammation associated enzymes such as cyclooxygenase (COX2) and nitric oxide synthase (iNOS), which were extensively studied in inflammation [14].

Herbal formula is characteristic of multiple herbs and has versatile pharmacological activities based on the single effect of multiple herbs as well as the compatibility effect of multiple traditional Chinese medicines, which is considered to play an important role in the treatment of diseases. CCSC, a Chinese herbal compound formula, consists of five traditional Chinese herbs, including Misai Kuching (*Clerodendranthus spicatus* (Thunb.), C.Y.Wu), North *Cordyceps* (*Cordyceps militaris* L. Link), Longan Arillus (*Dimocarpus longan* Lour.), Folium Ginseng (*Panax ginseng* C. A. Mey.), and Corni Fructus (*Cornus officinalis* Sieb. et Zucc.). The five herbs are widely used as food material and medicine in the clinic and daily life for the effect of "kidney-reinforcing" and "enhancing physical strength." Recent researches found that the five herbs have a variety of pharmacological activities, including antioxidant, antiaging, hepatoprotective, and immunomodulatory effects [15–18]. It should be noted that traditional herbs and spices also exist along with their active constituents. Researchers found that CCSC contained various active components, such as ginsenoside, loganin, cordycepin, rosmarinic acid, and uridine, which showed a variety of pharmacological activities, including antioxidant [19, 20], anti-inflammatory [21], and antifatigue [22]. However, no endeavor to date has been made to investigate the possible ameliorative effect of CCSC in liver and kidney injury induced by D-gal.

In this study, we investigated the possible effect of CCSC in alleviating the liver and kidney injury in D-gal-treated mice by measuring the body weight, organ index, and histological lesion. Additionally, the effects of CCSC on oxidative stress-related enzyme levels and mRNA expression, the protein expression of iNOS, COX2, and p-p65, p65, p-I$\kappa$B$\alpha$, and I$\kappa$B$\alpha$ in NF-$\kappa$B signaling pathway were investigated to illuminate the possible underlying mechanisms.

## 2. Materials and Methods

*2.1. Drug and Chemical Reagents.* Misai Kuching, North Cordyceps, Longan Arillus, Folium Ginseng, and Corni Fructus were purchased from the Yunnan Chinese Herbal Medicine Department. These herbs were authenticated by one of our authors, Professor Ziren Su, Guangzhou University of Chinese Medicine (GZUCM). The voucher specimens (Yu 15-6-25) were kept at School of Chinese Materia Medica, GZUCM, for reference. D-gal and vitamin E (VE) were purchased from Sigma-Aldrich (St. Louis, USA). Commercial biochemical assay kits for the measurements of superoxide dismutases (SOD), catalase (CAT), glutathione peroxidase (GPx), malondialdehyde (MDA), alanine aminotransferase (ALT), aspartate transaminase (AST), blood urea nitrogen (BUN), and creatinine (CRE) were purchased from Nanjing Jiancheng Bioengineering Institute (Nanjing, China). Tween 80 was purchased from Sinopharm (Shanghai, China). All reagents used were of either analytical or chromatographic grade.

*2.2. Preparation of Plant Extract.* The mixtures (CCSC) of dried Misai Kuching (300 g), North Cordyceps (100 g), Longan Arillus (300 g), Corni Fructus (250 g), and Folium Ginseng (150 g) were ground into powders and soaked in distilled water at room temperature for 30 min, followed by refluxing with distilled water (ratio: 1 g/10 mL) for 2 h. After filtration, the extraction procedure was repeated twice. The filtered extracts were pooled and evaporated under reduced pressure. To analyze the chemical composition, CCSC was dissolved in 50% methanol. For pharmacological tests, CCSC was dissolved in distilled water containing 1% Tween 80 solution.

*2.3. HPLC-Electrospray Ionization-MS Analysis.* HPLC experiments were conducted on a Shimadzu (Kyoto, Japan) HPLC system consisting of an LC-20AD quaternary solvent delivery system, an SIL-20AC autosampler, and a CTO-20AC column oven. The extracts were mixed with methanol and water (ratio: 1 : 1 v/v) and filtered through 0.22 $\mu$m microporous membrane prior to high performance liquid chromatography-electrospray ionization-MS (HPLC-ESI-MS/MS) analysis. The Kromasil KR100-5C18 column (250 mm × 4.6 mm, E17096) was applied for chromatographic separations. The mobile phase was composed of A (acetonitrile) and B (water) with a linear gradient elution: 0–20 min, 5–10% A; 20–40 min, 10–18% A; 40–65 min, 18% A; 65–80 min, 18–30% A; 80–85 min, 30–35% A; 85–95 min, 35–40% A; 95–100 min, 40–45% A; 100–110 min, 45–90%; 110–120 min, 90%. The injection volume was 10 $\mu$L at a flow rate of 0.4 mL/min. The column oven temperature was maintained at 25°C.

A Triple TOF™ 5600 system equipped with an electrospray ionization (ESI) source for mass detection and data processing was achieved with Multiquant™ Software system (AB SCIEX, CA, USA). The following parameter settings were used: ion spray voltage floating, −4500 kV; ion source heater, 500°C; curtain gas, 35 psi; ion source gas 1, 55 psi; and ion source gas 2, 55 psi. Mass analyzer scanned from 100 to 1500 *mz*. The MS-MS spectra were recorded in auto-MS-MS mode. The CE was −5 eV, and the CP was −100 eV in the MS/MS experiment. Mass spectra were simultaneously acquired using electrospray ionization in the positive and negative ionization modes.

*2.4. Animals and Treatment Procedure.* Male Kunming (KM) mice (18–22 g) were obtained from the Laboratory Animal Services Centre of GZUCM. After acclimatization for one week under constant conditions of temperature (23±1°C) and humidity (40–60%) on a 12 h light/dark cycle with free access to food and water, the animals were randomly divided into 6 groups ($n = 10$): control group, D-gal group (200 mg/kg), CCSC-L group (200 mg/kg), CCSC-M group (400 mg/kg), CCSC-H group (800 mg/kg), and VE group (80 mg/kg, the positive control). Except for the control, mice received a daily subcutaneous injection of D-gal at a dose of 200 mg/kg, while those in the control group received an injection of the same volume of physiological saline (0.9% NaCl). At the same time, mice in the treatment groups were administered orally with CCSC (200, 400, and 800 mg/kg/day) and VE (80 mg/kg/day)

TABLE 1: Primer sequences.

| Gene | Sequence | Product size | Accession number |
|---|---|---|---|
| 18S RNA | CCTGGATACCGCAGCTAGGA GCGGCGCAATACGAATGCCCC | 112 bp | NR_003286 |
| SOD1 | GTCGGCTTCTCGTCTTGCTC GCTTTCATCGCCATGCTTCC | 80 bp | NM_011434.1 |
| CAT | CGTCCGTCCCTGCTGTCTCA CTGCTCCTTCCACTGCTTCATC | 109 bp | NM_009804.2 |
| GPx1 | CGGGACCCTGAGACTTAGAGC GAAGGCATACACGGTGGACTG | 191 bp | NM_008160.6 |

The constitutive gene 18S was used as an internal control.

dissolved in distilled water containing 1% Tween 80 solution, respectively. Meanwhile, mice in the control and D-gal groups were given an equal volume of distilled water containing 1% Tween 80 solution without CCSC. All drugs (CCSC, VE, and D-gal) and vehicle were given daily to the animals between 4:30 a.m. and 6:00 a.m. for 8 weeks in a volume of 10 mL/kg body weight. The body weight and food intake of the animals were measured weekly.

*2.5. Body Weight and Organ Indexes Measurement.* During the entire experiment, body weights were measured every week. After 8 weeks, the mice were sacrificed, and the spleens, thymi, kidneys, and livers were carefully dissected out, washed with cold sterile physiological saline, and weighed. Their weights relative to the final body weight were calculated as organ indexes. Then, the liver and kidney were stored immediately at −80°C for the sequent biochemical measurements, western blotting analysis, and quantitative real-time PCR analysis.

*2.6. Biochemical Assays.* For biochemical analysis, 10% (w/v) tissue homogenate was prepared in sodium phosphate buffer (0.1 M PBS, pH 7.4) containing a protease inhibitor cocktail (Sigma-Aldrich), using a homogenizer at the speed of 4000 rpm for 3 min. The homogenate was centrifuged at 3000 rpm for 15 min at 4°C. The supernatants were collected for biochemical analysis. The protein concentrations were measured by BCA (bicinchoninic acid) method using bovine serum albumin as a standard. The activities of SOD, CAT, and GPx, as well as the levels of MDA in liver and kidney, were determined by the assay kit according to its provider's instructions.

*2.7. Determination of Liver and Kidney Functions.* Blood samples were collected from the mice eye socket after 8 weeks. The plasma was prepared by centrifugation at 3000 rpm for 10 min at 4°C. An automatic biochemistry analyzer (RT-2100, Rayto Shenzhen Rayto Life Science Co., Ltd., China) was used to measure the contents of ALT, AST, CRE, and BUN in serum according to the assay kit providers' instructions.

*2.8. Quantitative Real-Time PCR Analysis.* Total RNA was extracted from liver and kidney tissues using Trizol Reagent

(Invitrogen Life Technologies, Carlsbad, CA, USA) according to the manufacturer's instructions. The total RNA was digested with RNase-free DNase for 30 min at 42°C. Two $\mu$g of the total RNA was used for cDNA synthesis using real-time quantitative PCR SYBR Green Master (Rox). Concentrations of reagents used were determined according to the manufacturer's instructions. The transcript of the constitutive gene 18S was used as an internal control. The sequences of the primers were listed in Table 1. The reaction mixture was subjected to PCR to amplify the sequences to obtain the desired primers. Amplification was performed with 45 cycles of denaturation at 95°C for 10 s, annealing at 60°C for 30 s, and extension at 72°C for 30 s. Relative gene expression was calculated by $2^{-\Delta\Delta CT}$ method using cycle time values and data for normalization. The changes in the gene expression ratio were calculated using BioPhotometer plus data analysis software.

*2.9. Western Blotting Analysis.* The tissue proteins were separated by electrophoresis on sodium dodecyl sulfate- (SDS-) polyacrylamide gels and transferred to polyvinylidene difluoride (PVDF) membranes (Millipore, Temecula, CA) using a semidry transfer system. The membranes were first incubated in blocking solution (5% skim milk) and then incubated overnight at 4°C with the primary antibodies of iNOS, COX2, I$\kappa$B$\alpha$, p-I$\kappa$B$\alpha$, p65, p-p65, and $\beta$-actin (Sigma, St. Louis, MO, USA). The $\beta$-actin was used as internal control. Immunoblots were incubated with the corresponding secondary antibody conjugated with horseradish peroxidase for 1 h. Membranes were developed using an electrochemiluminescence kit (Merck, China). The density of the immunoreactive bands was analyzed using Image J software (National Institutes of Health, Bethesda, MD, USA).

*2.10. Histopathological Assessment.* For histological assessment, the liver and kidney tissues were fixed in formalin and then embedded in paraffin. Tissues 5 $\mu$m thick were taken, placed onto glass slides, deparaffinized, and stained with hematoxylin eosin (H&E). All tissue sections were observed under a microscope (Nikon Corporation, Tokyo, JP).

*2.11. Statistical Analysis.* Statistical analysis was performed with GraphPad Prism 5 (GraphPad Software, Inc.) software. Data were expressed as means ± standard deviation (SD).

TABLE 2: Peak assignment of aqueous extracts of CCSC using HPLC-ESI-MS/MS in positive and negative ionization modes.

| Number | RT (min) | Molecular weight | HPLC-ESI-MS | | Fragment ions | Identified compounds |
|---|---|---|---|---|---|---|
| | | | [M + H]$^+$ $m/z$ | [M − H]$^-$ $m/z$ | | |
| 1 | 7.8 | 198.05 | — | 197.04 | 135, 123 | Salvianic acid |
| 2 | 8.6 | 170.02 | — | 169.01 | 125, 107 | Gallic acid |
| 3 | 9.5 | 244.07 | — | 243.06 | 200, 152, 147, 110 | Uridine |
| 4 | 12.0 | 283.09 | — | 282.08 | 150, 133 | Guanosine |
| 5 | 21.6 | 251.10 | 252.11 | — | 136, 119 | Cordycepin |
| 6 | 34.3 | 388.14 | 389.14 | — | 227.1, 209, 195.1, 149 | Verbenalin |
| 7 | 37.0 | 180.04 | — | 179.03 | 135, 117 | Caffeic acid |
| 8 | 38.6 | 270.05 | — | 269.04 | 251, 179, 161, 135 | Baicalein |
| 9 | 42.6 | 390.15 | — | 389.14 | 227, 127 | Loganin |
| 10 | 44.9 | 358.13 | 359.13 | — | 197, 179, 151, 127 | Sweroside |
| 11 | 48.3 | 360.08 | — | 359.07 | 197, 179, 161, 135, 123 | Rosmarinic acid |
| 12 | 83.9 | 472.36 | 473.36 | — | 464, 416, 360, 351 | 2$\alpha$-Hydroxy-ursolic acid |
| 13 | 84.9 | 800.49 | — | 799.48 | 637, 475.4 | Ginsenoside Rg1 |
| 14 | 84.9 | 946.55 | — | 945.54 | 783, 637, 475 | Ginsenoside Re |
| 15 | 97.7 | 374.10 | — | 373.09 | 179, 135 | Methyl rosmarinate |

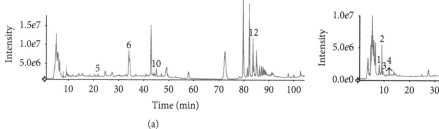

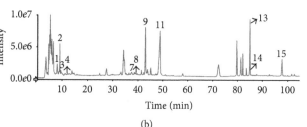

(a)                                                                   (b)

FIGURE 1: HPLC-ESI-MS/MS base peak chromatograms of the aqueous extracts of the CCSC recorded at positive ion mode (a) and negative ion mode (b). Peak numbers follow those listed in Table 2.

Differences among groups were analyzed by one-way analysis of variance (ANOVA) followed by Dunnett's test. A value of $P < 0.05$ or $P < 0.01$ was considered statistically significant.

## 3. Results

### 3.1. Separation and Identification Compounds of CCSC with HPLC-ESI-MS/MS.
The HPLC-ESI-MS/MS analysis was carried out in both negative and positive ionization modes. The HPLC-ESI base peak chromatograms in the positive mode (a) and negative mode (b) are shown in Figure 1. The identities, retention times (RT), molecular weight and observed molecular ions ([M + H]$^+$ $mz$/[M − H]$^-$ $mz$), and fragment ions for individual compounds are presented in Table 2. By comparing their retention time and recorded literatures, 15 compounds were identified. Peaks numbered 1–15 represented salvianic acid, gallic acid, uridine, guanosine, cordycepin, verbenalin, caffeic acid, baicalein, loganin, sweroside, rosmarinic acid, 2$\alpha$-hydroxy-ursolic acid, ginsenoside Rg1, ginsenoside Re, and methyl rosmarinate, respectively.

### 3.2. Effect of CCSC on Body Weights and Organ Indexes.
As shown in Table 3, at the beginning of the experiment, we did not find any differences in the mean body weight compared with the control mice ($P > 0.05$). However, at the end of the experiment, the mean body weight of D-gal-treated mice was significantly lower than the control, CCSC, and VE treatment groups. Organ indexes, including liver, kidney, thymus, and spleen, showed significant decrease in the D-gal-treated mice compared with control mice ($P < 0.05$ or $P < 0.01$). Administration of CCSC and VE restored the liver, kidney, thymus, and spleen indexes in a dose-dependent manner. These results suggested that CCSC could improve body weight and organ condition of D-gal-treated mice.

### 3.3. Effect of CCSC on Biochemistry Index.
As shown in Figures 2(a), 2(b), and 2(c), the SOD, CAT, and GPx activities of liver and kidney in the D-gal group decreased significantly ($P < 0.05$) compared with the control group. Moreover, our results (Figure 2(d)) also showed that the level of MDA in mice liver and kidney in the D-gal treatment group was significantly higher than that in the control group ($P < 0.01$).

TABLE 3: Effects of CCSC on the body weight and organ index in D-gal-treated mice (mean values and standard deviations, $n = 10$ per group).

| Group | Weight (g) | | Organ index (mg/g) | | | |
|---|---|---|---|---|---|---|
| | Initial | Final | Liver | Kidney | Thymus | Spleen |
| Control | 20.9 ± 1.29 | 34.21 ± 1.51 | 3.64 ± 0.21 | 1.04 ± 0.09 | 1.95 ± 0.23 | 3.33 ± 0.13 |
| D-gal | 20.0 ± 0.68 | 30.58 ± 1.09## | 3.29 ± 0.08## | 0.93 ± 0.09## | 1.49 ± 0.19## | 2.80 ± 0.10## |
| VE | 20.1 ± 0.85 | 32.98 ± 1.49** | 3.60 ± 0.25 | 1.03 ± 0.11* | 1.92 ± 0.35** | 3.11 ± 0.21** |
| CCSC-L | 19.7 ± 0.62 | 33.28 ± 1.36** | 3.65 ± 0.25* | 1.02 ± 0.08* | 1.70 ± 0.34 | 3.04 ± 0.12** |
| CCSC-M | 20.1 ± 0.35 | 33.76 ± 1.71** | 3.68 ± 0.34 | 1.05 ± 0.07** | 1.99 ± 0.22** | 3.05 ± 0.11** |
| CCSC-H | 19.9 ± 0.67 | 33.69 ± 1.61** | 3.55 ± 0.25 | 1.07 ± 0.09** | 1.78 ± 0.23* | 3.26 ± 0.26** |

## $P < 0.01$ compared to the control group. * $P < 0.05$ and ** $P < 0.01$ compared to the D-gal group.

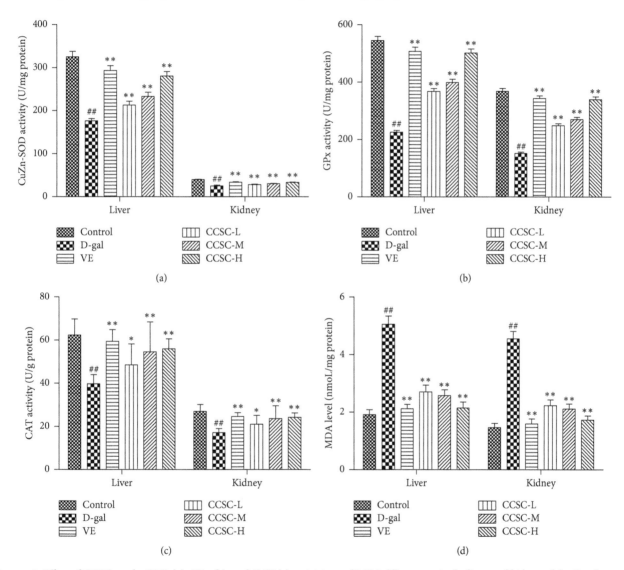

FIGURE 2: Effect of CCSC on the SOD (a), GPx (b), and CAT (c) activities and MDA (d) content in the liver and kidney of the D-gal-treated mice. Results are expressed as a mean ± SD ($n = 10$). ## $P < 0.01$ as compared with the control group. * $P < 0.05$ and ** $P < 0.01$ as compared with the D-gal group.

However, the SOD, CAT, and GPx activities were significantly ($P < 0.01$) restored and the MDA level was attenuated by CCSC and VE in a dose-dependent manner. The results suggested that CCSC treatment could significantly improve SOD, CAT, and GPx activities and decreased MDA level in D-gal-treated mice.

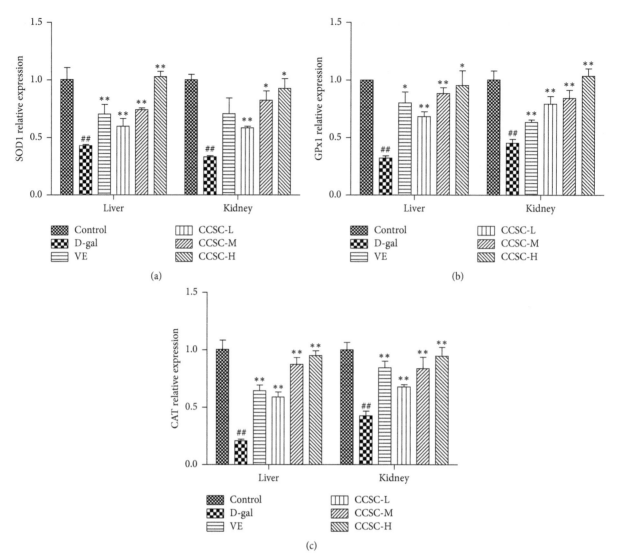

FIGURE 3: Effect of CCSC on mRNA expressions of SOD1 (a), CAT (b), and Gpx1 (c) in the liver and kidney of the D-gal-treated mice. Results are expressed as a mean ± SD ($n = 10$). $^{##}P < 0.01$ as compared with the control group. $^{*}P < 0.05$ and $^{**}P < 0.01$ as compared with the D-gal group.

*3.4. Quantitative Real-Time PCR Analysis.* As for the gene expression, SOD1, CAT, and GPx were significantly downregulated in the D-gal group compared with the control group, while they were significantly upregulated after administration of CCSC in a dose-dependent manner ($P < 0.05$ or $P < 0.01$, Figure 3). As a conventional antioxidant, VE was also observed to significantly upregulate these related gene expressions in D-gal-treated mice. Interestingly, the result showed that both CCSC-M (400 mg/kg) and CCSC-H (800 mg/kg) groups showed more potent effects in upregulating the hepatic and renal mRNA expressions of SOD1, CAT, and GPx than VE group.

*3.5. Determinations of ALT, AST, BUN, and CRE Levels.* Table 4 showed that the levels of AST, ALT, CRE, and BUN significantly increased after D-gal treatment compared with the control group. However, this increase was significantly suppressed by CCSC and VE ($P < 0.05$ or $P < 0.01$)

treatment. In addition, CCSC-L (200 mg/kg) exhibited superior suppressive effect on AST and ALT levels in liver than CCSC-M (400 mg/kg) and CCSC-H (800 mg/kg), while, in kidney, CCSC significantly suppressed the levels of CRE and BUN in a dose-dependent manner.

*3.6. Western Blotting Analysis.* The expression of iNOS, COX2, IκBα, p-IκBα, p65, and p-p65 in total proteins of the liver and kidney tissues of D-gal-treated mice was analyzed by western blotting analysis. As shown in Figure 4, the protein levels and the mean optical densities of iNOS and COX2 were higher in the D-gal-treated mice than the control group. However, CCSC and VE treatments caused a reduction in the protein levels and the mean densities of iNOS and COX2 in a dose-dependent manner. In Figure 5, our results clearly exhibited that CCSC group significantly increased IκBα level and decreased levels of p-IκBα, p65, and p-p65 in D-gal-treated liver and kidney tissues with the decreased

TABLE 4: Effects of CCSC on liver and kidney functions in D-gal-treated mice.

| | Liver function | | Kidney function | |
| --- | --- | --- | --- | --- |
| | ALT (U/L) | AST (U/L) | BUN ($\mu$moL/L) | CRE ($\mu$moL/L) |
| Control | $31.48 \pm 0.85$ | $107.54 \pm 2.75$ | $5.44 \pm 0.39$ | $25.63 \pm 2.03$ |
| D-gal | $64.41 \pm 1.48^{\#\#}$ | $163.62 \pm 2.04^{\#\#}$ | $16.47 \pm 0.49^{\#\#}$ | $82.36 \pm 2.45^{\#\#}$ |
| VE | $37.21 \pm 1.00^{**}$ | $111.44 \pm 3.13^{**}$ | $9.78 \pm 0.62^{**}$ | $43.00 \pm 2.59^{**}$ |
| CCSC-L | $36.93 \pm 0.99^{**}$ | $112.10 \pm 3.06^{**}$ | $11.01 \pm 1.24^{**}$ | $43.88 \pm 3.19^{**}$ |
| CCSC-M | $40.72 \pm 1.09^{**}$ | $117.14 \pm 2.74^{**}$ | $9.38 \pm 0.51^{**}$ | $41.74 \pm 1.99^{**}$ |
| CCSC-H | $43.73 \pm 1.17^{**}$ | $119.55 \pm 2.89^{**}$ | $8.89 \pm 0.85^{**}$ | $35.15 \pm 2.81^{**}$ |

Mean values and standard deviations, $n = 10$ per group. $^{\#\#}P < 0.01$ compared to the control group. $^{**}P < 0.01$ compared to the D-gal group.

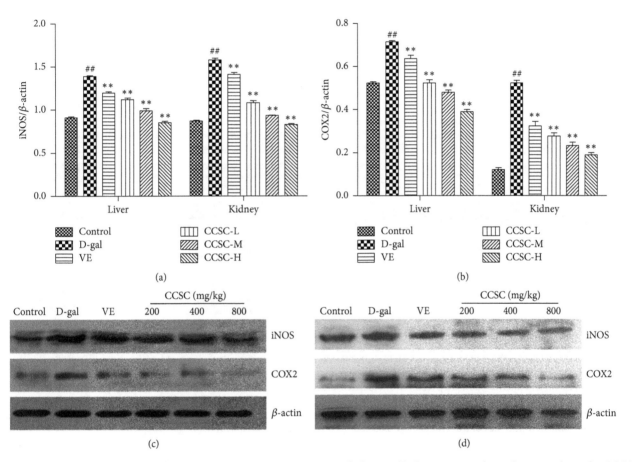

FIGURE 4: Western blotting analysis of iNOS and COX2 protein expression in the liver and kidney tissues. Relative density analysis of iNOS (a) and COX2 (b) and the representative images of expression of iNOS and COX2 in the liver (c) and kidney (d) tissues. The relative protein level between the tested target protein and internal standard $\beta$-actin was calculated and labeled on the $y$-axis. The bands are from a representative blot. Lane-1: control group; lane-2: D-gal-treated group; lane-3: VE-treated group (80 mg/kg); lane-4: CCSC-L-treated group (200 mg/kg); lane-5: CCSC-M-treated group (400 mg/kg); lane-6: CCSC-H-treated group (800 mg/kg). Values are expressed as mean $\pm$ SD in each group. $^{\#\#}P < 0.01$ as compared with the control group; $^{**}P < 0.01$ as compared with the D-gal group, $n = 3$.

ratio of p-I$\kappa$B$\alpha$ to I$\kappa$B$\alpha$. However, p-p65 versus p65 exhibited no significant differences both in liver and kidney tissues compared with D-gal group. Furthermore, our result showed that CCSC group in liver and kidney all showed more potent effect in downregulating the protein expression of iNOS, COX2, p65, p-p65, and p-I$\kappa$B$\alpha$ and upregulating I$\kappa$B$\alpha$ expression than VE (Figures 4(c), 4(d), 5(c), and 5(d)). It was noteworthy that high dose of CCSC-H (800 mg/kg) group exhibited particularly strong effect in downregulating and

upregulating the protein expression of iNOS, COX2, p65, p-p65, p-I$\kappa$B$\alpha$, or I$\kappa$B$\alpha$, restoring these protein levels almost to the level of the control group in both liver and kidney.

*3.7. Histopathological Analysis.* In the D-gal-treated mice, the histopathological examination of liver tissue revealed mussily arranged hepatic cord, binucleation of hepatocytes, and a large number of inflammatory cell infiltrations when compared to the control group (Figure 6(a)). However, in

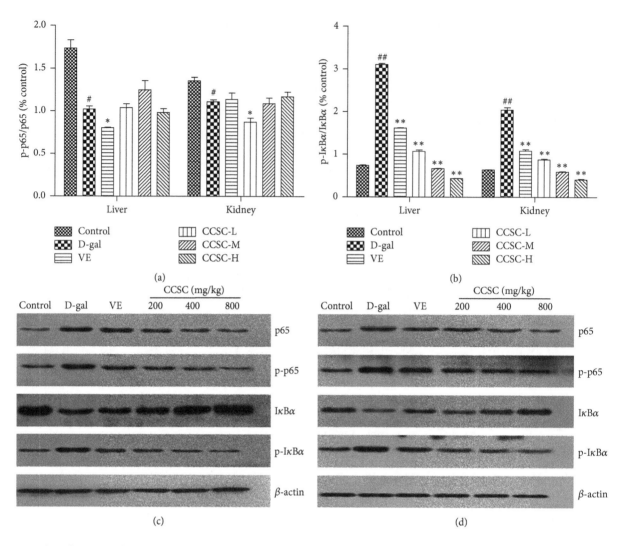

FIGURE 5: Effect of CCSC on the protein expression of NF-$\kappa$B pathway. Relative density analysis of p-p65/p65 (a) and p-I$\kappa$B$\alpha$/I$\kappa$B$\alpha$ (b) and the representative images of p-I$\kappa$B$\alpha$, I$\kappa$B$\alpha$, p-p65, and p65 expression in the liver (c) and kidney (d) tissues. The relative protein level between the tested target protein and internal standard $\beta$-actin was calculated and labeled on the $y$-axis. The bands are from a representative blot. Lane-1: control group; lane-2: D-gal-treated group; lane-3: VE-treated group (80 mg/kg); lane-4: CCSC-L-treated group (200 mg/kg); lane-5: CCSC-M-treated group (400 mg/kg); lane-6: CCSC-H-treated group (800 mg/kg). Values are expressed as mean ± SD in each group. $^{\#}P < 0.05$ and $^{\#\#}P < 0.01$ as compared with the control group; $^{*}P < 0.05$ and $^{**}P < 0.01$ as compared with the D-gal group, $n = 3$.

CCSC treatment groups, neatly arranged hepatic cord, fewer inflammatory infiltrations, and binucleation of hepatocytes were observed in liver tissues (Figures 6(d), 6(e), and 6(f)). On the other hand, the histopathological examination of kidney tissue showed that, in D-gal group, glomerulus showed obviously atrophy or even disappeared, balloon widened cavity, and drop of epithelial cells could occur in renal proximal convoluted tubules as compared with control group. However, CCSC and VE treatment significantly attenuated the glomerular atrophy and decreased the balloon widened cavity (Figures 7(c), 7(d), 7(e), and 7(f)).

## 4. Discussion

It has been shown that D-gal-treated mice were found similar to those of natural aging [23]. At high levels, D-gal could cause the metabolism of sugar in disorder and lead to the accumulation in the cell and induce osmotic stress and produce reactive oxygen species (ROS). Oxidative damage caused by reactive oxygen species (ROS) is expected to play a role in age-related changes in tissues, such as liver, brain, and kidney. D-gal treatment was also reported to cause inflammatory reactions and apoptotic and necrotic changes in the organs of animals and therefore has been widely used to establish an aging model for antiaging research and organ injured model [5, 24, 25].

It was reported that different ingredients potentiated each other's effect [26]. In traditional Chinese medicine, plant extracts from different herbs in a formula may contain different ingredients, which may play a different role in treating the same disease. CCSC, a traditional Chinese medicine compound recipe consisting of five food material

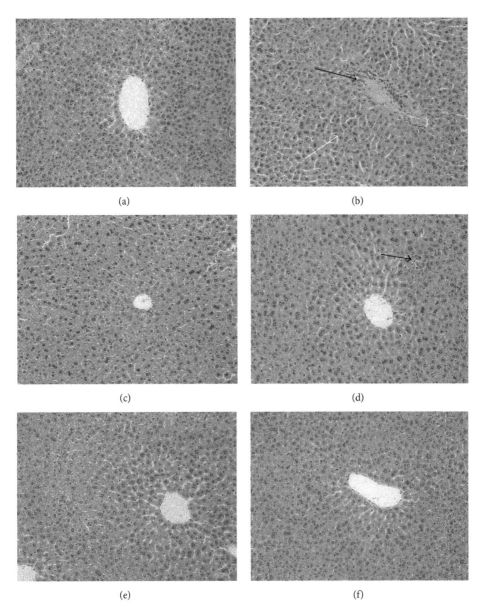

FIGURE 6: Histopathological appearance of liver in groups (H&E staining 200x). (a) Control group, (b) D-gal (200 mg/kg) group, (c) VE (80 mg/kg) group, (d) CCSC-L (200 mg/kg) group, (e) CCSC-M (400 mg/kg) group, and (f) CCSC-H (800 mg/kg) group. Inflammatory infiltration (black arrow), hepatic cord arranged mussily (yellow arrow), and binucleation of hepatocytes (blue arrow).

and medicine herbs, including Misai Kuching, North Cordyceps, Longan Arillus, Folium Ginseng, and Corni Fructus, has various pharmacological effects. Misai Kuching, a well-known medicine, is commonly used as herbal tea for diuresis, to treat rheumatism, diabetes, urinary lithiasis, oedema, eruptive fever, influenza, hepatitis, jaundice, biliary lithiasis, and hypertension [27, 28]. North Cordyceps, a precious medicinal herb widely distributed in China, is high in medicinal and nutritious components than Cordyceps and easy in cultivation and cheaper than Cordyceps [29]. North Cordyceps is widely used in functional food and healthcare products in China and exhibits various bioactive effects including regulating the immune function, invigorating the kidney, inhibition of cancer cell, deferring consenescence,

and increasing storage of glycogen and antifatigue [30]. HPLC-ESI-MS/MS results indicated that CCSC consisted of many components, such as uridine, cordycepin, loganin, rosmarinic acid, ginsenoside Rg1, and Re. Zhang et al. found that rosmarinic acid has effect on liver and kidney antioxidant enzymes, lipid peroxidation, and tissue ultrastructure in aging mice [20]. Cordycepin attenuated age-related oxidative stress and ameliorated antioxidant capacity in rats [31]. Loganin exhibited anti-inflammatory effect via inhibiting NF-κB activation [21]. Uridine and ginsenosides Rg1 and Re were also found to have various effects, such as antioxidant and antifatigue [19, 22, 32, 33].

Kidney and liver are two important organs in metabolism system. Their functions are declined gradually due to their

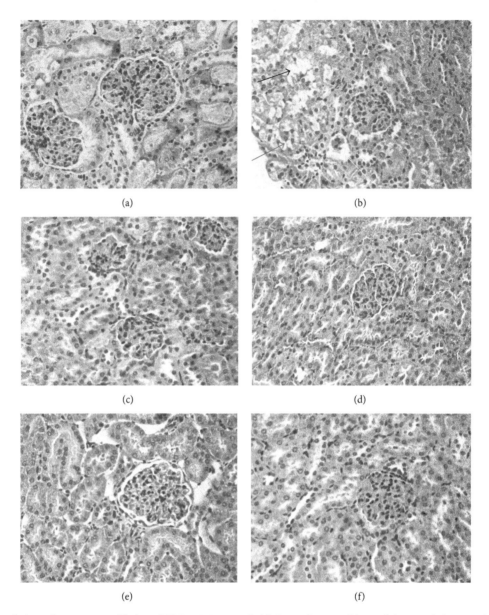

FIGURE 7: Histopathological appearance of kidney (H&E staining 400x). (a) Control group, (b) D-gal (200 mg/kg) group, (c) VE (80 mg/kg) group, (d) CCSC-L (200 mg/kg) group, (e) CCSC-M (400 mg/kg) group, and (f) CCSC-H (800 mg/kg) group. Atrophy (yellow arrow), balloon widened cavity (red arrow), and drop of epithelial cells in renal proximal convoluted tubules (black arrow).

structure atrophy with age. Recent studies showed that chronic administration of D-gal induced a mimetic aging effect in various tissues of rodents, such as liver, kidney, and brain. For the immune system, thymus and spleen, two important immune organs, also presented physiological diminution by D-gal treatment [34]. The present study clearly demonstrated that subcutaneous injection of D-gal at dose of 200 mg/kg/day for 8 weeks caused a severe aging-related appearance changes, including significant decrease in body weights and organ indexes. Meanwhile, kidney and liver were atrophied in D-gal-treated mice. However, CCSC supplement could partially reverse these deteriorating effects, increase both body weights and organ indexes, and as improve the

histopathologies of liver and kidney. The abovementioned observation suggested that CCSC could alleviate liver and kidney injury in D-gal-treated mice and the underlying molecular mechanisms were explored and described as follows.

Previous studies have shown that treatment with D-gal causes liver injury and dysfunction, followed by elevated activities or levels of serum enzymes [35]. AST, ALT, BUN, and CRE are commonly deemed as the key injury indicators for the liver and kidney [36–38]. The present study showed that AST, ALT, BUN, and CRE had higher levels in aged mice compared to the control group, which was in line with the previous report [39]. However, these increased levels were significantly decreased by CCSC and VE treatment, suggesting the protective effect of CCSC against D-gal-induced liver injury.

Oxidative stress could increase the generation of free radicals and could impair the antioxidant enzymes. A large number of studies revealed that the balance between ROS system and autoxidation system determined the degree of oxidative stress [40]. SOD is a superoxide radical scavenging factor that converted superoxide radicals to $H_2O_2$ [41]. CAT catalyses the decomposition of $H_2O_2$ into $H_2O$ and $O_2$ [42] and GPx reduces $H_2O_2$ or hydroperoxides to $H_2O$ and alcohol [42] where they are regarded as the first line of defense against the ROS generated during oxidative stress [43]. Meanwhile, MDA is one product of lipid peroxidation, whose content reflects the damage to the cell membrane [41]. The liver is a major organ involved in D-gal metabolism and D-gal treatment is found to increase hepatic MDA levels and cause DNA damage together with oxidative stress [5]. In the present work, subcutaneous injection of D-gal caused the oxidative stress, decreased the antioxidant enzymatic activity of SOD, CAT, and GPx, and increased the MDA level. However, supplementation of CCSC was observed to decrease the MDA level and restore the antioxidant defense system by increasing the activity of antioxidant enzymes and modulating the hepatic mRNA expressions of antioxidant enzymes in the livers of D-gal-treated mice in a dose-dependent manner, even stronger than the typical antioxidant VE. Taken together, CCSC administration protected the mouse liver against D-gal-induced hepatocyte oxidative stress via elevating multiple antioxidants gene expression and enhancing the antioxidant capacity. The results indicated that CCSC with antioxidant property might act as a potential candidate applicable for the antioxidant based functional formulae in complimentary or integrated therapy of age-related diseases.

On the one hand, oxidative stress could induce direct cellular and tissue damages; on the other hand, oxidative stress could activate transcription factors including NF-$\kappa$B pathway which regulate the expression of various inflammatory genes that could determine and maintain low-grade inflammation during aging and age-associated diseases [13]. The p65 protein is a key active component of NF-$\kappa$B. In most types of cells, NF-$\kappa$B dimers are transcriptionally inactive in cytoplasm due to the inhibitors of three I$\kappa$B isoforms (I$\kappa$B$\alpha$, I$\kappa$B$\beta$, and I$\kappa$B$\varepsilon$) [44]. I$\kappa$B degradation allows NF-$\kappa$B to translocate to the nucleus and bind DNA. In addition, under certain circumstances, NF-$\kappa$B dimers are activated and promote the phosphorylation of I$\kappa$B. The activated NF-$\kappa$B is translocated to the nucleus and regulates the proinflammatory gene expression such as iNOS and COX2 related to inflammatory, immune, fibrogenic, carcinogenic, and acute phase responses so as to cause tissue and organ damage following severe trauma [45, 46]. COX2-mediated inflammatory responses play important roles in biology and diseases such as renal function, nerve and brain function, ovarian and uterine function [47]. iNOS can consistently release high levels of nitric oxide (NO) and results in deleterious effects in both local and systemic inflammatory responses [48]. Therefore, inhibition of COX2, iNOS, and NF-$\kappa$B expression may be an effective strategy to suppress the inflammatory responses.

The present study showed that CCSC treatment not only significantly downregulated the protein expression of p-I$\kappa$B$\alpha$, NF-$\kappa$B p65, p-p65, iNOS, and COX2, but also obviously upregulated the I$\kappa$B$\alpha$ level in mice liver and kidney (Figures 4 and 5), suggesting that CCSC might exert anti-inflammatory effect via blocking the activation of NF-$\kappa$B signaling pathway and inhibiting iNOS and COX2 expression.

## 5. Conclusion

The present study demonstrated that CCSC could attenuate D-gal-induced liver and kidney injury in mice and the mechanism might be intimately associated with attenuating lipid peroxidation, renewing the activities of antioxidant enzymes, enhancing the antioxidant enzyme gene expression, and suppressing inflammatory response.

## Competing Interests

The authors declare that there are no competing interests.

## Authors' Contributions

Cailan Li and Zhizhun Mo contributed equally to this work.

## Acknowledgments

This work was supported by grants from the Guangdong Natural Science Foundation (2015A030310217), Science and Technology Planning Project of Guangzhou (no. 201300000145), Ph.D. Programs Foundation of Ministry of Education of China (no. 20134425110009), Science and Technology Innovation Project of Guangdong Provincial Department of Education (no. 2013KJCX0045), Development and Industrialization Planning Project of Guangdong Province (nos. 2013B090600007 and 2013B090600026), Science and Technology Planning Project of Guangdong Province (nos. 2014A020221042 and 2013A022100001), Dongguan International Scientific and Technological Cooperation Project (no. 201350810200151), and College Students' Innovative Entrepreneurial Training of Guangdong Province (no. 201410572067).

## References

[1] J. Lu, Y.-L. Zheng, D.-M. Wu, L. Luo, D.-X. Sun, and Q. Shan, "Ursolic acid ameliorates cognition deficits and attenuates oxidative damage in the brain of senescent mice induced by D-galactose," *Biochemical Pharmacology*, vol. 74, no. 7, pp. 1078–1090, 2007.

[2] S.-C. Ho, J.-H. Liu, and R.-Y. Wu, "Establishment of the mimetic aging effect in mice caused by D-galactose," *Biogerontology*, vol. 4, no. 1, pp. 15–18, 2003.

[3] M. Lei, X. Hua, M. Xiao, J. Ding, Q. Han, and G. Hu, "Impairments of astrocytes are involved in the d-galactose-induced brain aging," *Biochemical and Biophysical Research Communications*, vol. 369, no. 4, pp. 1082–1087, 2008.

[4] A. Liu, Y. Ma, and Z. Zhu, "Protective effect of selenoarginine against oxidative stress in D-galactose-induced aging mice,"

*Bioscience, Biotechnology and Biochemistry*, vol. 73, no. 7, pp. 1461–1464, 2009.

[5]  Z.-F. Zhang, S.-H. Fan, Y.-L. Zheng et al., "Purple sweet potato color attenuates oxidative stress and inflammatory response induced by d-galactose in mouse liver," *Food and Chemical Toxicology*, vol. 47, no. 2, pp. 496–501, 2009.

[6]  K. V. Anand, M. S. Mohamed Jaabir, P. A. Thomas, and P. Geraldine, "Protective role of chrysin against oxidative stress in D-galactose-induced aging in an experimental rat model," *Geriatrics and Gerontology International*, vol. 12, no. 4, pp. 741–750, 2012.

[7]  H.-L. Chen, C.-H. Wang, Y.-W. Kuo, and C.-H. Tsai, "Antioxidative and hepatoprotective effects of fructo-oligosaccharide in d-galactose-treated Balb/cJ mice," *British Journal of Nutrition*, vol. 105, no. 6, pp. 805–809, 2011.

[8]  B. V. Ramana, V. V. Kumar, P. N. R. Krishna, C. S. Kumar, P. U. M. Reddy, and T. N. Raju, "Effect of quercetin on galactose-induced hyperglycaemic oxidative stress in hepatic and neuronal tissues of Wistar rats," *Acta Diabetologica*, vol. 43, no. 4, pp. 135–141, 2006.

[9]  H. Nakanishi and Z. Wu, "Microglia-aging: roles of microglial lysosome- and mitochondria-derived reactive oxygen species in brain aging," *Behavioural Brain Research*, vol. 201, no. 1, pp. 1–7, 2009.

[10]  S. Khurana, M. Piche, A. Hollingsworth, K. Venkataraman, and T. C. Tai, "Oxidative stress and cardiovascular health: therapeutic potential of polyphenols," *Canadian Journal of Physiology and Pharmacology*, vol. 91, no. 3, pp. 198–212, 2013.

[11]  J. R. Speakman and C. Selman, "The free-radical damage theory: accumulating evidence against a simple link of oxidative stress to ageing and lifespan," *BioEssays*, vol. 33, no. 4, pp. 255–259, 2011.

[12]  S. Sreelatha, P. R. Padma, and M. Umadevi, "Protective effects of Coriandrum sativum extracts on carbon tetrachloride-induced hepatotoxicity in rats," *Food and Chemical Toxicology*, vol. 47, no. 4, pp. 702–708, 2009.

[13]  D. M. Dambach, S. K. Durham, J. D. Laskin, and D. L. Laskin, "Distinct roles of NF-κB p50 in the regulation of acetaminophen-induced inflammatory mediator production and hepatotoxicity," *Toxicology and Applied Pharmacology*, vol. 211, no. 2, pp. 157–165, 2006.

[14]  S. Uwe, "Anti-inflammatory interventions of NF-κB signaling: potential applications and risks," *Biochemical Pharmacology*, vol. 75, no. 8, pp. 1567–1579, 2008.

[15]  D. L. Chen, H. M. Long, H. M. Zhang, N. Li, and S. H. Liu, "In vitro antioxidant and mitochondria protective activities of clerodendranthus spicatus extracts," *Natural Product Research and Development*, vol. 26, no. 3, pp. 392–397, 2014.

[16]  Y. Luo, "Effects of Ginsenoside on immune function in fowls," 2003.

[17]  H. Liu and H.-Q. Xu, "Fructus Corni pharmacology and its main components research," *Journal of Nanjing TCM Univiersity*, vol. 19, no. 4, pp. 254–256, 2003.

[18]  Z.-Q. Jiang, Y. Li, L.-H. Jiang, H. Gu, and M.-Y. Wang, "Hepatoprotective effects of extracts from processed corni fructus against D-galactose-induced liver injury in mice," *Journal of Chinese Medicinal Materials*, vol. 36, no. 1, pp. 85–89, 2013.

[19]  C. R. Hwang, S. H. Lee, G. Y. Jang et al., "Changes in ginsenoside compositions and antioxidant activities of hydroponic-cultured ginseng roots and leaves with heating temperature," *Journal of Ginseng Research*, vol. 38, no. 3, pp. 180–186, 2014.

[20]  Y. Zhang, X. Chen, L. Yang, Y. Zu, and Q. Lu, "Effects of rosmarinic acid on liver and kidney antioxidant enzymes, lipid peroxidation and tissue ultrastructure in aging mice," *Food and Function*, vol. 6, no. 3, pp. 927–931, 2015.

[21]  M.-J. Kim, G.-S. Bae, I.-J. Jo et al., "Loganin protects against pancreatitis by inhibiting NF-κB activation," *European Journal of Pharmacology*, vol. 765, pp. 541–550, 2015.

[22]  L. J. Chen, Y. Wang, D. L. Cai et al., "Compatible effect of ginsenoside Rg1 and 1,6-fructose diphosphate on anti-fatigue," *Amino Acids & Biotic Resources*, vol. 32, no. 4, pp. 58–62, 2010.

[23]  B. Chen, Y. Zhong, W. Peng, Y. Sun, and W.-J. Kong, "Age-related changes in the central auditory system: comparison of D-galactose-induced aging rats and naturally aging rats," *Brain Research*, vol. 1344, pp. 43–53, 2010.

[24]  Y. Ren, X. Yang, X. Niu, S. Liu, and G. Ren, "Chemical characterization of the avenanthramide-rich extract from oat and its effect on d-galactose-induced oxidative stress in mice," *Journal of Agricultural and Food Chemistry*, vol. 59, no. 1, pp. 206–211, 2011.

[25]  G.-X. Mao, H.-B. Deng, L.-G. Yuan, D.-D. Li, Y.-Y. Y. Li, and Z. Wang, "Protective role of salidroside against aging in a mouse model induced by D-galactose," *Biomedical and Environmental Sciences*, vol. 23, no. 2, pp. 161–166, 2010.

[26]  L.-T. Yi, Q. Xu, Y.-C. Li, L. Yang, and L.-D. Kong, "Antidepressant-like synergism of extracts from magnolia bark and ginger rhizome alone and in combination in mice," *Progress in Neuro-Psychopharmacology and Biological Psychiatry*, vol. 33, no. 4, pp. 616–624, 2009.

[27]  W. Sumaryono, P. Proksch, V. Wray, L. Witte, and T. Hartmann, "Qualitative and quantitative analysis of the phenolic constituents from *Orthosiphon aristatus*," *Planta Medica*, vol. 57, no. 2, pp. 176–180, 1991.

[28]  Y. Tezuka, P. Stampoulis, A. H. Banskota et al., "Constituents of the Vietnamese medicinal plant Orthosiphon stamineus," *Chemical & Pharmaceutical Bulletin*, vol. 48, no. 11, pp. 1711–1719, 2000.

[29]  H. Qh, "North Cordyceps is eligible for replacing Cordyceps sinensis," *China Food Newspaper*, vol. 6, pp. 1–2, 2013.

[30]  R. R. M. Paterson, "Cordyceps: a traditional Chinese medicine and another fungal therapeutic biofactory?" *Phytochemistry*, vol. 69, no. 7, pp. 1469–1495, 2008.

[31]  T. Ramesh, S.-K. Yoo, S.-W. Kim et al., "Cordycepin (3′-deoxyadenosine) attenuates age-related oxidative stress and ameliorates antioxidant capacity in rats," *Experimental Gerontology*, vol. 47, no. 12, pp. 979–987, 2012.

[32]  I. B. Krylova, V. V. Bulion, E. N. Selina, G. D. Mironova, and N. S. Sapronov, "Effect of uridine on energy metabolism, LPO, and antioxidant system in the myocardium under conditions of acute coronary insufficiency," *Bulletin of Experimental Biology and Medicine*, vol. 153, no. 5, pp. 644–646, 2012.

[33]  G.-D. Huang, J. Mao, and Z. Ji, "Evaluation of ginsenoside Rg1 as a potential antioxidant for preventing or ameliorating progression of atherosclerosis," *Tropical Journal of Pharmaceutical Research*, vol. 12, no. 6, pp. 941–948, 2013.

[34]  J. A. Knight, "The biochemistry of aging," *Advances in Clinical Chemistry*, vol. 35, pp. 1–62, 2001.

[35]  Z.-F. Zhang, J. Lu, Y.-L. Zheng et al., "Purple sweet potato color protects mouse liver against d-galactose-induced apoptosis via inhibiting caspase-3 activation and enhancing PI3K/Akt pathway," *Food and Chemical Toxicology*, vol. 48, no. 8-9, pp. 2500–2507, 2010.

[36] H. Nyblom, U. Berggren, J. Balldin, and R. Olsson, "High AST/ALT ratio may indicate advanced alcoholic liver disease rather than heavy drinking," *Alcohol and Alcoholism*, vol. 39, no. 4, pp. 336–339, 2004.

[37] H. Nyblom, E. Björnsson, M. Simrén, F. Aldenborg, S. Almer, and R. Olsson, "The AST/ALT ratio as an indicator of cirrhosis in patients with PBC," *Liver International*, vol. 26, no. 7, pp. 840–845, 2006.

[38] A. Wang, Z. Xiao, L. Zhou, J. Zhang, X. Li, and Q. He, "The protective effect of atractylenolide I on systemic inflammation in the mouse model of sepsis created by cecal ligation and puncture," *Pharmaceutical Biology*, vol. 54, no. 1, pp. 146–150, 2016.

[39] N. Gagliano, F. Grizzi, and G. Annoni, "Mechanisms of aging and liver functions," *Digestive Diseases*, vol. 25, no. 2, pp. 118–123, 2007.

[40] B. Poljsak, D. Šuput, and I. Milisav, "Achieving the balance between ROS and antioxidants: when to use the synthetic antioxidants," *Oxidative Medicine and Cellular Longevity*, vol. 2013, Article ID 956792, 11 pages, 2013.

[41] A. Kowald, A. Hamann, S. Zintel, S. Ullrich, E. Klipp, and H. D. Osiewacz, "A systems biological analysis links ROS metabolism to mitochondrial protein quality control," *Mechanisms of Ageing and Development*, vol. 133, no. 5, pp. 331–337, 2012.

[42] H. Chen, M. Yu, M. Li et al., "Polymorphic variations in manganese superoxide dismutase (MnSOD), glutathione peroxidase-1 (GPX1), and catalase (CAT) contribute to elevated plasma triglyceride levels in Chinese patients with type 2 diabetes or diabetic cardiovascular disease," *Molecular and Cellular Biochemistry*, vol. 363, no. 1-2, pp. 85–91, 2012.

[43] S.-J. Tsai and M.-C. Yin, "Anti-oxidative, anti-glycative and anti-apoptotic effects of oleanolic acid in brain of mice treated by D-galactose," *European Journal of Pharmacology*, vol. 689, no. 1–3, pp. 81–88, 2012.

[44] X. Dolcet, D. Llobet, J. Pallares, and X. Matias-Guiu, "NF-kB in development and progression of human cancer," *Virchows Archiv*, vol. 446, no. 5, pp. 475–482, 2005.

[45] Y. Kotake, H. Sang, T. Miyajima, and G. L. Wallis, "Inhibition of NF-$\kappa$B, iNOS mRNA, COX2 mRNA, and COX catalytic activity by phenyl-N-tert-butylnitrone (PBN)," *Biochimica et Biophysica Acta—Molecular Cell Research*, vol. 1448, no. 1, pp. 77–84, 1998.

[46] A. S. Baldwin Jr., "The NF-$\kappa$B and I$\kappa$B proteins: new discoveries and insights," *Annual Review of Immunology*, vol. 14, pp. 649–681, 1996.

[47] R. N. Dubois, S. B. Abramson, L. Crofford et al., "Cyclooxygenase in biology and disease," *FASEB Journal*, vol. 12, no. 12, pp. 1063–1073, 1998.

[48] K. Müller-Decker, G. Manegold, H. Butz et al., "Inhibition of cell proliferation by bacterial lipopolysaccharides in TLR4-positive epithelial cells: independence of nitric oxide and cytokine release," *Journal of Investigative Dermatology*, vol. 124, no. 3, pp. 553–561, 2005.

# 12

# Intravenous Mistletoe Treatment in Integrative Cancer Care: A Qualitative Study Exploring the Procedures, Concepts, and Observations of Expert Doctors

**Gunver S. Kienle,[1,2] Milena Mussler,[1] Dieter Fuchs,[3] and Helmut Kiene[1]**

[1]Institute for Applied Epistemology and Medical Methodology, University of Witten/Herdecke, Zechenweg 6, 79111 Freiburg, Germany
[2]Center for Complementary Medicine, Institute for Environmental Health Sciences and Hospital Infection Control, University Medical Center Freiburg, Breisacher Strasse 115B, 79106 Freiburg, Germany
[3]Department of Theology, Caritas Sciences, University of Freiburg, Werthmannplatz 3, 79098 Freiburg, Germany

Correspondence should be addressed to Gunver S. Kienle; gunver.kienle@ifaemm.de

Academic Editor: Konrad Urech

*Background.* Mistletoe therapy (MT) is widely used in patient-centered integrative cancer care. The objective of this study was to explore the concepts, procedures, and observations of expert doctors, with a focus on intravenous MT. *Method.* A qualitative interview study was conducted with 35 highly experienced doctors specialized in integrative and anthroposophic medicine. Structured qualitative content analysis was applied. For triangulation, the results were compared with external evidence that was systematically collected, reviewed, and presented. *Results.* Doctors perform individualized patient assessments that lead to multimodal treatment approaches. The underlying goal is to help patients to live with and overcome disease. Mistletoe infusions are a means of accomplishing this goal. They are applied to stabilize disease, achieve responsiveness, induce fever, improve quality of life, and improve the tolerability of conventional cancer treatments. The doctors reported long-term disease stability and improvements in patients' general condition, vitality, strength, thermal comfort, appetite, sleep, pain from bone metastases, dyspnea in pulmonary lymphangitis carcinomatosa, fatigue, and cachexia; chemotherapy was better tolerated. Also patients' emotional and mental condition was reported to have improved. *Conclusion.* Individualized integrative cancer treatment including MT aims to help cancer patients to live well with their disease. Further research should investigate the reported observations.

## 1. Introduction

Mistletoe treatment (MT) is an essential part of integrative cancer care [1–5]. It is mostly used to improve quality of life (QoL), increase the tolerability of chemotherapy, and exert a possible benefit on tumor control and survival. Mistletoe extracts (MEs) contain a variety of biologically active compounds such as lectins, viscotoxins, oligo- and polysaccharides [6, 7], and triterpene acids [8]. They are cytotoxic, have strong apoptosis-inducing effects [9–11], enhance the cytotoxicity of anticancer drugs [12, 13], stimulate the immune system, possess DNA-stabilizing properties in mononuclear cells, and enhance endorphins *in vivo* [14, 15]. When injected into tumor-bearing animals, MEs inhibit and decrease tumor growth [14, 15]. In clinical practice,

MEs are usually applied subcutaneously, starting with low doses that increase according to tolerability and local skin reactions or to lectin content. Various clinical studies have shown improvements in the QoL of cancer patients. A recent randomized controlled trial (RCT) found a highly statistical significant benefit of survival for patients with advanced pancreatic cancer [16]. Other studies have been inconsistent in this regard [17, 18]. Case reports and series have reported regressions of different tumor types after high-dose local applications of MEs [14, 19–25].

Despite the extensive body of scientific information, practicing physicians and experts have expressed the view that MEs are applied differently in clinical trials (i.e., in a highly standardized manner according to producer guidelines) than clinical reality, particularly when applied by highly experienced experts within an integrative setting.

ME treatment for cancer was largely developed by medical doctors, mostly within the context of anthroposophic medicine (AM), a healthcare approach that provides an integrative, multimodal, system-based cancer care [26]. Therapies and MT are individually applied, tailored to the specific medical condition and complaints of the patient; to his or her emotional, mental, spiritual, and social needs; and to his or her respective goals. Although global effectiveness studies have assessed individualized treatment applications [27–30], they do not provide detailed insights and covered only a small area. It remains unresolved whether such an individual way of applying MT brings about better results for patients, what those results are, and what characterizes such an individual treatment. It is of further interest to determine whether a study of concepts and internal evidence of highly experienced doctors can give rise to appropriate research and therapy development.

A qualitative study was conducted to gain insight into the concepts, goals, procedures, and observations associated with individualized cancer care; the long-term care of severely ill patients; the mental, emotional, and spiritual aspects involved; the sources of experts' knowledge and judgments; and whether the results convey clues for the further development of ME treatment. Interviews were conducted with highly experienced doctors. The study unearthed a wealth of information that is currently being published. One result was that physicians often stress the importance and potential of intravenous application of MEs, which differs from normal subcutaneous ME treatment and is a hardly known off-label type of intervention.

Therefore, the presented study aimed to focus on ME application as an intravenous infusion. It posed the following questions.

(i) Why are MEs applied as an intravenous infusion? What are the reasons, goals, and situations involved?

(ii) How are the MEs applied? What are the procedures, differences, commonalities, and safety aspects?

(iii) What do doctors observe? What are the benefits and risks?

(iv) What are the concepts?

(v) How do these results compare with external evidence?

## 2. Methods

A qualitative guideline-based interview study was carried out with doctors highly experienced in integrative cancer care and MT in order to assess the doctors' concepts, procedures, experiences, and observations [31, 32]. The study was approved by the Ethics Committee of the University of Freiburg.

*2.1. Sample.* Participants were purposively sampled [33, 34]. The selection criteria included a spectrum of different therapy approaches, preparation methods, and doctors' medical specializations, treatment contexts (e.g., hospital or office-based practice and palliative or curative patients), ages, and countries. The doctors were contacted and received information about the study aims and interview durations and were asked to prepare oncological case examples.

*2.2. Interviews.* The interviews were conducted by two researchers (GK and MM) between 2009 and 2012. GK is a medical doctor and researcher and well known in the fields of integrative cancer care, AM, and MT. MM is a psychologist and researcher. All of the interviews were conducted face-to-face. Anonymity and high confidentiality were ensured, which enabled open communication. Most of the interviews took place in the work setting of the respective doctors. A few were conducted at the research institute or within the context of a congress. All interviews were carried out in a quiet undisturbed room. All doctors consented to digital audio recording except for one, whose interview consisted of field notes.

All of the interviews started with a warm-up question. The doctors then provided one or two case examples to give an uninfluenced account of their procedures, concepts, and observations. A guideline with interview questions was used as a checklist to ensure completeness of content and to follow up on certain topics [35]. It was constructed with input from the literature and external experts. Interview topics ranged from patient assessment to choosing mistletoe applications, preparations, host trees and doses, monitoring and adjusting treatments, time aspects, treatment goals, effectiveness, specific constellations, symptoms and complaints related to cancer disease, psychological and spiritual issues, additional therapies and influences, safety aspects, and new insights. The doctors were asked to concretize their answers and illustrate them using case examples. At the end of the interviews, each doctor was asked to fill in a short sheet with sociodemographic information. All of the interviews were transcribed by staff members of the research institute according to the approach suggested by Kuckartz [36]. The interviews were sent to the participants for member validation [33] and member checks were maintained throughout the different stages of the research process [32, 35]. After data collection from the 35 interviews was completed, it was assumed that no further relevant areas of information would be found [33].

*2.3. Content Analysis.* We used qualitative content analysis according to Mayring [31] and charting techniques of the thematic framework approach of Ritchie [33] to analyze the data. Data analysis was predominantly conducted by GK and MM using MAXQDA computer software [36] to manage the data, code and extract text passages, and search the text. Two other researchers took part in team meetings (HK, a researcher and medical doctor, and DF, a psychologist and experienced qualitative researcher). Analysis was done in close exchange between the researchers and its steps were documented.

We conducted two pilot interviews. We then discussed and specified the guidelines (e.g., put questions into the past tense to access observations) and conducted further interviews while starting initial analysis. In the first step, we read the interviews, noted the codes (open coding), and then combined the data with the codes from the interview guidelines [31]. Second, the domains for data extraction and further analyses were defined and extracted for each doctor (axial coding) [31]. In analyzing the doctors' intravenous applications, contents related to actual treatment procedures, QoL observations, tumor behavior, courses of disease, symptoms, psychological issues, and safety were extracted and their core meaning was summarized in a circular process to condense the given information. Words and phrases from the participants' own languages were used to stay as close to the original interview text as possible, and relevant quotes were kept alongside to ground the extracted themes in data [33]. Publications and literature referrals of the interviewees were included in charts to make what was said more explicit (explication) [31]. The charts were reviewed, discussed, and corrected by at least two researchers. The condensed information was merged into one chart covering all of the participants to find key themes (vertical analysis) [31], such as the doctors' reasons for applying ME infusions, proceedings, observations, and treatment concepts (selective coding).

All doctors were asked whether they would participate in publishing case reports. In the process, their patients' charts were checked and the patients and other attending physicians were contacted. Furthermore, several of the interviewees had published articles or books that served as additional sources of information for their reports.

The doctors received the interview transcripts and final analysis results before publication. The results contained anonymized codes instead of names so that the doctors could revise them. The codes were removed before publication.

For triangulation, the results were compared with external evidence. Clinical studies and trials on intravenous MT were systematically collected as reported elsewhere [14, 17, 37–39]. The inclusion criteria were (1) prospective or retrospective studies or trials, with or without control groups; (2) study populations made up of cancer patients; (3) intervention groups treated with intravenous infusions of MEs; (4) clinically relevant outcome parameters; (5) completion of the study; and (6) published or unpublished status. Studies were excluded if they only measured toxicity or tolerability (phase I trial), only measured immune stimulation, or were not conducted on cancer patients. There were no language restrictions. Earlier systematic reviews provided a quality assessment of these studies [14, 17, 37–39]. It was not possible to collect case reports in a completely systematic way, as they were usually published not in peer-reviewed journals but in other journals, books, brochures, and so forth. The case reports collected were therefore confined to those published by interviewees.

## 3. Results

Thirty-five interviews were conducted. Ten doctors could not be interviewed due to organizational problems (two), lack of response (four), illness (one), or unwillingness to present therapeutic intimacies in public (three). The interviews lasted between 100 and 297 (mean 171) minutes.

3.1. The Sample. Table 1 shows the characteristics of the interviewed doctors. All of the doctors worked within an integrative treatment context, usually as part of a team of caregivers. They all worked in or collaborated with cancer centers or conventional experts (oncologists, surgeons, radiotherapists, etc.). Close collaboration within the team and other attending physicians was given significant consideration. Patient assessment was based on a precise diagnosis of tumor, stage, histology, symptoms, and relevant clinical, laboratory, and imaging evaluations. It included other relevant present and past conditions and complaints; functional, emotional, cognitive, social, and biographical issues; and goals and priorities to generate a whole "picture" of each patient [40]. Assessment was prioritized and a multimodal treatment approach tailored to the individual patient was pursued [40]. This also applied to MT and intravenous MT cases (Figure 1), which were individualized and adapted to the patient's diagnosis, condition, and evolving goals and later adjusted accordingly [40].

The doctors illustrated their reports with numerous case examples and some were published. Their arguments were usually critical and self-critical. Most of the doctors were careful or resistant to drawing any causal conclusions or generalizations. They reflected basic methodological principles, such as the difficulties involved in making assessments without control groups, and the presence of confounders and possible biases such as a "positivity bias," in which case they would pass their own positive attitude onto their patients. They frequently referred to the results of clinical trials or other research. They were sometimes critical of mistletoe and its effects.

3.2. General Concepts. The interviewed doctors' global therapeutic concept underlying MT and AM cancer care was to enable patients to overcome disease, if possible, or to live *with* their disease and achieve a good condition in the long term even if the disease progressed. This global concept was associated with the following goals: tumor control and symptom relief; acceptance and good tolerability of standard cancer treatments; strengthening (i.e., physical, emotional, and mental strength; vitality; immune system); improving responsiveness and agility; gaining autonomy, also from the disease (acceptance, peace, perspectives, and being less bothered); the ability to recover (sleep, appetite, and restructuring); and the beneficial effects of overcoming a crisis, particularly fever (Figure 2).

3.3. Reasons for Applying Mistletoe Infusions. Doctors applied ME as intravenous infusion in the following situations, particularly to enhance the subcutaneous MT effect using larger doses without causing local reactions:

(i) Lack of response under subcutaneous treatment, when "*nothing changes anymore*," to regenerate responsiveness.

(ii) Stabilization and support in advanced, progressing, metastasizing diseases, when patients are in a critical situation or appear devitalized and when their "*strength flows out*," to invigorate, strengthen, and

TABLE 1: Sample characteristics: doctors using MT and integrative cancer care.

| | Number | Years Median (range) |
| --- | --- | --- |
| Doctors | 35 | |
| Men | 30 | |
| Women | 5 | |
| Age (years) | | 55 (40–84) |
| Specialty of doctor[*] | | |
| Oncology, hematology | 8 | |
| Internal medicine, pulmonology, or gastroenterology | 17 | |
| General practitioner | 12 | |
| Pediatrician | 3 | |
| Gynecology | 1 | |
| Neurology | 1 | |
| Research doctor | 1 | |
| Work experience as a physician | | 26 (11–57) |
| Cancer patients treated with ME/year: median (range) | 270 (13–1,000) | |
| Using intravenous ME application | 29 | |
| Regularly | 3 | |
| Rarely | 6 | |
| Setting | | |
| Hospital or outpatient clinic | 21 | |
| Resident doctor | 14 | |
| Working in or collaborating with cancer centers | 35 | |
| Country of workplace | | |
| Germany | 22 | |
| Switzerland | 6 | |
| England, France, Sweden, Italy, Czech Republic, Egypt, Peru | 1 from each country | |

[*]Some doctors had several specialties and are mentioned twice.

consolidate patients ("*get ground under one's feet*") and to stabilize the tumor situation.

(iii) High-risk patients who have relapsed or are at risk of relapsing.

(iv) To induce a fever reaction, stimulate the immune system, and raise the patient's temperature and feelings of warmth, to support recovery after adjuvant tumor treatment, and "*to structure the chaos again.*"

(v) Specific tumor situations such as gastric cancer with poor prognosis, prostate cancer and bone metastases, and advanced lung cancer and plasmacytoma not treated with chemotherapy.

(vi) Improvement of QoL in general and in particular situations, such as pain, especially from bone metastases, fatigue, and dyspnea in lymphangitis carcinomatosa of the lung, and tumor cachexia, to improve the tolerability of chemotherapy.

(vii) High-dose mistletoe induction in mistletoe-naïve patients, to elicit a fever response, start therapy with an intense high-dose concept, reduce tumor burden, decelerate tumor growth, stimulate the immune system before surgery or chemotherapy, and support

patients in advanced, metastatic, and critical or palliative condition.

*3.4. Side Effects and Safety Aspects.* Doctors reported that hypersensitivity (pseudoallergic, rarely allergic) might occur more often under intravenous than subcutaneous treatment. Its symptoms, which include shivering, dyspnea and asthma, erythema, partly patchy or blistered, and cardiovascular reactions, are usually self-limited and occasionally require intervention. In addition to dose, this reaction was observed to be "*strictly dependent on dripping speed of the infusion [...] When it is too fast, I can provoke a reaction in about everybody*" (general practitioner). To prevent these reactions, the drip rate of the infusion has to be slow and the patient must be instructed not to accelerate the infusion on his or her own, or the dose must be decreased and increased only carefully, the preparation changed (e.g., from Abnoba to Helixor), and primary high-dose MT must be confined to patients with no previous mistletoe contact. When the safety aspects were taken into regard these reactions were rarely observed and intravenous MT was safe in high doses. When patients continued to develop pseudoallergic reactions, infusion therapy was terminated.

Additional reported side effects included self-limited skin blistering under high-dose induction, cellulitis in a patient

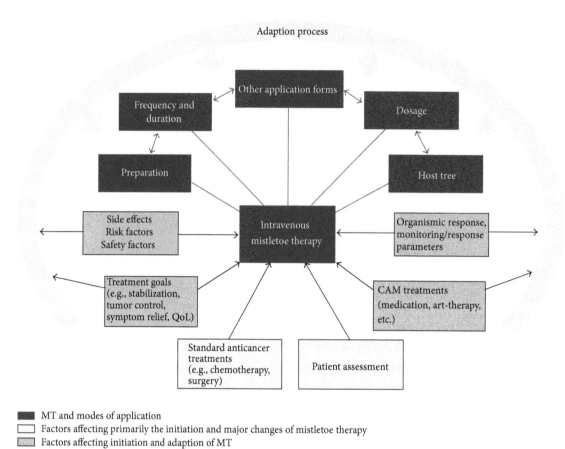

FIGURE 1: Intravenous mistletoe therapy: factors for choices and adaptions.

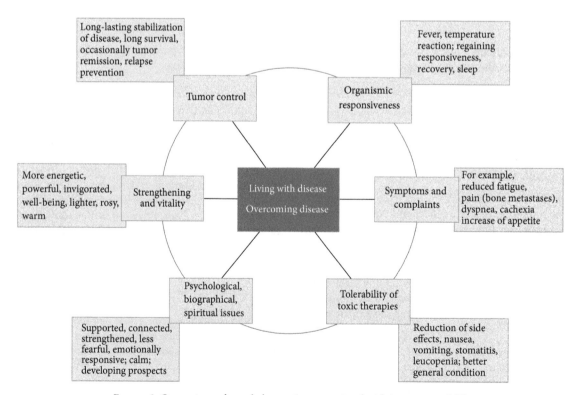

FIGURE 2: Concepts, goals, and observations associated with intravenous MT.

*Abnoba Viscum*
Characteristics:
(i) Favored for an initial high-dose fever-inducing treatment, combining i.v. and s.c. application.
Application:
Infusions added to a subcutaneous application:
(i) Low starting dose between 0.2 and 10 mg (rarely 20–40 mg) or last subcutaneous dose.
(ii) Stepwise dose increase, depending on the tolerability, up to 20–40 mg or to 160–200 mg as a maintenance dose.
(iii) Mostly applied weekly.
For high-dose therapy induction (no prior mistletoe contact):
(i) Infusions are started on three consecutive days (Fraxini 40–80–160 mg), combined with subcutaneous injection to induce fever (e.g., 10 mg day 1 or 3 or else) and, if possible, also intratumoral application.
(ii) A subcutaneous treatment and weekly or monthly infusions usually follow.
*Helixor*
Characteristics:
(i) Favored because of its good tolerability.
(ii) In progressive disease.
(iii) To support tolerability of chemotherapy.
(iv) To relieve pain from bone metastases and fatigue.
Application
(i) Mali is often used in the host tree, such as in cachectic and metastatic situations. Pini is also used occasionally.
(ii) Mostly a low starting dose of 100, 200 or 300 mg, stepwise increased up to 600 mg, depending on tolerability.
(iii) Rarely increased up to 5–7 g.
(iv) A 5–10 mg initial dose in very sensitive patients, increased up to 50–100 mg.
Daily application in weak patients and patients at the progressive disease stage, decreased to biweekly application later.
For pain, 3-4 infusions are given on consecutive days. Three infusions per week are administered for fatigue.
*Iscador*
Characteristics
(i) Favored for repeated fever induction or temperature response.
Application
(i) For fever induction, the dosage has to be high enough and infusion time long enough. For instance: Iscador M or Qu, 5 mg ("Spezial") followed by a stepwise increase to 20–40 mg.
(ii) Host trees may be combined.
(iii) Applied once or twice per week initially and eventually every second week.
(iv) Daily infusions are too strenuous.

Box 1: Examples of how the doctors applied infusions with different preparations.

who had received an epithelial growth factor before MT, phlebitides in children, and flushes and resurgence of old injection sites. Fever induction and high-dose application could be very strenuous and tiring ("*they are worn out*"). Initial shivering, flu-like symptoms, and acute-phase reaction could occur. Strong emotional reactions were also induced ("*tears to flow*"). However, these reactions were of short duration, and the patients' well-being, strength, and mood subsequently improved tremendously, like "*a phoenix from the ashes.*"

Infusions are predominantly done in hospitals, special daybeds, or well-suited office-based practices under supervision of a physician and a skilled staff. Some of the doctors interviewed rarely used intravenous applications because external circumstances did not allow for it or the doctors found it too risky. An emergency case and medications to handle potential hypersensitivity should be available. Patients were informed about therapy, safety aspects, side effects, and their off-label status and signed informed consent sheets.

The doctors regarded high-dose fever-inducing infusions to be inappropriate for weak, end-stage patients and children with advanced disease and poor condition during chemotherapy or if the patients felt too worn out, had no emotional resources, or could not tolerate fever and shivering. Some doctors also considered patients suffering from brain tumors, tumor compression, liver metastases, or tumor fever as inappropriate for intravenous treatment.

*3.5. Application, Preparations, Dose, and Time Aspects.* Preparations (Box 1) were chosen depending on the therapeutic goal, the patient's situation, the working context, and personal preferences of the doctors. Doses depended on preparation, the patient's condition, and the therapeutic goal. Infusions continued for 1–4 hours. Treatment durations varied and could last for years, until death or until the patients improved.

*3.6. Fever.* The frequency, quality, and time course of fever responses differ with different ME preparations.

*Iscador* infusions repeatedly induce fever after about 2 hours, accompanied by influenza-like symptoms, chills, shivering, and feeling unwell. When high temperature is reached, the patients feel comfortable, appear rosy, and start to sweat. Fever goes up to about 39°C, lasts for approximately 3 hours, and then drops again, so that outpatients can go home on the same day. Slower infusions can cause higher fever responses.

*AbnobaViscum* infusions do not induce fever alone, but only when combined with a subcutaneous injection (which alone can also induce fever). Fever can usually be elicited only 3-4 times, and only in patients without prior MT. It rises 6–12 hours after subcutaneous injection, up to 39,5–39,8°C, lasts for about 8–24 hours, and is gone after 2-3 days. It is exhausting, sometimes accompanied by headaches, and patients have to recover before receiving the next dose.

Regarding *Helixor* some doctors did not observe a fever response, while others did, albeit inconsistently. The response may depend on very high dosages. Temperature rises after 3-4 hours up to 38–40°C or just 0.5–1°C, measurable only with appropriate instruments. The fever is easier to endure, and patients feel more relaxed and well and may not notice it at all.

Infusions are sometimes combined with whole-body hyperthermia to prolong and intensify the fever period. Fever can rise up to 41.8°C and patients may be exhausted for 2 days. Patients are supported to better handle the fever, increase their well-being, and relieve the side effects.

*3.7. Observations of QoL.* The doctors described that patients experience an improved QoL and well-being under intravenous mistletoe infusion: patients regularly become "*more powerful*" and "*feel lighter.*" When the patients struggle with increasing weakness in advanced stages, they feel more energetic, dynamic, stronger, and "*invigorated*" with mistletoe infusions and can stay in a good condition for a long time, despite their progressive disease. Patients experience improved inner strength in addition to physical condition and fitness. Their condition becomes stable and "*recovery is activated.*" The patients become warmer, sleep better, have better appetites, start to eat again, and shift from catabolism to anabolism. Their skin becomes rosy. These effects were described as intense and extensive."*It is a wonderful therapy. I would do it myself and also give exactly that to my mother*" (gastroenterologist). "*After 5 days the patient reports: I feel much more powerful, I can get up again, I can go for walks twice as long as before. [...] If somebody says, 'I can only walk three steps from my bed into the kitchen and then I'm tired', then I can expect that they are more mobile again after one week of inpatient treatment and that they can walk again without support to a certain degree. If they say, 'I can only walk with a walking aid,' then I want to see that they eventually can at least walk again with crutches*" (internist).

These improvements are reported for about 50% to 80% of patients and about 20% to 30% of children and to be repeatable. Pausing intravenous infusions, on the other side, can lead to a deterioration of the patients' condition. In terms of care of dying patients, some of the doctors considered infusions as ineffective; others reported that well-being still improves and that "*calm and light [comes] into the situation*" (oncologist).

Pain caused by bone metastases was reported to improve reliably and substantially. The pain does not subside all at once and might even increase for a short time, but it resolves after the third or fourth infusion. Connected functions might also improve. For instance, patients no longer require walking aids. Prior associated freezing and chilling give way to a pleasant feeling of warmth after infusions. It was observed that X-rays showed sclerosis of the metastases (with osteolytic destabilizing metastases always receiving radiotherapy). Visceral pain does not or only modestly improve in a similar way, and opiates could not be replaced. Rather, the emaciation experienced through exhausting pain is relieved.

Fatigue, such as chemotherapy-associated fatigue, was described to also improve substantially and frequently within 2–4 weeks. This necessitates two to three infusions per week.

An improvement of QoL during chemotherapy was reported in about 50–80% of patients receiving a mistletoe infusion. General tolerability and the vitality and mood of the patients increase, and levels of asthenia, fatigue, mucositis, nausea, vomiting, and leucopenia decrease. Dose adaptions and premature terminations of chemotherapy become less likely.

The doctors reported that the emotional and mental levels of the patients stabilize and strengthen and that their moods improve. Patients become emotionally responsive, find inner peace and calmness, are less anxious, feel at ease ("*secure*"), feel confident, and develop prospects for the future ("*to have perspectives and will power*" [gastroenterologist]). The doctors used the following terms to describe the changes: "*emotional coat of warmth,*" "*sun,*" "*light,*" "*brightness,*" "*rest in,*" and "*connect with themselves.*"

*3.8. Observations in regard to Tumor Control.* The doctors indicated that tumor control was very difficult to assess in individual patients. However, many of the doctors illustrated via numerous case examples that high-dose treatments with intravenous infusions were followed by a long-lasting stabilization of the disease and a much longer-term survival than predicted, with good condition and QoL (Box 2). For instance, patients with peritoneal disseminated ovarian cancer lived for years under stable conditions with repeated intravenous MT (Helixor) ("*They actually should have already died a long time ago and they are still alive*" [general practitioner]). Sometimes the condition improved after changing the mistletoe preparation or host trees or combining it with other remedies (Box 3).

Relevant tumor reduction with infusions was not expected and not observed by most of the doctors. Still, some physicians did observe durable tumor remissions with intravenous infusions, mostly in combination with other application forms (Box 4), which seemed to augment the tumor responses. For instance, long-lasting tumor remissions were achieved in Merkel cell carcinoma, breast cancer, primary cutaneous B-cell lymphoma (which have also been published [19, 20, 24]), head and neck cancers, and others. One doctor perceived intravenous MT as a "*turning point*" in courses with recurrent relapses ("*There are many examples of this kind where you have the impression that again it was a turning point*" [general practitioner]). However, the doctors also indicated that a clear differentiation from the spontaneous course of disease was not often possible.

(i) A patient with breast cancer, lymphangiosis carcinomatosa and shortness of breath declined chemotherapy and received mistletoe infusions (Iscador) every 3 weeks. Each time, this substantially improved her breathing for a period of 2 weeks. She lived five years after diagnosis of lymphangiosis and 10 years since diagnosis of breast cancer. (General practitioner)

(ii) One patient with a huge inoperable colorectal carcinoma, metastases in the liver and lymph nodes and an additional renal cell cancer was first treated with intratumoral and subcutaneous applications. The tumor became harder and encapsulated. Due to gastrointestinal bleeding, the tumor, which had a weight of 5-6 kg, was removed (R0). After recovery from postoperative septic complications, the patient received MT subcutaneously and intravenously. His condition improved and stabilized. The patient returned to work despite his liver and bone metastases and lived for at least 3 more years until he died of a sudden cardiac arrest. (Internist)

(iii) A patient over 70 years old with a partly resected metastatic sigmoid colon cancer (T4) refused chemotherapy. She received infusions (Helixor, rhythmic dosages 100–500 mg) and lived well for 6 more years. She later also agreed to a temporary oral capecitabine treatment. The ultrasound showed an encapsulation of the tumor. After 6 years, the tumor induced heavy bleeding in the sigma and the patient died. (General practitioner)

(iv) One patient with a large pseudomyxoma peritonei, encircling large parts of the colon, had been treated with multiple operations, hyperthermia, chemotherapy and anthroposophic medicine. The tumor led to a rectovaginal fistula. The patient was then treated with fever-inducing mistletoe infusions (Iscador M spezial, 5 mg). A CT scan showed a slight improvement, and the fistula closed up temporarily. The patient lived with her disease for 15 years and was still alive at the time of the interview. (Oncologist)

(v) One patient with advanced inoperable prostate cancer and bone metastases (one in the pelvis at a size of 10 cm) received intravenous and partly intratumoral MT, and partly hormones and chemotherapy; he survived 12 years. (Neurologist, intensive care specialist)

(vi) Another patient with prostate cancer and lymph node metastases had received hormone treatment (bicalutamid, goserelin), which led to a reduction in PSA levels. After about 5 months, he engaged in a new partnership and gave great importance to his sexual function and thus terminated hormone treatment. After some months of increasing the PSA levels, an intravenous MT (Helixor M, 10–1500 mg) was started, intensifying the previous standard subcutaneous application. This led to a stabilization of PSA levels for 1 year. (Oncologist)

(vii) A patient had a rapidly growing glioblastoma at an initial size of 15 cm. Due to the rapid growth, the patient's first surgery was followed by re-surgery after only 2 weeks, and the subsequent radiotherapy terminated after 4 weeks. As this point, the tumor was already larger than its size before the first surgery. Mistletoe infusions were started and the situation stabilized. The patient lived for 1 more year. (Neurologist, intensive care specialist)

Box 2: Case illustrations of favorite course of disease under MT infusions, as reported by interviewed doctors.

(i) A patient with advanced, progressive non-small-cell lung cancer, lymphangiosis carcinomatosa, multiple metastases and pericardial effusion who had undergone prior palliative chemotherapies developed massive shortness of breath and pain. Her previous intravenous infusions with Iscador were changed to Helixor. Her condition unexpectedly improved drastically. She was able to go home and lived well for 3 more months. After a fall and injury, her condition deteriorated and she died. (General practitioner)

(ii) A patient with plasmocytoma received weekly infusions (Helixor P, 100–300 mg), inducing fever (38-39°C). Her condition and protein levels improved and became stable. The proteins later increased again, and a fever reaction could no longer be induced. Infusions were changed to an Abnoba preparation with high-dose intravenous (40–80 mg) and subcutaneous (10 mg) application. For 3 years, up to the interview, the patient was in good condition, was working and lived a very active life. (Average survival in untreated plasmocytoma is 3.5 years). (Internist) Another doctor described the stabilization of condition and bone manifestations in advanced plasmocytoma for periods of 6-7 years under regular mistletoe infusions. (Oncologist)

(iii) A patient with colon cancer and extensive liver metastases was expected to die soon. Different mistletoe applications had made no difference. Mistletoe infusion was combined with Helleborus niger, which was followed by a stabilization of the disease for several months with good QoL. (Internist)

Box 3: Case illustrations of favorite course of disease under infusions with changing ME preparations or combinations, as presented by interviewed doctors.

(i) A patient with metastatic, chemotherapy-resistant, very advanced esophageal cancer and a survival prognosis of 4 months was treated with mistletoe infusions twice per week for 5 years and had a complete tumor remission. The patient survived for more than 20 years up to the interview. (General practitioner, oncologist)

(ii) The residual tumor after the fourth surgical resections of recurrent breast cancer disappeared under treatment with mistletoe infusions alone. Since then the patient lived about 9 years. (General practitioner)

(iii) A patient with a cancer of unknown primary, a rapidly growing squamous cell carcinoma, peritoneal carcinosis and a very poor prognosis received weekly mistletoe infusions (Helixor A, 100–500 mg). He had a stable condition for 1,5 years, and the CT scan showed regression of some of the tumors. The tumors progressed again thereafter, and the infusions were switched to another host tree (Helixor M). The situation stabilized again, with further partial regressions in the CT scan, and remained as such at the time of the interview (about 9 months later). (Oncologist)

(iv) A patient with fungating locally recurrent breast cancer received MEs as peritumoral injections and intravenous infusions. The tumor regressed repeatedly for at least 2 years. (Internist)

(v) A patient with stomach cancer (removed by gastrectomy), liver and lymph node metastases and a depressed mood refused all standard oncological treatments. Her survival prognosis was 9 months. Her condition improved under mistletoe infusions alone (Abnoba Viscum Qu). She gained weight, vitality and enjoyment of life, and her depressive symptoms subsided. After some months, the liver metastases progressed, but now the patient agreed to chemotherapy (capecitabin oxaliplatin), which induced a partial remission. Mistletoe infusions were continued weekly, and the patient remained in a stable condition for 8 years. At the time of the interview, she had consulted the physician following a seizure, when a brain tumor or metastasis were suspected. (Oncologist) Another patient with colon cancer was treated with the same intravenous MT by the same physician, but similar good results could not be replicated. (Oncologist)

(vi) In a patient with leukemia mistletoe (Helixor) infusions had no remarkable influence on controlling lymphocytosis. However, previously frequent infections (lung) became less frequent and healed more easily and extensive fatigue vanished. (Oncologist)

Box 4: Case illustrations regarding tumor response and favorite course of disease under MT infusions.

*3.9. External Evidence.* Treatment of cancer patients with intravenous infusions with MEs has been investigated in four RCTs, one matched-pair study (see Table 2), and ten retrospective studies (see Table 3). Their methodological quality has been assessed elsewhere [14, 17, 37–39]. Three of the RCTs investigated the influence of MT infusion on tolerability of chemotherapy [41–43]. The fourth RCT [44] and matched-pair study [45] investigated its influence on surgery-induced suppression of the granulocyte function and NK-cell activity. Two of the studies investigated just a single infusion [44, 45]. One RCT also assessed survival [42]. The trials had small sample sizes and some lacked detailed information. The retrospective studies assessed the application of MT infusions in everyday practice, predominantly in patients with advanced, inoperable, and recurrent disease, but also partly in patients subsequent to surgery or radiotherapy. Most of the studies were published in the 1940s and 1950s, had methodological weaknesses, and investigated preparations no longer used in cancer therapy.

In terms of QoL, most of the trials reported an improved tolerability of chemotherapy, fewer side effects, a better general condition, and decreased anxiety. The retrospective studies mostly investigated patients with advanced metastatic disease. They described an improved subjective and general condition following intravenous MT; improved mental states; increases in well-being and initiative; a reduction of or freedom from symptoms despite disease progression; reductions of pain and fatigue; increases in weight, appetite, and physical strength; and better performance. Some of the studies also reported tumor remissions, partly in combination with intratumoral application and, in one study, with radiotherapy. The reported side effects were short-term fever and flu-like symptoms.

Studies investigating the safety of the intravenous application of MEs or recombinant mistletoe lectins found good tolerability and no toxicity [46–51]. One recent observational study assessed 475 cancer patients who had received 6,028 intravenous ME applications. Twenty-two patients had reported 32 adverse drug reactions (ADRs) of mild or moderate severity. ADRs were more frequent in early rather than advanced stages. ADRs were less frequent in intravenous than in subcutaneous application [52].

Several case reports on the intravenous infusion of MEs have been published, including some by the doctors interviewed in this study, and mostly exhibited a good reporting quality in accordance with the current CARE guidelines [53]. These cases mostly described tumor remissions and improvements of general condition during intravenous applications that were often combined with subcutaneous application and, if possible, intratumoral mistletoe intervention [19, 20, 54, 55].

## 4. Discussion

Doctors use individually applied intravenous MT to stabilize disease, improve QoL and general condition, strengthen patients, support tumor control, and relieve symptoms. The application is individually adapted. In a wider context the general therapeutic goal is to strengthen the patients' whole

TABLE 2: Randomized and nonrandomized controlled clinical trials on intravenous mistletoe treatment in cancer.

| Author, year | Site | Stage | Intervention (evaluable patients) | Survival | Immune parameters | Quality of life |
|---|---|---|---|---|---|---|
| Büssing et al. 2008 [41] | Breast | No data | (i) (5-Fu) EC, Iscador (32) (ii) (5-Fu) EC (33) | | Granulocyte function, lymphocytes: no difference | Reduction of EC-related side effects: nausea, constipation, pain, stomatitis.* EORTC C30, BR 23: no difference |
| Schink et al. 2007 [44] | Colon, rectum | II–IV | (i) Surgery, Iscador$^\S$ (11) (ii) Surgery (11) | | Decreased surgery-induced suppression of NK-cell activity* | |
| Büssing et al. 2005 [45] | Breast (suspected) | | (i) Surgery, Iscador$^\S$ (47) (ii) Surgery (51) | | Decreased surgery-induced suppression of granulocyte function* | |
| Cazacu et al. 2003 [42] | Colon, rectum | Dukes C and D | (i) Surgery, 5-Fu, Isorel (29) (ii) Surgery, 5-Fu (21) (iii) Surgery (14) | Median \| mean survival (months) | Dukes C \| D 25*\|17* 18\|7 17\|15 | 5-FU side effects (% of pat.) 0% 19% QoL: ↑, data not shown |
| Heiny 1991 [43] | Breast | Progredient | (i) VEC, Eurixor (21) (ii) VEC, placebo (19) | | | QoL ↑*, anxiety ↓*, leucopenia ↓*. No effect on thrombocytes |

§: single infusion. EC: epirubicin, cyclophosphamide; 5-Fu: 5-fluorouracil; V: vindesine; NK-cells: natural killer cells; ↑: increase; ↓: decrease; *statistically significant superior compared with control group.

constitution, including physical, vegetative, emotional, spiritual, and social dimensions, and to enable them to overcome or live with their disease and improve their physical, emotional, and mental condition despite life-threatening or progressing disease and potentially harmful treatments. Inducing fever is considered important, based on the conceptual background of AM and on data about the restorative and preventive function of high feverous infections and the historic success of fever therapy with bacterial toxins [19, 20, 56, 57]. The therapeutic concepts are based on a holistic understanding of the human organism [26, 58].

The different therapeutic components are considered to comprise a *therapeutic system* that synergizes effects and thus enhances the chances of health improvement [26, 59–61]. Cancer disease and treatment are understood within the holistic paradigm [62, 63]. Great emphasis is also put on the active participation, autonomy, and self-responsibility of the patient [26, 38].

The therapeutic goals, concepts, and observations voiced by the doctors interviewed in this study are consistent with the reasons given by patients for consulting AM doctors. In addition to having their disease and symptoms treated, patients seek to strengthen their physical constitution and immune systems to better cope with the side effects of conventional treatments and improve their chances of being cured. They also seek a holistic approach (integration of psychic, spiritual, and biographical issues) and want to take greater responsibility for themselves and actively participate in treatment [30, 38, 64, 65].

The therapeutic goals, concepts, and observations identified in this study closely matched the problems, concerns, and needs of cancer patients in general. Patients often feel weak or tired, lack energy, or suffer from fatigue [66, 67]. Persistent chill and feeling too cold are underrecognized and underexplored forms of patient distress [68] that are presumably relevant for tumor control [69]. Disturbed sleep, pain, impaired taste or appetite, anorexia, and depression are additional problems [66, 67, 70, 71]. On the emotional level, substantial emotional distress—the sixth vital sign [72]—can be induced by diagnosis and treatment [73, 74]. Being younger and more educated increases a patient's risk of distress [75]. The ability to have a normal life without being too restricted by symptoms and to feel autonomous and in control of situations connected to one's personal life and treatment situation is essential [76, 77]. Functional limitations such as not being able to continue usual routines or daily life tasks and an inability to carry out important roles together with existential concerns are sources of suffering, particularly for palliative patients [75]. The needs of these patients often stay unmet and are underrepresented in the markers of good conventional oncology care, at least in Germany [78]. Therefore, a systematic approach toward

TABLE 3: Single-arm retrospective studies of intravenous mistletoe treatment in cancer.

| Author, year | Preparation | Cotherapy[i] | Tumor site[ii] | Tumor behaviour | $n$[iii] | Quality of life |
|---|---|---|---|---|---|---|
| Wolf et al. 1994 [88] | Isorel | | Diverse | | 25 | Improved condition and mood, decreased pain and depression |
| Wolf 1987 [89] | Isorel | | Diverse | Remissions | 60 | Improved subjective condition, appetite, digestion, weight gain |
| Brück 1950, 1954 [90, 91] | Plenosol | It | Diverse | Remissions | 5 | Improved general condition, well-being, symptom-free |
| Tosetti 1954 [92] | Plenosol | It, vitamins | Gynecologic | | 60 | Improved general condition, weight gain |
| Rupp and Siegert 1952 [93] | Plenosol | | Breast, cervix | | 50 | Improved condition |
| Meythaler and Händel 1952 [94] | Plenosol | | Diverse | Remissions | 78 | Improved condition, appetite, mood, physical strength, weight gain, decreased fatigue |
| Stehberger 1951 [95] | Plenosol | RT | Diverse | | ~40 | Improved condition, weight gain, able to work again |
| Röseler 1952 [96] | Plenosol | It, surgery | Breast, gynecologic | Remissions | 68 | Improved physical strength, symptom-free despite progressing, disseminated disease |
| Wasmuht 1944 [97] | Plenosol | It, RT | ENT | Remissions | 21 | |
| Kraft 1940 [98] | Plenosol | It | Diverse | Remissions | 27 (50) | Improved general condition, appetite, able to work again |

[i]It: intratumoral application of mistletoe extract; RT: radiotherapy; [ii]mostly advanced, inoperable, and recurrent; [iii]$n$: number of patients.

individualized integrative care can complement conventional cancer care in a meaningful way.

The results from our interviews are consistent with the results from clinical mistletoe studies that have reported an improved general condition and mental state, decreased symptoms in patients with advanced disease, or improved tolerability of chemotherapy (see Tables 2 and 3). Other qualitative studies interviewing cancer patients about their experiences with MT or AM have reported similar issues: stronger vitality, enhanced autonomy, increased hope, better disease acceptance, and personal achievements such as new prospects, professional life changes, capacity to make own decisions and establish priorities, and improved self-confidence and strength [79–82]. Case reports have described condition stabilization or tumor remission, mostly under combined intravenous and subcutaneous and intratumoral ME application [19, 20, 54, 55].

Compared with the literature, this study illustrates a larger range of observations related to vitality, regaining strength and well-being, and condition stabilization and covers observation periods that last up to many years and decades. The safety aspects reported by the interviewed doctors provided more details than clinical studies [46–52].

*4.1. Strengths and Weaknesses.* The main strength of this study is the richness of information, arising directly from everyday clinical practice and from doctors who took care of their patients, often over years or even decades. Therefore, this study provides information about what may be pursued and possibly achieved in patients who are constrained by a serious life-threatening or life-limiting disease and are often suffering to a great extent. Additional strengths include the range of participants (achieved through purposive sampling), reflecting different specializations, countries, settings, and ages among other characteristics; the extensive interviews (up to 5 hours in duration); the amount of information gathered about complex therapy systems and treatment processes; the trusting and open atmosphere established through confidentiality; and the reputation of the researchers.

This study also has limitations. First, it presents only the views of doctors. The perspectives of patients were not evaluated and the treatment process was not directly observed. Both would have been important complements to the doctors' reports. In principle, however, other qualitative studies interviewing patients and patient surveys have reported similar outcomes. Patients judged AM cancer care in an AM hospital as particularly positive with regard to emotional effects, quality of human relations, and cognitive-spiritual effects, but also with regard to the effects on tumors and the body, mostly with reference to patients' recovery and general improvement. Their compliance with AM was high [27, 28]. In a British study, patients gave favorable acknowledgment of the time given to consultations, the quality of those consultations, the thoroughness involved in exploring medical and biographical histories, the combined conventional/AM approach, good and dialogue-like communication, care and personal encouragement, the holistic nature of the patient-centered approach, the benefits of individually tailored treatment, the facilitation of personal learning and development, and their personal involvement in the management of their illnesses [82]. Furthermore, patients' satisfaction with AM care has generally been high and their therapeutic expectations were fulfilled [30, 38, 83–85].

Other limitations include the confounding element of the integrative treatment setting which, as the doctors pointed out, impeded causal attributions to MT in most cases. Furthermore, our doctors, given their high levels of expertise in complementary and conventional cancer care and associated devices, may not be representative of the average caregiver. Many of the doctors had positive and empathic attitudes which possibly provided further additional support [86, 87]. However, although the doctors were careful when drawing causal conclusions and discussing the variety of confounders, they were certain about some specific therapeutic benefits of the intravenous application of MEs and made clear safety recommendations. Therefore, these benefits may be achieved in other therapeutic contexts as well and their further investigation is worthwhile. However, clear generalizations and the frequency of therapeutic effects are beyond the methods of this study.

Further research questions emerging from our results should be investigated in future clinical studies, including the influence of intravenous applications of MEs on (1) increasing weakness in progressive disease; (2) cancer-related fatigue; (3) pain caused by bone metastases; (4) tolerability of chemotherapy; (5) dyspnea in lymphangitis carcinomatosa of the lung; (6) tumor cachexia; (7) disease stabilization; and (8) tumor recurrence in high-risk patients. Secondary outcomes should include tumor control and patient survival, if possible. Furthermore, the effects and improvement of thermal comfort should be assessed in addition to functional abilities and issues of inner and outer autonomy. Close attention must be paid to the described individualization of treatment and safety aspects. A comparison of individualized treatment with standardized application or placebo administration would be a warranted treatment objective for later trials. If some of the presented observations are validated or replicated in clinical trials, they may contribute to the healthcare of cancer patients and help to relieve their suffering.

## 5. Conclusions

Individualized integrative cancer treatment including MT aims to help cancer patients to live well with their disease in many ways. According to the experiences of interviewed doctors, intravenous MT may particularly support patients in advanced stages and help stabilize and improve QoL and meet important needs and distresses of patients and help to positively affect a patient's tumor situation. Further research should investigate the reported observations.

## Competing Interests

IFAEMM has received restricted research grants, honorariums, and travel expenses from Weleda, Abnoba, and Helixor. None of this funding had any influence on the design, conduction, analysis, and publication of the study.

## Authors' Contributions

Gunver S. Kienle, Milena Mussler, Dieter Fuchs, and Helmut Kiene contributed to study design. Gunver S. Kienle and Milena Mussler carried out interviews and analyzed the data. Dieter Fuchs and Helmut Kiene participated in data analysis. All authors approved the final paper.

## Acknowledgments

The authors thank the participants in this interview study for their detailed and insightful responses. The authors also thank the Society of Anthroposophic Doctors in Germany (GAÄD) and *Arbeitsgruppe niedergelassener Ärzte in Deutschland* for their collaboration in designing and conducting the study. The authors are grateful to the Society of Anthroposophic Doctors in Germany (GAÄD), Software AG Stiftung, Mahle Stiftung, Zukunftsstiftung Gesundheit/Christophoros Stiftungsfond, Hauschka-Stiftung, Abnoba, Helixor, Weleda/Hiscia, and the families and friends of cancer patients for financially supporting this work.

## References

[1] P. A. Fasching, F. Thiel, K. Nicolaisen-Murmann et al., "Association of complementary methods with quality of life and life satisfaction in patients with gynecologic and breast malignancies," *Supportive Care in Cancer*, vol. 15, no. 11, pp. 1277–1284, 2007.

[2] A. Molassiotis, J. A. Scott, N. Kearney et al., "Complementary and alternative medicine use in breast cancer patients in Europe," *Supportive Care in Cancer*, vol. 14, no. 3, pp. 260–267, 2006.

[3] A. Molassiotis, P. Fernandez-Ortega, D. Pud et al., "Use of complementary and alternative medicine in cancer patients: a European survey," *Annals of Oncology*, vol. 16, no. 4, pp. 655–663, 2005.

[4] *Arzneiverordnungs-Report 2008*, Springer, Berlin, Germany, 2008.

[5] E. Petru, P. Schmied, and C. Petru, "Komplementäre Maßnahmen bei Patientinnen mit gynäkologischen Malignomen unter

Chemo- und Hormontherapie—Bestandsaufnahme und kritische Überlegungen für die Praxis," *Geburtshilfe und Frauenheilkunde*, vol. 61, no. 2, pp. 75–78, 2001.

[6] E. A. Mueller and F. A. Anderer, "A Viscum album oligosaccharide activating human natural cytotoxicity is an interferon γ inducer," *Cancer Immunology Immunotherapy*, vol. 32, no. 4, pp. 221–227, 1990.

[7] C. Y. Klett and F. A. Anderer, "Activation of natural killer cell cytotoxicity of human blood monocytes by a low molecular weight component from viscum album extract," *Drug Research*, vol. 39, no. 12, pp. 1580–1585, 1989.

[8] S. Jäger, K. Winkler, U. Pfüller, and A. Scheffler, "Solubility studies of oleanolic acid and betulinic acid in aqueous solutions and plant extracts of *Viscum album* L.," *Planta Medica*, vol. 73, no. 2, pp. 157–162, 2007.

[9] J. Eggenschwiler, L. von Balthazar, B. Stritt et al., "Mistletoe lectin is not the only cytotoxic component in fermented preparations of *Viscum album* from white fir (*Abies pectinata*)," *BMC Complementary and Alternative Medicine*, vol. 7, no. 1, article 14, 2007.

[10] A. Büssing and M. Schietzel, "Apoptosis-inducing properties of *Viscum album* L. extracts from different host trees, correlate with their content of toxic mistletoe lectins," *Anticancer Research*, vol. 19, no. 1, pp. 23–28, 1999.

[11] U. Elsässer-Beile, S. Lusebrink, U. Grussenmeyer, U. Wetterauer, and W. Schultze-Seemann, "Comparison of the effects of various clinically applied mistletoe preparations on peripheral blood leukocytes," *Arzneimittel-Forschung/Drug Research*, vol. 48, no. 12, pp. 1185–1189, 1998.

[12] I. Siegle, P. Fritz, M. McClellan, S. Gutzeit, and T. E. Mürdter, "Combined cytotoxic action of *Viscum album* agglutinin-1 and anticancer agents against human A549 lung cancer cells," *Anticancer Research*, vol. 21, no. 4, pp. 2687–2691, 2001.

[13] H. Bantel, I. H. Engels, W. Voelter, K. Schulze-Osthoff, and S. Wesselborg, "Mistletoe lectin activates caspase-8/FLICE independently of death receptor signaling and enhances anticancer drug-induced apoptosis," *Cancer Research*, vol. 59, no. 9, pp. 2083–2090, 1999.

[14] G. S. Kienle and H. Kiene, *Die Mistel in der Onkologie—Fakten und konzeptionelle Grundlagen*, Schattauer Verlag, Stuttgart, Germany, 2003.

[15] A. Büssing, *Mistletoe. The Genus Viscum*, Hardwood Academic Publishers, Amsterdam, The Netherlands, 2000.

[16] W. Tröger, D. Galun, M. Reif, A. Schumann, N. Stanković, and M. Milićević, "*Viscum album* [L.] extract therapy in patients with locally advanced or metastatic pancreatic cancer: a randomised clinical trial on overall survival," *European Journal of Cancer*, vol. 49, no. 18, pp. 3788–3797, 2013.

[17] G. S. Kienle and H. Kiene, "Complementary cancer therapy: a systematic review of prospective clinical trials on anthroposophic mistletoe extracts," *European Journal of Medical Research*, vol. 12, no. 3, pp. 103–119, 2007.

[18] G. S. Kienle, A. Glockmann, M. Schink, and H. Kiene, "*Viscum album* L. extracts in breast and gynaecological cancers: a systematic review of clinical and preclinical research," *Journal of Experimental and Clinical Cancer Research*, vol. 28, article 79, 2009.

[19] M. Orange, A. Lace, M. P. Fonseca, B. H. von Laue, S. Geider, and G. S. Kienle, "Durable regression of primary cutaneous B-cell lymphoma following fever-inducing mistletoe treatment: two case reports," *Global Advances in Health and Medicine*, vol. 1, no. 1, pp. 18–25, 2012.

[20] M. Orange, M. Fonseca, A. Lace, H. B. von Laue, and S. Geider, "Durable tumour responses following primary high dose induction with mistletoe extracts: two case reports," *European Journal of Integrative Medicine*, vol. 2, no. 2, pp. 63–69, 2010.

[21] A. Scheffler, H. Mast, S. Fischer, and H. R. Metelmann, "Komplette remission eines mundhöhlenkarzinoms nach alleiniger mistelbehandlung," in *Grundlagen der Misteltherapie Aktueller Stand der Forschung und klinische Anwendung*, R. Scheer, H. Becker, and P. A. Berg, Eds., pp. 453–466, Hippokrates Verlag GmbH, Stuttgart, Germany, 1996.

[22] A. Kirsch, "Successful treatment of metastatic malignant melanoma with *Viscum album* extract (Iscador® M)," *Journal of Alternative and Complementary Medicine*, vol. 13, no. 4, pp. 443–445, 2007.

[23] G. Seifert, C. Tautz, K. Seeger, G. Henze, and A. Laengler, "Therapeutic use of mistletoe for CD30+ cutaneous lymphoproliferative disorder/lymphomatoid papulosis," *Journal of the European Academy of Dermatology and Venereology*, vol. 21, no. 4, pp. 558–560, 2007.

[24] P. G. Werthmann, D. Helling, P. Heusser, and G. S. Kienle, "Tumour response following high-dose intratumoural application of *Viscum album* on a patient with adenoid cystic carcinoma," *BMJ Case Reports*, 2014.

[25] P. G. Werthmann, G. Sträter, H. Friesland, and G. S. Kienle, "Durable response of cutaneous squamous cell carcinoma following high-dose peri-lesional injections of *Viscum album* extracts—a case report," *Phytomedicine*, vol. 20, no. 3-4, pp. 324–327, 2013.

[26] G. S. Kienle, H. Albonico, E. Baars, H. J. Hamre, P. Zimmermann, and H. Kiene, "Anthroposophic medicine: an integrative medical system originating in Europe," *Global Advances in Health and Medicine*, vol. 2, no. 6, pp. 20–31, 2013.

[27] P. Heusser, S. B. Braun, M. Bertschy et al., "Palliative in-patient cancer treatment in an anthroposophic hospital: II. Quality of life during and after stationary treatment, and subjective treatment benefits," *Forschende Komplementärmedizin*, vol. 13, no. 3, pp. 156–166, 2006.

[28] P. Heusser, S. B. Braun, R. Ziegler et al., "Palliative in-patient cancer treatment in an anthroposophic hospital. I. Treatment patterns and compliance with anthroposophic medicine," *Forschende Komplementärmedizin*, vol. 13, no. 2, pp. 94–100, 2006.

[29] H. J. Hamre, C. Becker-Witt, A. Glockmann, R. Ziegler, S. N. Willich, and H. Kiene, "Anthroposophic therapies in chronic disease: the Anthroposophic Medicine Outcomes Study (AMOS)," *European Journal of Medical Research*, vol. 9, no. 7, pp. 351–360, 2004.

[30] M. Arman, A.-S. Hammarqvist Anne-Sofie, and A. Kullberg, "Anthroposophic health care in Sweden-a patient evaluation," *Complementary Therapies in Clinical Practice*, vol. 17, no. 3, pp. 170–178, 2011.

[31] P. Mayring, *Qualitative Inhaltsanalyse*, Beltz, Weinheim, Germany, 2010.

[32] A. Broom, "Using qualitative interviews in CAM research: a guide to study design, data collection and data analysis," *Complementary Therapies in Medicine*, vol. 13, no. 1, pp. 65–73, 2005.

[33] J. L. J. Ritchie, *Qualitative Research Practice. A Guide for Social Science Students and Researchers*, Sage, London, UK, 2003.

[34] M. Q. Patton, *Qualitative Research and Evaluation Methods*, Sage, Thousand Oaks, Calif, USA, 2002.

[35] U. Flick, *Qualitative Sozialforschung*, Rowohlt, 2007.

[36] U. Kuckartz, *Einführung in die Computergestützte Analyse Qualitativer Daten*, Sozialwissenschaftler, Wiesbaden, Germany, 2007.

[37] G. S. Kienle, F. Berrino, A. Büssing, E. Portalupi, S. Rosenzweig, and H. Kiene, "Mistletoe in cancer-a systematic review on controlled clinical trials," *European Journal of Medical Research*, vol. 8, no. 3, pp. 109–119, 2003.

[38] G. S. Kienle, H. Kiene, and H. U. Albonico, *Anthroposophic Medicine: Effectiveness, Utility, Costs, Safety*, Schattauer, Stuttgart, Germany, 2006.

[39] G. S. Kienle and H. Kiene, "Influence of *Viscum album* L (European Mistletoe) extracts on quality of life in cancer patients: a systematic review of controlled clinical studies," *Integrative Cancer Therapies*, vol. 9, no. 2, pp. 142–157, 2010.

[40] G. S. Kienle, M. Mussler, D. Fuchs, and H. Kiene, "Individualized integrative cancer care in anthroposophic medicine: a qualitative study of the concepts and procedures of expert doctors," *Integrative Cancer Therapies*, In press.

[41] A. Büssing, U. Brückner, U. Enser-Weis et al., "Modulation of chemotherapy-associated immunosuppression by intravenous application of *Viscum album* L. extract (Iscador): a randomised phase II study," *European Journal of Integrative Medicine*, vol. 1, supplement 1, pp. 2–3, 2008.

[42] M. Cazacu, T. Oniu, C. Lungoci et al., "The influence of Isorel on the advanced colorectal cancer," *Cancer Biotherapy & Radiopharmaceuticals*, vol. 18, no. 1, pp. 27–34, 2003.

[43] B. M. Heiny, "Additive Therapie mit standardisiertem Mistelextrakt reduziert die Leukopenie und verbessert die Lebensqualität von Patientinnen mit fortgeschrittenem Mammakarzinom unter palliativer Chemotherapie (VEC-Schema)," *Krebsmedizin*, vol. 12, pp. 1–14, 1991.

[44] M. Schink, W. Tröger, A. Dabidian et al., "Mistletoe extract reduces the surgical suppression of natural killer cell activity in cancer patients. A randomized phase III trial," *Research in Complementary Medicine*, vol. 14, no. 1, pp. 9–17, 2007.

[45] A. Büssing, M. Bischof, W. Hatzmann et al., "Prevention of surgery-induced suppression of granulocyte function by intravenous application of a fermented extract from *Viscum album* L. in breast cancer patients," *Anticancer Research*, vol. 25, no. 6, pp. 4753–4758, 2005.

[46] E. Böcher, C. Stumpf, A. Büssing, and M. Schietzel, "Prospektive Bewertung der Toxizität hochdosierter Viscum album L.-Infusionen bei Patienten mit progredienten Malignomen," *Zeitschrift für Onkologie*, vol. 28, no. 4, pp. 97–106, 1996.

[47] A. Büssing, C. Stumpf, R. T. Stumpf, H. Wutte, and M. Schietzel, "Therapiebegleitende untersuchung immunologischer parameter bei tumor-patienten nach hochdosierter intravenöser applikation von Viscum album L.-Extrakten," *Zeitschrift für Onkologie*, vol. 28, no. 2, pp. 54–59, 1996.

[48] P. Schöffski, I. Breidenbach, J. Krauter et al., "Weekly 24 h infusion of aviscumine (rViscumin): a phase I study in patients with solid tumours," *European Journal of Cancer*, vol. 41, no. 10, pp. 1431–1438, 2005.

[49] P. Schöffski, S. Riggert, P. Fumoleau et al., "Phase I trial of intravenous aviscumine (rViscumin) in patients with solid tumors: a study of the European Organization for research and treatment of cancer new drug development group," *Annals of Oncology*, vol. 15, no. 12, pp. 1816–1824, 2004.

[50] K. R. Wiebelitz and A. M. Beer, "Intravenöse Hochdosis-Misteltherapie—Klinische Ergebnisse, Laborparameter, unerwünschte Ereignisse in einer Fallserie von 107 Anwendungen an 17 Patienten," in *Die Mistel in der Tumortherapie 3 Aktueller Stand der Forschung und Klinische Anwendung*, R. Scheer, S. Alban, H. Becker et al., Eds., pp. 295–314, KVC Verlag, Essen, Germany, 2013.

[51] G. S. Kienle, R. Grugel, and H. Kiene, "Safety of higher dosages of *Viscum album* L. in animals and humans—systematic review of immune changes and safety parameters," *BMC Complementary and Alternative Medicine*, vol. 11, no. 1, article 72, 2011.

[52] M. L. Steele, J. Axtner, A. Happe, M. Kröz, H. Matthes, and F. Schad, "Safety of intravenous application of mistletoe (*Viscum album* L.) preparations in oncology: an observational study," *Evidence-Based Complementary and Alternative Medicine*, vol. 2014, Article ID 236310, 10 pages, 2014.

[53] J. J. Gagnier, G. Kienle, D. G. Altman, D. Moher, H. Sox, and D. Riley, "The CARE guidelines: consensus-based clinical case report guideline development," *Journal of Clinical Epidemiology*, vol. 67, no. 1, pp. 46–51, 2014.

[54] F. Schad, M. Kröz, M. Girke, H. P. Lemmens, D. Brauer, and B. Matthes, "Intraläsionale und kombinierte subkuta-intravenöse Misteltherapie bei einem Patienten mit Kolonkarzinom," *Der Merkurstab*, vol. 52, no. 9, pp. 399–406, 1999.

[55] J. Gutsch, "Außergewöhnlicher Krankheitsverlauf bei metastasierendem Mammakarzinom unter Misteltherapie nach pseudoallergischer Reaktion," in *Die Mistel in der Tumortherapie Grundlagenforschung und Klinik*, R. Scheer, R. Bauer, H. Becker, P. A. Berg, and V. Fintelmann, Eds., pp. 379–387, KVC Verlag, Essen, Germany, 2001.

[56] G. S. Kienle, "Fever in cancer treatment: Coley's therapy and epidemiologic observations," *Global Advances in Health and Medicine*, vol. 1, no. 1, pp. 92–100, 2012.

[57] U. Hobohm, "Healing heat: harnessing infection to fight cancer," *American Scientist*, vol. 97, no. 1, pp. 34–41, 2009.

[58] P. Heusser and G. S. Kienle, "Anthroposophic medicine, integrative oncology, and mistletoe therapy of cancer," in *Integrative Oncology*, D. Abrams and A. Weil, Eds., pp. 560–588, Oxford University Press, New York, NY, USA, 2014.

[59] M. Girke, *Innere Medizin: Krankheitsbilder und therapeutische Konzepte der Anthroposophischen Medizin*, Natur Mensch Medizin, Bad Boll, Germany, 2010.

[60] G. Soldner and H. M. Stellmann, *Individuelle Pädiatrie: Leibliche, Seelische und Geistige Aspekte in Diagnostik und Beratung; Anthroposophisch-Homöopathische Therapie*, Wissenschaftliche Verlagsgesellschaft, Stuttgart, Germany, 2007.

[61] IOM (Institute of Medicine), *Integrative Medicine and the Health of the Public: A Summary of the February 2009 Summit*, The National Academies Press, Washington, DC, USA, 2009.

[62] G. Kienle and H. Kiene, "From reductionism to holism: systems-oriented approaches in cancer research," *Global Advances in Health and Medicine*, vol. 1, no. 5, pp. 68–77, 2012.

[63] G. S. Kienle and H. Kiene, "'Beyond reductionism'—zur Notwendigkeit komplexer, organischer Ansätze in der Tumorimmunologie und Onkologie," in *Die Mistel in der Onkologie*, G. S. Kienle and H. Kiene, Eds., pp. 333–432, Schattauer, Stuttgart, Germany, 2003.

[64] A. Laengler, C. Spix, G. Seifert, S. Gottschling, N. Graf, and P. Kaatsch, "Complementary and alternative treatment methods in children with cancer: a population-based retrospective survey on the prevalence of use in Germany," *European Journal of Cancer*, vol. 44, no. 15, pp. 2233–2240, 2008.

[65] E. von Rohr, S. Pampallona, B. van Wegberg et al., "Attitudes and beliefs towards disease and treatment in patients with advanced cancer using anthroposophical medicine," *Onkologie*, vol. 23, no. 6, pp. 558–563, 2000.

[66] A. H. Kamal, J. Bull, D. Kavalieratos, D. H. Taylor Jr., W. Downey, and A. P. Abernethy, "Palliative care needs of patients with cancer living in the community," *Journal of Oncology Practice*, vol. 7, no. 6, pp. 382–388, 2011.

[67] V. Lidstone, E. Butters, P. T. Seed, C. Sinnott, T. Beynon, and M. Richards, "Symptoms and concerns amongst cancer outpatients: identifying the need for specialist palliative care," *Palliative Medicine*, vol. 17, no. 7, pp. 588–595, 2003.

[68] K. M. Kokolus, C.-C. Hong, and E. A. Repasky, "Feeling too hot or cold after breast cancer: is it just a nuisance or a potentially important prognostic factor?" *International Journal of Hyperthermia*, vol. 26, no. 7, pp. 662–680, 2010.

[69] K. M. Kokolus, M. L. Capitano, C.-T. Lee et al., "Baseline tumor growth and immune control in laboratory mice are significantly influenced by subthermoneutral housing temperature," *Proceedings of the National Academy of Sciences of the United States of America*, vol. 110, no. 50, pp. 20176–20181, 2013.

[70] O. G. Palesh, J. A. Roscoe, K. M. Mustian et al., "Prevalence, demographics, and psychological associations of sleep disruption in patients with cancer: University of Rochester Cancer Center-community clinical oncology program," *Journal of Clinical Oncology*, vol. 28, no. 2, pp. 292–298, 2010.

[71] M. R. Irwin, R. E. Olmstead, P. A. Ganz, and R. Haque, "Sleep disturbance, inflammation and depression risk in cancer survivors," *Brain, Behavior, and Immunity*, vol. 30, pp. S58–S67, 2013.

[72] B. D. Bultz and J. C. Holland, "Emotional distress in patients with cancer: the sixth vital sign," *Community Oncology*, vol. 3, no. 5, pp. 311–314, 2006.

[73] L. E. Carlson and B. D. Bultz, "Efficacy and medical cost offset of psychosocial interventions in cancer care: making the case for economic analyses," *Psycho-Oncology*, vol. 13, no. 12, pp. 837–849, 2004.

[74] L. E. Carlson, M. Angen, J. Cullum et al., "High levels of untreated distress and fatigue in cancer patients," *British Journal of Cancer*, vol. 90, no. 12, pp. 2297–2304, 2004.

[75] H. M. Chochinov, T. Hassard, S. McClement et al., "The landscape of distress in the terminally ill," *Journal of Pain and Symptom Management*, vol. 38, no. 5, pp. 641–649, 2009.

[76] T. G. Thomsen, S. R. Hansen, and L. Wagner, "Prioritising, downplaying and self-preservation: processes significant to coping in advanced cancer patients," *Open Journal of Nursing*, vol. 2, no. 2, pp. 48–57, 2012.

[77] T. G. Thomsen, S. R. Hansen, and L. Wagner, "How to be a patient in a palliative life experience? A qualitative study to enhance knowledge about coping abilities in advanced cancer patients," *Journal of Psychosocial Oncology*, vol. 29, no. 3, pp. 254–273, 2011.

[78] K. Hermes-Moll, G. Klein, R. E. Buschmann-Maiworm et al., "WINHO-Qualitätsindikatoren für die ambulante onkologische Versorgung in Deutschland," *Zeitschrift für Evidenz, Fortbildung und Qualität im Gesundheitswesen*, vol. 107, no. 8, pp. 548–559, 2013.

[79] M. Brandenberger, A. P. Simões-Wüst, M. Rostock, L. Rist, and R. Saller, "An exploratory study on the quality of life and individual coping of cancer patients during mistletoe therapy," *Integrative Cancer Therapies*, vol. 11, no. 2, pp. 90–100, 2012.

[80] M. Arman, A. Rehnsfeldt, M. Carlsson, and E. Hamrin, "Indications of change in life perspective among women with breast cancer admitted to complementary care," *European Journal of Cancer Care*, vol. 10, no. 3, pp. 192–200, 2001.

[81] M. Arman, A. Ranheim, A. Rehnsfeldt, and K. Wode, "Anthroposophic health care—different and home-like," *Scandinavian Journal of Caring Sciences*, vol. 22, no. 3, pp. 357–366, 2008.

[82] J. Ritchie, J. Wilkinson, M. Gantley, G. Feder, Y. Carter, and J. Formby, *A Model of Integrated Primary Care: Anthroposophic Medicine*, vol. 158, National Centre for Social Research Department of General Practice and Primary Care, St. Bartholomew's and the Royal London School of Medicine and Dentistry, Queen Mary, University of London, London, UK, 2001.

[83] B. M. Esch, F. Marian, A. Busato, and P. Heusser, "Patient satisfaction with primary care: an observational study comparing anthroposophic and conventional care," *Health and Quality of Life Outcomes*, vol. 6, article 74, 2008.

[84] G. S. Kienle, A. Glockmann, R. Grugel, H. J. Hamre, and H. Kiene, "Klinische Forschung zur Anthroposophischen Medizin—Update eines Health Technology Assessment-Berichts und Status Quo," *Forschende Komplementärmedizin*, vol. 18, pp. 269–282, 2011.

[85] E. B. Koster, R. R. S. Ong, R. Heybroek, D. M. J. Delnoij, and E. W. Baars, "The consumer quality index anthroposophic healthcare: a construction and validation study," *BMC Health Services Research*, vol. 14, article 148, 2014.

[86] B. D. Jani, D. N. Blane, and S. W. Mercer, "The role of empathy in therapy and the physician-patient relationship," *Forschende Komplementärmedizin*, vol. 19, no. 5, pp. 252–257, 2012.

[87] S. W. Mercer, D. Reilly, and G. C. M. Watt, "The importance of empathy in the enablement of patients attending the Glasgow Homoeopathic Hospital," *British Journal of General Practice*, vol. 52, no. 484, pp. 901–905, 2002.

[88] P. Wolf, N. Freudenberg, and M. Konitzer, "Analgetische und stimmungsaufhellende Wirkung bei Malignom-Patienten unter hochdosierter Viscum album-Infusionstherapie (Vysorel)," *Deutsche Zeitschrift für Onkologie*, vol. 26, no. 2, pp. 52–54, 1994.

[89] P. Wolf, "Erfahrungsbericht über eine rhythmische Infusionstherapie mit einem Viscum-album-Präparat in einer allgemeinen Praxis," *Erfahrungsheilkunde*, vol. 36, no. 12, pp. 836–838, 1987.

[90] D. Brück, "Kasuistischer beitrag zur karzinombehandlung mit plenosol," *Hippokrates*, no. 3, pp. 76–79, 1950.

[91] D. Brück, "Plenosoltherapie des Karzinoms in der Praxis," *Hippokrates. Zeitschrift für praktische Heilkunde*, vol. 25, no. 3, pp. 80–82, 1954.

[92] K. Tosetti, "Mistelextrakt und vitamin A in der behandlung der weiblichen genitalkarzinome," *Zentralblatt für Gynäkologie*, no. 13, pp. 509–514, 1954.

[93] L. Rupp and A. Siegert, "Über die wirkung des plenosols bei collum- und mamma-carcinom-rezidiven," *Therapie der Gegenwart*, no. 7, pp. 251–255, 1952.

[94] F. Meythaler and F. Händel, "Die Karzinombehandlung mit Plenosol," *Deutsche Medizinische Wochenschrift*, vol. 77, no. 43, pp. 1319–1323, 1952.

[95] W. Stehberger, "Über die bisherigen erfahrungen mit der I.V. plenosoltherapie bei carcinomkranken," *Therapiewoche*, no. 1, pp. 581–582, 1951.

[96] W. B. Röseler, "Über die nachbehandlung operierter oder bestrahlter kollumkarzinomkranker mit dem mistelextrakt

plenosol," *Zentralblatt für Gynäkologie*, no. 48, pp. 1905–1912, 1952.

[97] M. Wasmuht, *Erfahrungen Über die Behandlung von Krebskranken mit Mistelextrakt*, Albert-Ludwigs-Universität Freiburg, Freiburg im Breisgau, Germany, 1944.

[98] P. Kraft, "Praktische Erfahrungen über die Behandlung der Krebskrankheit mit Mistelextrakten," *Münchner Medizinische Wochenschrift*, no. 50, pp. 1395–1399, 1940.

# 13

# Tanreqing Injection Attenuates Lipopolysaccharide-Induced Airway Inflammation through MAPK/NF-κB Signaling Pathways in Rats Model

**Wei Liu, Hong-li Jiang, Lin-li Cai, Min Yan, Shou-jin Dong, and Bing Mao**

*Pneumology Group, Department of Integrated Traditional Chinese and Western Medicine, West China Hospital, Sichuan University, Chengdu 610041, China*

Correspondence should be addressed to Bing Mao; maobing2013@yeah.net

Academic Editor: Sergio R. Ambrosio

*Background.* Tanreqing injection (TRQ) is a commonly used herbal patent medicine for treating inflammatory airway diseases in view of its outstanding anti-inflammatory properties. In this study, we explored the signaling pathways involved in contributions of TRQ to LPS-induced airway inflammation in rats. *Methods/Design.* Adult male Sprague Dawley (SD) rats randomly divided into different groups received intratracheal instillation of LPS and/or intraperitoneal injection of TRQ. Bronchoalveolar Lavage Fluid (BALF) and lung samples were collected at 24 h, 48 h, and 96 h after TRQ administration. Protein and mRNA levels of tumor necrosis factor- (TNF-) $\alpha$, Interleukin- (IL-) $1\beta$, IL-6, and IL-8 in BALF and lung homogenate were observed by ELISA and real-time PCR, respectively. Lung sections were stained for p38 MAPK and NF-κB detection by immunohistochemistry. Phospho-p38 MAPK, phosphor-extracellular signal-regulated kinases ERK1/2, phospho-SAPK/JNK, phospho-NF-κB p65, phospho-IKKα/β, and phospho-IκB-α were measured by western blot analysis. *Results.* The results showed that TRQ significantly counteracted LPS-stimulated release of TNF-α, IL-1β, IL-6, and IL-8, attenuated cells influx in BALF, mitigated mucus hypersecretion, suppressed phosphorylation of NF-κB p65, IκB-α, IKKα/β, ERK1/2, JNK, and p38 MAPK, and inhibited p38 MAPK and NF-κB p65 expression in rat lungs. *Conclusions.* Results of the current research indicate that TRQ possesses potent exhibitory effects in LPS-induced airway inflammation by, at least partially, suppressing the MAPKs and NF-κB signaling pathways, in a general dose-dependent manner.

## 1. Introduction

Tanreqing injection (TRQ) is a widely used classical compound herbal recipe for several decades in China. It is composed of water soluble natural extractives from five crude herbal plants, namely, Radix Scutellariae Baicalensis, Fel Selenarcti, Cornu Naemorhedi, Flos Lonicerae, and Forsythiae Fructus [1], and is a mixture of about 12 main active pharmaceutical ingredients including *chlorogenic acid, caffeic acid, luteoloside, forsythiaside, forsythin, forsythigenol, baicalin, wogonoside, wogonin, salidroside,* and *ursodeoxycholic acid* [2]. Clinical evidence has supported the minimal toxicity and side effects of TRQ [3, 4]. With its predominant antibacterial and antiviral actions being proved by modern pharmacologic studies [5, 6], TRQ is predominately used for acute inflammatory lung diseases including acute upper respiratory tract

infections [7], pneumonia [3, 8, 9], acute COPD [4, 10, 11], SARS (Serious Acute Respiration Symptom) [12, 13], A/H1N1 flu [14, 15], A/H7N9 flu [16], and the recently mentioned Middle East Respiratory Syndrome (National Health and Family Planning Commission of China, http://www.nhfpc.gov.cn/).

Stimulation of MAPKs and IKK/IκB/NF-κB pathways is common phenomena in many types of inflammation response. Targeting the pathways has been considered as an effective therapeutic approach to mitigate progression of numbers of inflammatory disorders, such as the classical neutrophil-predominant airway inflammation induced by Lipopolysaccharide (LPS) [17]. The involvement of the ubiquitous nuclear transcription factor NF-κB in the pathogenesis of the LPS-induced inflammatory response has been well recognized [18]. LPS liberates and activates NF-κB mostly through IκB kinase- (IKK-) dependent phosphorylation and subsequent degradation of IκB-α [19]. The liberated NF-κB dimers are crucial for regulating transcription of diverse genes coding for cytokines including TNF-α, IL-1β, IL-6, and IL-8 [20, 21], which together contribute to the upregulation of inflammatory responses. Similar to IKK/IκB-α/NF-κB pathway, the mitogen-activated protein kinase (MAPK) pathway is also activated during an LPS-challenged inflammatory condition [22]. The three subfamilies, extracellular regulated kinases (ERK1/2), c-Jun N-terminal kinases (JNK), and p38 MAP kinases, have been implicated in the release of proinflammatory cytokines [23, 24] and the activation of NF-κB [25].

Prior studies have given consistent results on the ability of TRQ to alleviate LPS-induced inflammation through multiple actions including scavenging excessive oxygen free radicals, suppressing the activation and expression of NF-κB, decreasing serum NO level, and downregulating the expression of Caspase-3 and Bcl-2/Fas gene [12, 13, 26–28]. Collectively, no efforts have been done to understand the pathways that are involved in its effect. Since MAPKs and NF-κB pathway has been highlighted during the LPS-induced inflammatory disorders, we hypothesize that protective actions of TRQ are likely, at least partially, due to its regulations on the two pathways. In the present study, we attempted to elucidate the anti-inflammatory potential of TRQ on LPS-induced airway inflammation in rat models by investigating the pivotal molecular basis involved in the two classical signaling pathways.

## 2. Material and Methods

*2.1. Animals and Drugs.* 75 male specific-pathogen-free (SPF) grade SD rats (10–12 weeks old, initially weighing 180–220 g) were raised under SPF conditions on a 12 h light/dark cycle at a temperature of 22 ± 2°C with free access to food and water. Protocol of this experiment was approved by the Animal Care and Use Committee of West China Hospital and the investigation conformed to the "Guide for the Care and Use of Laboratory Animals" [29]. SD rats used for the experiment were obtained from Jianyang Animal and Science Co., Ltd. (Sichuan, China). Tanreqing injection was purchased from Shanghai Kai Bao Pharmaceutical Co., Ltd. (Shanghai, China).

*2.2. Experimental Groups and Protocol.* Rats were randomly divided into four groups ($n = 15$ per group): (a) control group: rats receiving sterile saline; (b) LPS group: rats receiving intratracheal instillation (i.t.) of LPS + intraperitoneal injection (i.p.) of sterile saline; (c) low dose TRQ group: rats receiving LPS i.t. + 2.8 mL/kg TRQ i.p.; and (d) high dose TRQ group: rats receiving LPS i.t. + 5.6 mL/kg TRQ i.p. LPS (Sigma, St. Louis, MO, USA) was administered intratracheally during inspiration once at baseline, at a dose of 240 μg/rat. TRQ would be injected 1 h before LPS administration at baseline and then every 24 hours.

*2.3. Bronchoalveolar Lavage Fluid (BALF) and Tissue Extraction.* On 24 h, 48 h, and 96 h, which have been previously

reported as optimal time points to observe the anti-inflammatory activity of TRQ [28], rats were intraperitoneally anaesthetised with 4% sodium pentobarbital (40 mg/kg) and then exsanguinated from the abdominal aorta. The chest cavity was opened by a midline incision to expose and cannulate the trachea. The right lobe of the lung was ligated at the hilus of the lung, and the left lung was immediately lavaged three times with 2 mL ice sterile saline through the tracheostomy tube. Fluid recovery was always above 90% of the original volume. Pooled BALF samples were centrifuged and the supernatants were collected and stored at −80°C for cytokine ELISA. The deposited cells were resuspended for total leukocyte count and the differential leukocyte classification, counting 500 cells from each rat. An experienced investigator who was independent of experimental operations did all the enumerations based on standard morphological criteria. The right middle lobe of the lung was preserved in 4% paraformaldehyde for 24 h at 4°C for histology and histochemical studies. The right posterior lobe of the lung was snap preserved in liquid nitrogen and stored at −80°C for mRNA and protein analysis.

*2.4. Enzyme-Linked Immunosorbent Assay (ELISA).* Quantitation of cytokines in the supernatants of undiluted BALF and lung homogenate was determined by ELISA technique, according to the manufacturer's instructions. Three replicates were carried out for each of the different treatments. Rat IL-1β ELISA kit was purchased from Shanghai ExCell Biology Company (Shanghai, China) (Cat. Number: ER008-96; Sensitivity: 15 pg/mL; Assay Range: 31.25~2000 pg/mL). Rat CXCL-1/CINC-1 ELISA kit (rat analogue of human IL-8) (Cat. Number: RCN100; Sensitivity: 1.3 pg/mL; Assay Range: 7.8~500 pg/mL), Rat IL-6 ELISA kit (Cat. Number: R6000B; Sensitivity: 0.7 pg/mL; Assay Range: 3.1~700 pg/mL), and Rat TNF-α ELISA kit (Cat. Number: RTA00; Sensitivity: 5 pg/mL; Assay Range: 12.5~800 pg/mL) were purchased from USA R&D Systems (Minneapolis, MN, USA). Samples were applied to wells of 96-well polystyrene microtiter plates that were precoated with specific monoclonal antibodies before incubation, and then wells were washed five times, followed by incubation with the respective HRP-conjugated polyclonal antibodies. After the repeat of aspiration and washing steps, the substrate solutions and stop solutions were added one after another. The optical density of each well was determined at 450 nm using a microplate reader (Bio-Rad, Richmond, CA) within 30 minutes.

*2.5. Histopathology and Immunohistochemistry.* Fixed specimen was rinsed in PBS, dehydrated, and embedded in paraffin according to standard procedures and serially sectioned at 4 micrometer. Then sections were stained with haematoxylin and eosin (H&E) and Alcian blue (AB)/periodic acid-Schiff (PAS) for general morphology evaluation, which were subsequently practiced by a pathologist who was blinded to group allocation under a light microscopy. The evaluation of inflammation lesions was performed using a subjective numeric scale ranging from 0 to 10, which comprises three scoring parts including peribronchial/peribronchiolar inflammation score, perivascular inflammation score, and alveolar inflammation score. Peribronchial/peribronchiolar and perivascular inflammations were individually scored from 0 to 4, representing normal (score 0), mild inflammation (score 1, <25%), moderate inflammation (score 2, 25–50%), severe inflammation (score 3, 50–75%), and very severe inflammation (score 4, >75%), respectively [30]. Alveolar inflammation was scored from 0 to 2 that represents normal (score 0), mild inflammation infiltration (score 1, few foci present), and severe inflammation infiltration (score 2, many foci present). The scores were then summed to give a total inflammatory score. Percentage of AB/PAS positively stained areas to the total area of bronchial epithelium was measured.

For p38 MAPK and NF-$\kappa$B immunohistochemical staining, paraffin-embedded sections were deparaffinized, rehydrated, and washed with distilled water. The monoclonal antibodies used were as follows: rabbit anti-p38 MAPK (1 : 400 dilution) and rabbit NF-$\kappa$B p65 (1 : 800 dilution). Both antibodies were purchased from Cell Signaling (Danvers, MA, USA). PBS was used to replace the primary antibody as a blank control. The mean optical density (IOD) was calculated by measuring 10 consecutive visual fields for each sample at a magnification of 400x, using an optical microscope equipped with an Image-Pro Plus software (version 6.0, Media Cybernetics, Silver Spring, MD, USA) by a pathologist who was blinded to the identity of the groups.

*2.6. RNA Extraction, Reverse Transcription, and Quantitative Real-time Polymerase Chain Reaction.* Frozen tissue was ground to a fine powder in liquid nitrogen. After the samples were thawed, total RNA was isolated from 30 mg lung tissue using the E.Z.N.ATM HP total RNA kit (Omega Biotech, Norcross, GA, USA) according to specific modifications to maximize RNA extraction. RNA pellets were ethanol-precipitated, washed, and resuspended in sterile ribonuclease-free water. RNA samples were reverse transcribed using the iScript cDNA synthesis kit (Bio-Rad Laboratories, Hercules, CA, USA) to synthesize the first-strand cDNA. Reverse transcription was then performed on 1 $\mu$L RNA sample by adding iScript reagents to a final reaction volume of 20 $\mu$L. The RNA samples were incubated in a Bio-Rad DNA Engine Peltier Thermal Cycler (Bio-Rad Laboratories, Inc., Hercules, CA, USA) at 25°C for 5 min and then reverse transcribed at 42°C for 30 min and, finally, the enzyme was denatured at 85°C for 5 min. Subsequently, the RNA concentrations were determined by measuring the absorbance at 260 and 280 nm, using a Nanodrop spectrophotometer (Montchanin, DE, USA).

PCR primers specific for selected target genes were predesigned and validated (Table 1). Gradient PCRs were used to determine the optimal annealing temperature and primer concentration. qPCR reactions had a final volume of 10 $\mu$L and contained 1 $\mu$L of cDNA, 0.5 $\mu$L of each primer, 5 $\mu$L Sso-Fast EvaGreen supermix (Bio-Rad Laboratories, Hercules, CA, USA), and 3 $\mu$L DEPC-treated sterile distilled water. The relative expression levels of mRNA of studied cytokines were

TABLE 1: The primer sequences.

| TNF-$\alpha$-forward | TGCTATCTCATACCAGGAGA |
| TNF-$\alpha$-reverse | GACTCCGCAAAGTCTAAGTA |
| IL-6-forward | TCTTGGGACTGATGTTGTTG |
| IL-6-reverse | TAAGCCTCCGACTTGTGAA |
| IL-1$\beta$-forward | GCAACTGTTCCTGAACTCAACT |
| IL-1$\beta$-reverse | ATCTTTTGGGGTCCGTCAACT |
| CXCL-1/CINC-1-forward | CTCCAGCCACACTCCAACAGA |
| CXCL-1/CINC-1-reverse | CACCCTAACACAAAACACGAT |
| $\beta$-actin-forward | CCT CAT GAA GAT CCT GAC CG |
| $\beta$-actin-reverse | ACC GCT CAT TGC CGA TAG TG |

calculated relative to $\beta$-actin. Each qPCR was performed in triplicate for the individual sample. The PCR program was initiated by a 30 s of enzyme activation at 95°C and then 5 s of cDNA denaturation at 95°C, followed by 40 cycles at 55°C for 20 s of annealing/extension using Roche LightCycler® 96 Real-Time PCR System. A melting-point curve was then measured, starting from 65°C and increasing by 4.4°C every second up to 95°C, to detect any nonspecific PCR products. Data was analysed using $2^{-\Delta\Delta Ct}$ method with actin as the reference gene.

*2.7. Western Blot Analysis.* Nuclear and cytosolic extracts were prepared using a Nuclear and Cytoplasmic Protein Extraction Kit (Beyotime Co., Jiangsu, China) according to the manufacturer's instructions. The concentration of the protein was measured using a bicinchoninic acid protein assay kit (Beyotime Co., Shanghai, China). A total of 50 ug of protein that resolved with 2x SDS-PAGE was transferred onto immunoblot polyvinylidene difluoride membranes (Bio-Rad Laboratories, Inc., Hercules, CA, USA). The blots were blocked with 5% BSA in Tris-buffered saline with 0.1% Tween (TBST) for 2 h at room temperature and were incubated overnight at 4°C with primary antibodies of phospho-p38 MAPK (1 : 1000), phospho-p65 (1 : 1000), phospho-ERK1/2 (1 : 1000), phosphor-IKK$\alpha$/$\beta$ (1 : 900), phospho-JNK (1 : 900), phospho-I$\kappa$B-$\alpha$ (1 : 800), and $\beta$-actin (1 : 2000). Blots were then washed three times for 5 min each in TBST and incubated with horseradish peroxidase-labeled secondary goat anti-rabbit antibody at room temperature. After washing for three times, membranes were visualized with Clarity Western ECL Substrate (Bio-rad, Hercules, CA, USA). Densitometry was carried out using Quantity One (version 4.6.2) quantitation software (Bio-Rad, Hercules, CA, USA). All primary antibodies were purchased from Cell Signaling Technology (Danvers, MA, USA). $\beta$-actin and secondary antibody were purchased from Santa Cruz Biotechnology (Santa Cruz, CA, USA).

*2.8. Statistical Analysis.* Continuous variables were presented as mean ± standard deviation (SD) of 3 independent experiments done in duplicate. One-way analysis of variance (ANOVA) was performed to calculate the significance between groups. Pair-wise comparisons of four data sets were performed using Fisher LSD tests. The Kruskal-Wallis nonparametric ANOVA test was used for variables that do not follow a normal distribution when comparing multiple groups. A $P$ value of less than 0.05 was considered statistically significant. All statistical analyses were processed using commercially available software package SPSS 20.0 (IBM SPSS Inc., Chicago, IL, USA).

# 3. Results

*3.1. TRQ Protects LPS-Induced Histopathological Damage of Rat Lungs.* Histopathological changes in rat lungs showed major difference in gross morphology between groups treated with and without TRQ. In non-LPS-exposed tissues sections, no obvious histological abnormalities were revealed (Figures 1(a)–1(c)). In contrast, intratracheal instillation of LPS induced an acute bronchopneumonia involving the focal areas of the main bronchus and also preterminal bronchioles, presented as prominent thickening of the airway epitheliums and the alveolar septa, conspicuous peribronchial inflammatory cell infiltration, and bronchiolar lumen obstruction by mucus and cell debris. In addition, some blood vessels in affected regions also thickened with a mixed inflammatory infiltrate of main neutrophils and less monocytes and lymphocytes (Figures 1(d)–1(f)). Low dose TRQ treatment failed to contribute to a remarkable alleviation of extensive inflammation with alveolar air spaces flooded with fibrinous exudate admixed with numerous neutrophils at 24 h (Figure 1(g)); however, high dose TRQ expressed noteworthy anti-inflammation property throughout the observing period (Figures 1(j)–1(l)). In general, inflammatory lesion scores decreased over time and they were effectively decreased by TRQ administration in a dose-dependent way (Figure 1(m)).

Besides, a noticeable and conspicuous increase in numbers of mucous cells and amounts of mucosubstances was detected along the airway surface epithelium in LPS group (Figures 2(d)–2(f)), verifying the exact link between airway inflammation and mucus production [31], while the goblet cell metaplasia and hyperplasia were rarely found in the main airways in control rats (Figures 2(a)–2(c)), with a faint positive AB/PAS staining area being detected. TRQ treatment significantly inhibited, though not fully abrogated, the mucus hypersecretion at each time point (Figures 2(g)–2(l)).

*3.2. TRQ Regulates LPS-Induced Leukocyte Accumulation in BALF.* As a potent stimulus for immune cell, LPS significantly recruited more cells at 24 h, and although the total cell amount decreased over time, it was always significantly higher than that in the control group. TRQ effectively accelerated the process of cell number decrease (Figure 3(a)). For the number of neutrophils, even low dose of TRQ effectively cut down the neutrophil release in BALF after LPS administration at 24 h (Figure 3(b)). The inhibitory effect of TRQ in macrophage accumulation started from 48 h, which was only in high dose group (Figure 3(c)). The number of lymphocytes in BALF enhanced observably after LPS administration, which was completely reversed by high dose TRQ at 24 h (Figure 3(d)).

*3.3. TRQ Attenuates LPS-Induced Proinflammatory Cytokines in BALF and Lungs.* Since they have been previously reported [32], protein release and mRNA upregulation of TNF-$\alpha$, IL-1$\beta$, IL-6, and CINC-1 were examined to determine the effect of TRQ. As expected, levels of selected cytokines were significantly elevated in BALF (Figure 4) and lung homogenate (Figure 5) 24 h after LPS inoculation. Although they were always significantly higher than those in the control groups, levels of TNF-$\alpha$, IL-6, and CINC-1 tended to rapidly decrease from 24 h, while levels of IL-1$\beta$ continued to be high at 48 h. Amounts of TNF-$\alpha$, IL-6, and CINC-1 were markedly reduced starting from 24 h after LPS exposure by even low dose of TRQ. Of interest, for IL-1$\beta$ a reduction was observed only in high dose TRQ group at 48 h. At the last time point, high dosage of TRQ successfully recovered levels of all cytokines to normal. Taken together, TRQ exerted a more potent and earlier effect on reversing the overproduction of IL-6, which was completely repressed at 48 h.

As for the qPCR results, CINC-1 was accumulated with mRNA levels peaking at 24 h and then declining. TNF-$\alpha$, IL-6, and IL-1$\beta$ mRNA reached a plateau at 24 h and continued to escalate until the end of the 48 hour study. These data demonstrated the complex patterns of cytokine gene expression and suggest that production of early mediators may augment continued expression of TNF-$\alpha$, IL-6, and IL-1$\beta$ mRNA. The mRNA induction for each cytokine was significantly mitigated or reversed by TRQ treatment (Figure 6).

*3.4. TRQ Modulates LPS-Induced Synthesis of Signaling Proteins in Rat Lungs.* Effect of TRQ on LPS-induced p38 MAPK and NF-$\kappa$B p65 expression in rat lungs was measured by immunohistochemistry. Results revealed that IOD value of areas positively stained by p38 MAPK and NF-$\kappa$B p65 monoclonal antibody in lung sections increased markedly at 24 h after LPS exposure, which could be significantly attenuated by TRQ in a dose-dependent way (Figures 7 and 8).

*3.5. TRQ Modulates LPS-Induced Phosphorylation of Signaling Proteins in MAPKs Pathway in Rat Lungs.* Western blot analysis on changes of prominent protein expressions involved in MAPKs pathway in rat lungs showed that stimulation with LPS resulted in a significant increase in the amount of phosphorylation of p38, JNK, and ERK1/2 compared with the control group at 24 h, which were markedly inhibited by an addition of TRQ (Figures 9(a) and 9(c)–9(e)). Except for phospho-JNK, a significant difference between the effects in different dosage of TRQ was observed in all indicators.

*3.6. TRQ Suppresses LPS-Induced Phosphorylation of Signaling Proteins in NF-$\kappa$B Pathway in Rat Lungs.* According to the results, stimulation with LPS alone for 24 h notably induced the strong signal of the immunostained band for phosphorylated p65, I$\kappa$B-$\alpha$, and IKK$\alpha$/$\beta$ in rat lungs, which were significantly decreased after TRQ treatment in a dosage-dependent manner, as expected (Figures 9(b) and 9(f)–9(h)).

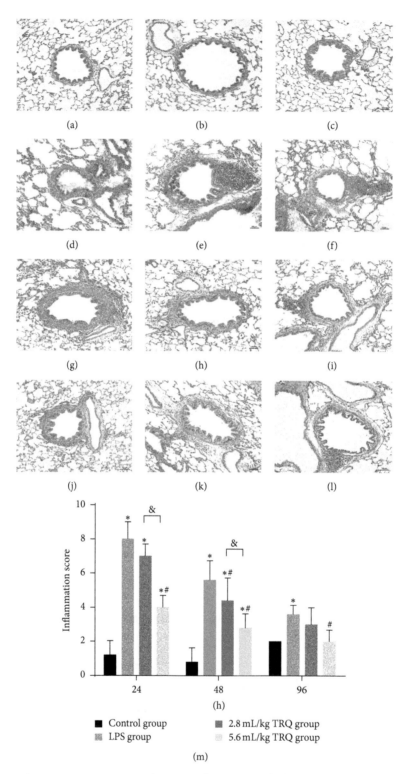

(a)　(b)　(c)

(d)　(e)　(f)

(g)　(h)　(i)

(j)　(k)　(l)

(m)

FIGURE 1: Histological changes in rat airways. Lung tissues from control rats at (a) 24 h, (b) 48 h, and (c) 96 h, rats exposed to LPS alone at (d) 24 h, (e) 48 h, and (f) 96 h, rats treated with LPS + TRQ 2.8 mL/kg at (g) 24 h, (h) 48 h, and (i) 96 h, and rats treated with LPS + TRQ 5.6 mL/kg at (j) 24 h, (k) 48 h, and (l) 96 h were all analysed by haematoxylin and eosin staining. Scale bars = 50 $\mu$m. (m) Lung inflammatory scores for rat airways. Values are expressed as mean ± SD. [*]$P < 0.05$ means significant difference from the control group; [#]$P < 0.05$ means significant difference from the LPS group and [&]$P < 0.05$ means significant difference between LPS + 2.8 mL/kg TRQ group and LPS + 5.6 mL/kg TRQ group.

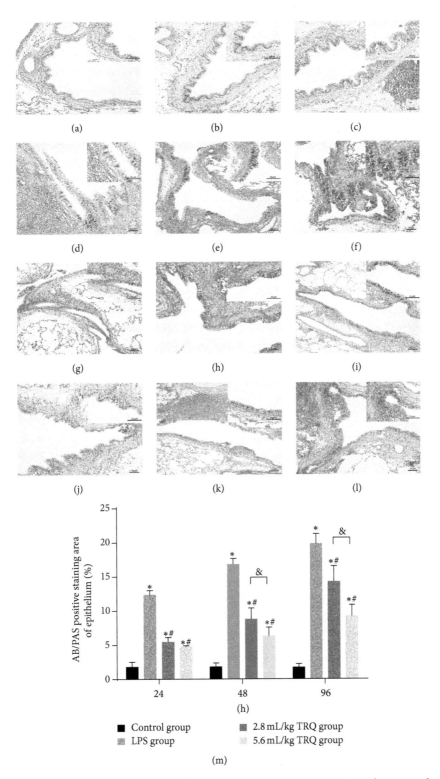

FIGURE 2: Changes of Alcian blue (AB)/periodic acid-Schiff (PAS) staining in rat airways. Lung tissues from control rats at (a) 24 h, (b) 48 h, and (c) 96 h, rats exposed to LPS alone at (d) 24 h, (e) 48 h, and (f) 96 h, rats treated with LPS + TRQ 2.8 mL/kg at (g) 24 h, (h) 48 h, and (i) 96 h, and rats treated with LPS + TRQ 5.6 mL/kg at (j) 24 h, (k) 48 h, and (l) 96 h were all analysed by AB/PAS staining. Scale bars = 50 $\mu$m; upper right insert: scale bars = 25 $\mu$m. (m) The percentage of AB/PAS positively staining area to total epithelial area in rat airways. Values are expressed as mean ± SD. $^*P < 0.05$ means significant difference from the control group; $^\#P < 0.05$ means significant difference from the LPS group and $^\&P < 0.05$ means significant difference between LPS + 2.8 mL/kg TRQ group and LPS + 5.6 mL/kg TRQ group.

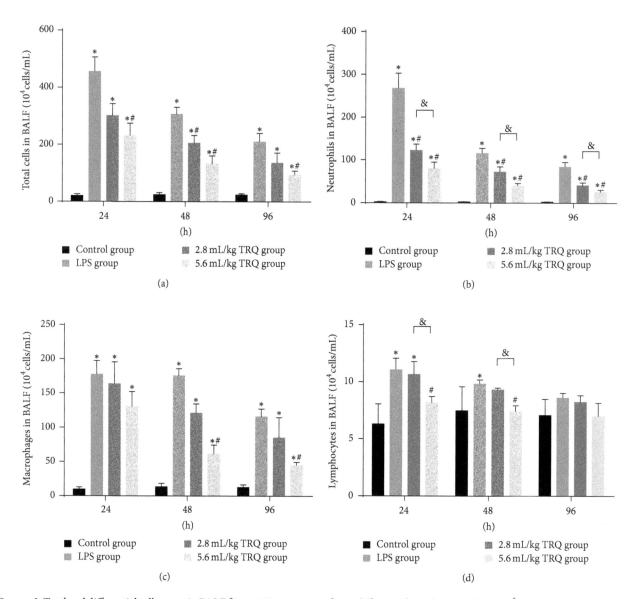

FIGURE 3: Total and differential cell counts in BALF. $^*P < 0.05$ means significant difference from the control group; $^#P < 0.05$ means significant difference from the LPS group and $^\&P < 0.05$ means significant difference between LPS + 2.8 mL/kg TRQ group and LPS + 5.6 mL/kg TRQ group.

## 4. Discussion

In recent decades, MAPKs and IKK/IκB-α/NF-κB p65 signaling pathways have attracted considerable attention as targets for inflammation inhibition. In the present study, we focused on the two pathways to tentatively explore the pharmacological mechanisms of TRQ, which, we hope, might in turn advance the drug development. Here we showed that TRQ effectively reduced the phosphorylation of pivotal factors in MAPKs and NF-κB signaling pathways, which contribute to significantly less recruitment and infiltration of immune cells in BALF and subsequent suppression on toxic cytokines release, realizing a promising mitigation on LPS-induced airway inflammation.

As prominent target cells of LPS, neutrophils and macrophages were dramatically induced in BALF after LPS stimulation. As for the neutrophil migration, LPS induces an enhanced chemokinesis by its direct effect on cells and an increased chemotaxis by indirect effects. For example, LPS challenge prominently enhances the level of IL-8, an essential CXC chemokine to attract neutrophils to sites of inflammation in the lung. Both direct and indirect effects are modulated by the coordinated action of ERK, p38 MAPK, and NF-κB pathways [33]. The pathways also contribute to macrophage migration. It has been demonstrated that LPS or TNF-α-induced activation of matrix metalloproteinases, key players in macrophage migration and invasion into foci inflammation, is controlled via ERK1/2, JNK, and

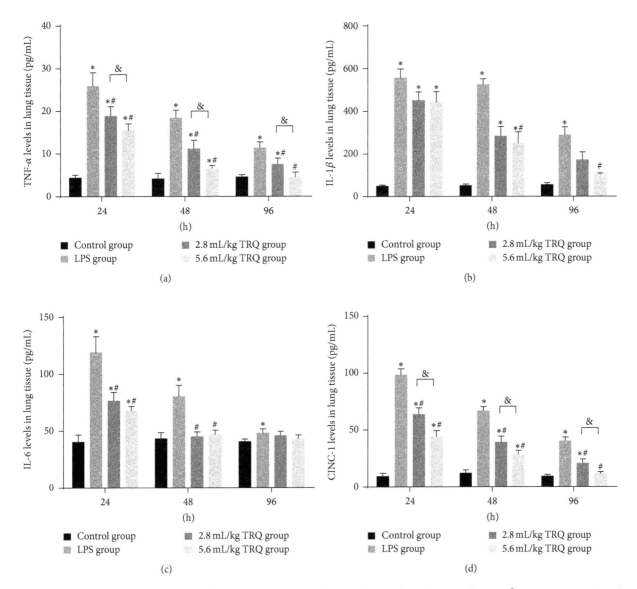

FIGURE 4: Levels of cytokines in lung tissues. $^*P < 0.05$ means significant difference from the control group; $^#P < 0.05$ means significant difference from the LPS group and $^&P < 0.05$ means significant difference between LPS + 2.8 mL/kg TRQ group and LPS + 5.6 mL/kg TRQ group.

IKK/NF-$\kappa$B pathway [34, 35]. Besides, the expression of MCP-1, another important chemokine for monocytes/macrophages, is stimulated by LPS via NF-$\kappa$B-dependent mechanism [36]. In particular, the involvement of lymphocytes was also observed after LPS treatment in this study. Previous data showed that lymphocytes present in lung played a role in immunopathology of inflammatory process in both humans and mice [37, 38]. More specifically, study of Dushianthan and colleagues [39] revealed a rapid infiltration of different T cells, including regulatory T cells (Tregs), NKT, and NK cells in human lungs in response to LPS, accompanied by a significant elevation of IL-17, a potent recruiter of neutrophils to inflammatory sites. They demonstrated that both lymphocyte released IL-17 and Tregs modulated the recruitment of neutrophils to the lung in LPS-induced ALI.

Therefore, the drastic rise of neutrophils in BALF may partly be attributed to the elevation of lymphocytes in this study.

It has been well characterized that LPS administration on rats leads to overproduction of cytokines from neutrophils and macrophages including IL-1$\beta$, IL-6, IL-8, and TNF-$\alpha$ [40–42] for up to 48 h [43], as a result of a series of MAPKs/NF-$\kappa$B signal transduction cascade. It has been demonstrated that pretreatment with TNF inhibitors led to a reduction in circulating IL-1, IL-6, and IL-8, suggesting an important role of TNF-$\alpha$ in the amplification of inflammatory response [44]. TNF helps neutrophils, monocytes, and lymphocytes recruitment and infiltration by inducing vasodilation and loss of vascular permeability [45] and triggering the secretion of chemokines [46] and cell adhesion molecules [47]. Similarly to TNF, IL-1$\beta$ is also mainly produced and

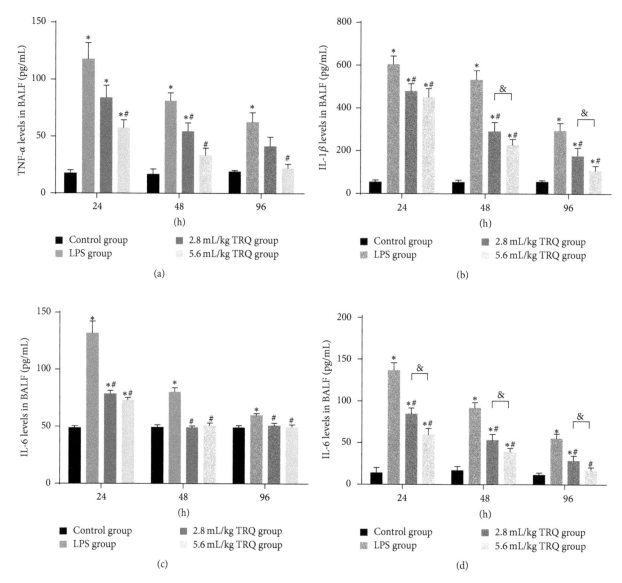

FIGURE 5: Levels of cytokines in BALF. $^*P < 0.05$ means significant difference from the control group; $^#P < 0.05$ means significant difference from the LPS group and $^&P < 0.05$ means significant difference between LPS + 2.8 mL/kg TRQ group and LPS + 5.6 mL/kg TRQ group.

released from monocytes/macrophages in the initiation of inflammatory process after endotoxin exposure. Released IL-1$\beta$ subsequently triggers further production of IL-1$\beta$ and other cytokines/chemokines by infiltrating cells and accounts for the perpetuation of inflammation. This may partially explain why IL-1$\beta$ keeps at high levels at 48 h after LPS instillation in our results. As a pleiotropic cytokine that possesses both pro- and anti-inflammation properties, IL-6 plays a key role in acute-phase of lung injury by affecting the release and functions of neutrophils and macrophages [48]. Time-course studies showed that induction of mRNA for IL-1$\beta$ and TNF-$\alpha$ occurred rapidly preceding that of IL-6 mRNA after LPS exposure [49]. Subsequently, depending on p38 MAPK and NF-$\kappa$B pathways, early produced IL-1$\beta$ and TNF-$\alpha$ induced IL-6 mRNA expression and more

IL-6 production. This may explain the continued rise in IL-6 mRNA level till 48 h. Therefore, it is noteworthy that a large proportion of LPS-stimulated IL-6 is actually indirectly induced by TNF-$\alpha$ and/or IL-1$\beta$ [50]. Inversely, endotoxin-induced IL-6 functions to downregulate its own inducers, TNF-$\alpha$ and IL-1$\beta$ on mRNA and protein levels [51, 52], with a negative feedback mechanism. As a result, the acute neutrophil and macrophage exudation would be diminished [53], realizing the protective role of IL-6 on endotoxin-induced inflammation [54]. Although nonnegligible amount of IL-6 is induced by TNF-$\alpha$ and IL-1$\beta$ in this condition, TNF-$\alpha$ and IL-1$\beta$ are both produced in a very rapid burst in response to LPS; therefore, the decrease of IL-6 levels here was likely not due to a secondary effect exerted by decline of TNF-$\alpha$ and IL-1$\beta$ levels, which should be ascribed to the effect from

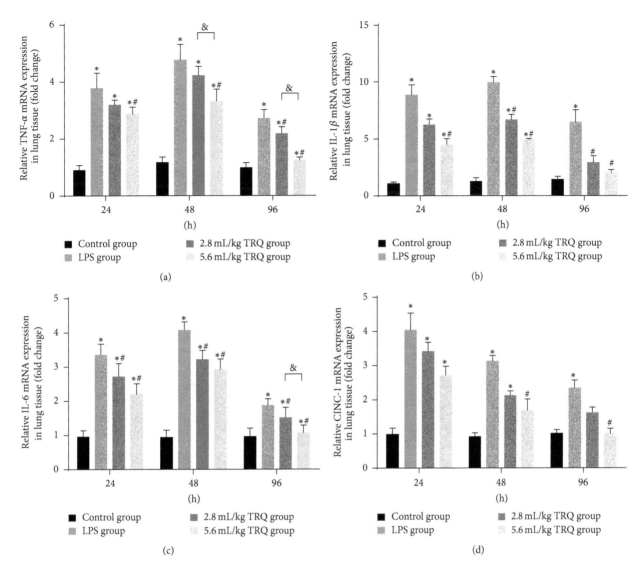

FIGURE 6: Changes in relative mRNA levels of cytokines in lung tissues. $^*P < 0.05$ means significant difference from the control group; $^\#P < 0.05$ means significant difference from the LPS group and $^\&P < 0.05$ means significant difference between LPS + 2.8 mL/kg TRQ group and LPS + 5.6 mL/kg TRQ group.

TRQ. Clinical trials demonstrated that TRQ administration showed a potent effect on lowering the levels of IL-1$\beta$, IL-6, IL-8, TNF-$\alpha$, and IL-17 in plasma of patients under acute pulmonary conditions [11, 55, 56], which was promisingly consistent with our results obtained from rat models.

To our knowledge, it is the first attempt to discover the underlying mechanism involving signaling pathways for the effect of TRQ. This present study had some limitations. Although pathogenesis of LPS-induced airway inflammation generally involves multiple signaling pathways, we only investigated MAPKs/NF-$\kappa$B pathways and only discussed its role in LPS-stimulated inflammations in vivo. If necessary, we will conduct more comprehensive work in the future to systematically evaluate its function in vitro and multiple pathways and also other pathogen-induced inflammation models.

## 5. Conclusion

In summary, this work demonstrated that TRQ dose-dependently attenuated LPS-induced neutrophils, macrophages, and lymphocytes infiltration and inhibited proinflammatory cytokines including TNF-$\alpha$, IL-1$\beta$, IL-6, and IL-8 on both mRNA transcription and protein synthesis levels, which were very beneficial to the resolution of inflammation. The therapeutic action of TRQ, in some degree, benefited from its inhibitory effect on the expressions of p38 MAPK and NF-$\kappa$B p65 in lungs by reducing phosphorylation of p38 MAPK, ERK1/2, IKK$\alpha$/$\beta$, I$\kappa$B-$\alpha$, and NF-$\kappa$B p65. All the present findings specified that the underlying mechanisms of the suppressive actions of TRQ on LPS-induced airway inflammation and mucus overproduction might be due to, at least in part, the suppression on MAPKs and NF-$\kappa$B signaling pathways.

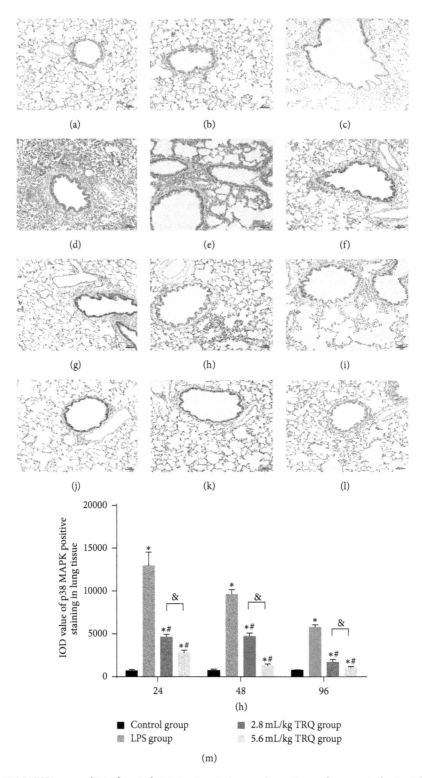

FIGURE 7: Changes in p38 MAPK immunohistochemical staining in rat airways. Lung tissues from control rats at (a) 24 h, (b) 48 h, and (c) 96 h, rats exposed to LPS alone at (d) 24 h, (e) 48 h, and (f) 96 h, rats treated with LPS + TRQ 2.8 mL/kg at (g) 24 h, (h) 48 h, and (i) 96 h, and rats treated with LPS + TRQ 5.6 mL/kg at (j) 24 h, (k) 48 h, and (l) 96 h were all analysed by haematoxylin and eosin staining. Scale bars 50 $\mu$m. (m) Integrated option density sum (IOD sum) value of positive p38 MAPK staining in rats. Values are expressed as mean ± SD. $^*P < 0.05$ means significant difference from the control group; $^#P < 0.05$ means significant difference from the LPS group and $^\&P < 0.05$ means significant difference between LPS + 2.8 mL/kg TRQ group and LPS + 5.6 mL/kg TRQ group.

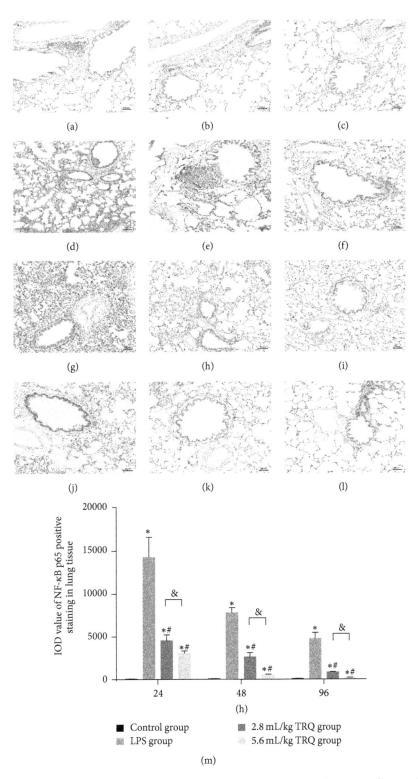

FIGURE 8: Changes in NF-κB p65 immunohistochemical staining in rat airways. Lung tissues from control rats at (a) 24 h, (b) 48 h, and (c) 96 h, rats exposed to LPS alone at (d) 24 h, (e) 48 h, and (f) 96 h, rats treated with LPS + TRQ 2.8 mL/kg at (g) 24 h, (h) 48 h, and (i) 96 h, and rats treated with LPS + TRQ 5.6 mL/kg at (j) 24 h, (k) 48 h, and (l) 96 h were all analysed by haematoxylin and eosin staining. Scale bars 50 μm. (m) Integrated option density sum (IOD sum) value of positive NF-κB p65 staining in rats. Values are expressed as mean ± SD. *P < 0.05 means significant difference from the control group; #P < 0.05 means significant difference from the LPS group and &P < 0.05 means significant difference between LPS + 2.8 mL/kg TRQ group and LPS + 5.6 mL/kg TRQ group.

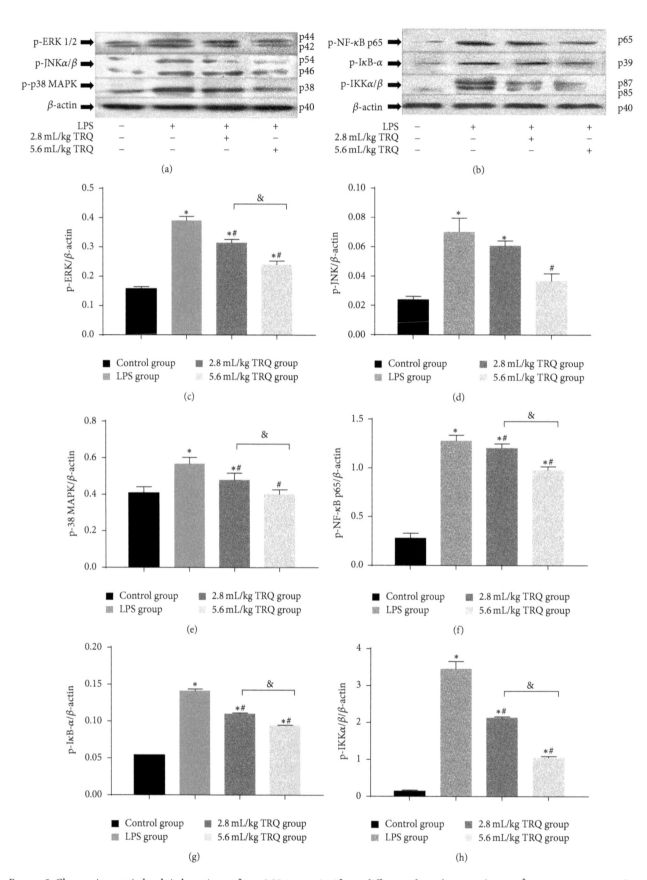

FIGURE 9: Changes in protein levels in lung tissues. $^*P < 0.05$ means significant difference from the control group; $^\#P < 0.05$ means significant difference from the LPS group and $^\&P < 0.05$ means significant difference between LPS + 2.8 mL/kg TRQ group and LPS + 5.6 mL/kg TRQ group.

## Competing Interests

The authors declare that they have no competing interests.

## Authors' Contributions

Wei Liu and Hong-li Jiang are co-first authors and they contributed equally to this work. Bing Mao contributed to the initiation of the study design. Wei Liu, Lin-li Cai, and Min Yan contributed to lab work implementation. Wei Liu contributed to the draft of the paper. Agreement on the final version was obtained from all authors.

## Acknowledgments

The current research is supported by the Administrative Bureau of Traditional Chinese Medicine in Sichuan province.

## References

[1] W. Li, L. Xing, L. Fang, J. Wang, and H. Qu, "Application of near infrared spectroscopy for rapid analysis of intermediates of Tanreqing injection," *Journal of Pharmaceutical and Biomedical Analysis*, vol. 53, no. 3, pp. 350–358, 2010.

[2] S.-Y. Liu, D.-S. Xue, J.-C. Pan, W.-M. Zhang, W.-L. Li, and H.-B. Qu, "Screening and identification of multiple components in Tanreqing injection using RP-HPLC combined with DAD and ESI-TOF/MS," *Chinese Journal of Natural Medicines*, vol. 12, no. 7, pp. 535–541, 2014.

[3] H.-L. Jiang, B. Mao, Y.-Q. Zhong, H.-M. Yang, and J.-J. Fu, "Tanreqing injection for community-acquired pneumonia: a systematic review of randomized evidence," *Zhong Xi Yi Jie He Xue Bao*, vol. 7, no. 1, pp. 9–19, 2009.

[4] W. Li, B. Mao, G. Wang et al., "A study of the mechanism of Qingre Huatan therapy in treatment of acute exacerbation of chronic obstructive pulmonary disease by improving airway inflammation and mucus hypersecretion," *Zhong Xi Yi Jie He Xue Bao*, vol. 6, no. 8, pp. 799–805, 2008.

[5] Y. Wang, T. Wang, J. Hu et al., "Anti-biofilm activity of TanRe-Qing, a Traditional Chinese Medicine used for the treatment of acute pneumonia," *Journal of Ethnopharmacology*, vol. 134, no. 1, pp. 165–170, 2011.

[6] Y. N. Li, *The Anti-Bacterial Effection of a Herbal Medicine-Tanreqing on the ESBLs Klebsiella Pneumoniae In Vivo*, Beijing Traditional Chinese Medicine, Beijing, China, 2012.

[7] T. Wu, X. Yang, X. Zeng, and P. Poole, "Traditional Chinese medicine in the treatment of acute respiratory tract infections," *Respiratory Medicine*, vol. 102, no. 8, pp. 1093–1098, 2008.

[8] S. He, X. Wen, and N. Xu, "Clinical research of Tanreqing joint Azithromycin sequential therapy in children with mycoplasma pneumoniae pneumonia," *China Medical Herald*, vol. 35, article 31, 2009.

[9] Y. X. Yu, "Effects of tanreqing injection on CRP, il-6 and TNF-α of patients with ventilator assoeiated pneumonia," *Journal of Emergency in Traditional Chinese Medicine*, vol. 18, no. 2, pp. 184–186, 2009.

[10] Y. Zhong, B. Mao, G. Wang et al., "Tanreqing injection combined with conventional western medicine for acute exacerbations of chronic obstructive pulmonary disease: a systematic review," *Journal of Alternative and Complementary Medicine*, vol. 16, no. 12, pp. 1309–1319, 2010.

[11] W. Li, B. Mao, G. Wang et al., "Effect of Tanreqing Injection on treatment of acute exacerbation of chronic obstructive pulmonary disease with Chinese medicine syndrome of retention of phlegm and heat in Fei," *Chinese Journal of Integrative Medicine*, vol. 16, no. 2, pp. 131–137, 2010.

[12] W. C. Liu and J. Zheng, "Research on the effect of Tanreqing injection on endotoxin-induced acute lung injury," *Journal of Shanxi medical university*, vol. 10, no. 05, pp. 489–492, 2006.

[13] P. T. Li, N. Zhang, X. L. Zhu et al., "Effect of the Tanreqing injection on the endotoxin-induced acute lung injury," *Chinese Pharmaceutical Journal*, vol. 5, no. 7, pp. 518–521, 2005.

[14] G. X. Kou, H. A. Han, M. M. Chen, F. M. Xiong, and D. Y. Luo, "Clinical observation of treatment effection of Tanreqing injection on H1N1 influenza with pneumonia," *Journal of Emergency in Traditional Chinese Medicine*, vol. 3, no. 6, pp. 872–876, 2011.

[15] W. B. Huang, M. Wu, and M. X. Huang, "BiPAP combined with Tanreqing injection on H1N1 influenza," *Zhejiang Journal of Integrated Traditional Chinese and Western Medicine*, vol. 21, no. 3, pp. 166–167, 2011.

[16] W. Kai, "Tanreqing injection as a treatment for H7N9 avian influenza," *Health News*, vol. 27, no. 5, p. 2, 2013.

[17] E.-B. Haddad, M. Birrell, K. McCluskie et al., "Role of p38 MAP kinase in LPS-induced airway inflammation in the rat," *British Journal of Pharmacology*, vol. 132, no. 8, pp. 1715–1724, 2001.

[18] T. Lawrence, "The nuclear factor NF-kappaB pathway in inflammation," *Cold Spring Harbor Perspectives in Biology*, vol. 1, no. 6, Article ID a001651, 2009.

[19] M. Karin and M. Delhase, "The IκB kinase (IKK) and NF-κB: key elements of proinflammatory signalling," *Seminars in Immunology*, vol. 12, no. 1, pp. 85–98, 2000.

[20] K. De Bosscher, W. Vanden Berghe, and G. Haegeman, "The interplay between the glucocorticoid receptor and nuclear factor-κB or activator protein-1: molecular mechanisms for gene repression," *Endocrine Reviews*, vol. 24, no. 4, pp. 488–522, 2003.

[21] C. Popa, M. G. Netea, P. L. C. M. van Riel, J. W. M. van der Meer, and A. F. H. Stalenhoef, "The role of TNF-α in chronic inflammatory conditions, intermediary metabolism, and cardiovascular risk," *Journal of Lipid Research*, vol. 48, no. 4, pp. 751–762, 2007.

[22] A. B. Carter, M. M. Monick, and G. W. Hunninghake, "Both Erk and p38 kinases are necessary for cytokine gene transcription," *American Journal of Respiratory Cell and Molecular Biology*, vol. 20, no. 4, pp. 751–758, 1999.

[23] J.-N. Dai, Y. Zong, L.-M. Zhong et al., "Gastrodin inhibits expression of inducible no synthase, cyclooxygenase-2 and proinflammatory cytokines in cultured LPS-Stimulated microglia via MAPK pathways," *PLoS ONE*, vol. 6, no. 7, article e21891, 2011.

[24] M. A. Ajmone-Cat, R. De Simone, A. Nicolini, and L. Minghetti, "Effects of phosphatidylserine on p38 mitogen activated protein kinase, cyclic AMP responding element binding protein and nuclear factor-κB activation in resting and activated microglial cells," *Journal of Neurochemistry*, vol. 84, no. 2, pp. 413–416, 2003.

[25] A. Israël, "The IKK complex: an integrator of all signals that activate NF-κB?" *Trends in Cell Biology*, vol. 10, no. 4, pp. 129–133, 2000.

[26] W. Yu, *Research on the Actions of the Tanreqing Injection on the Endotoxin-Induced Acute Lung Injury Mouse Models*, Nanchang Medical College, 2013.

[27] C. Zhu and X. M. Huang, "The protective effect of Tanreqing injection on ALI rats model," *Chinese Archives of Traditional Chinese Medicine*, vol. 19, no. 8, pp. 1743–1745, 2012.

[28] S. Dong, Y. Zhong, K. Yang, X. Xiong, and B. Mao, "Intervention effect and dose-dependent response of Tanreqing injection on airway inflammation in lipopolysaccharide-induced rats," *Journal of Traditional Chinese Medicine*, vol. 33, no. 4, pp. 505–512, 2013.

[29] National Research Council, *Guide for the Care and Use of Laboratory Animals*, National Research Council, Washington, DC, USA, 8th edition, 2011.

[30] E. G. Barrett, J. A. Wilder, T. H. March, T. Espindola, and D. E. Bice, "Cigarette smoke-induced airway hyperressponsiveness is not dependent on elevated immunoglobulin and eosinophilic inflammation in a mouse model of allergic airway disease," *American Journal of Respiratory and Critical Care Medicine*, vol. 165, no. 10, pp. 1410–1418, 2002.

[31] J. A. Voynow, S. J. Gendler, and M. C. Rose, "Regulation of mucin genes in chronic inflammatory airway diseases," *American Journal of Respiratory Cell and Molecular Biology*, vol. 34, no. 6, pp. 661–665, 2006.

[32] J. J. Haddad and S. C. Land, "Amiloride blockades lipopolysaccharide-induced proinflammatory cytokine biosynthesis in an IκB-α/NF-κB-dependent mechanism. Evidence for the amplification of an antiinflammatory pathway in the alveolar epithelium," *American Journal of Respiratory Cell and Molecular Biology*, vol. 26, no. 1, pp. 114–126, 2002.

[33] K. Aomatsu, T. Kato, H. Fujita et al., "Toll-like receptor agonists stimulate human neutrophil migration via activation of mitogen-activated protein kinases," *Immunology*, vol. 123, no. 2, pp. 171–180, 2008.

[34] W.-C. Huang, G. B. Sala-Newby, A. Susana, J. L. Johnson, and A. C. Newby, "The IKK complex: an integrator of all signals that activate NF-κB?" *PLoS ONE*, vol. 7, no. 8, Article ID e42507, 2012.

[35] M. Y. Murray, T. P. Birkland, J. D. Howe et al., "Macrophage migration and invasion is regulated by MMP10 expression," *PLoS ONE*, vol. 8, no. 5, Article ID e63555, 2013.

[36] S. Akira, K. Takeda, and T. Kaisho, "Toll-like receptors: critical proteins linking innate and acquired immunity," *Nature Immunology*, vol. 2, no. 8, pp. 675–680, 2001.

[37] P. G. Holt, D. H. Strickland, M. E. Wikström, and F. L. Jahnsen, "Regulation of immunological homeostasis in the respiratory tract," *Nature Reviews Immunology*, vol. 8, no. 2, pp. 142–152, 2008.

[38] P. A. Greenberger, "7. Immunologic lung disease," *The Journal of Allergy and Clinical Immunology*, vol. 121, no. 2, supplement 2, pp. S393–S418, 2008.

[39] A. Dushianthan, R. Cusack, V. Goss, M. Grocott, and A. Postle, "S58 surfactant phospholipid kinetics in patients with Acute Respiratory Distress Syndrome (ARDS)," *Thorax*, vol. 67, supplement 2, article A30, 2012.

[40] F. Hayashi, T. K. Means, and A. D. Luster, "Toll-like receptors stimulate human neutrophil function," *Blood*, vol. 102, no. 7, pp. 2660–2669, 2003.

[41] K. Asehnoune, D. Strassheim, S. Mitra, J. Y. Kim, and E. Abraham, "Involvement of reactive oxygen species in toll-like receptor 4-dependent activation of NF-κB," *Journal of Immunology*, vol. 172, no. 4, pp. 2522–2529, 2004.

[42] A. K. Mankan, M. W. Lawless, S. G. Gray, D. Kelleher, and R. McManus, "NF-κB regulation: the nuclear response," *Journal of Cellular and Molecular Medicine*, vol. 13, no. 4, pp. 631–643, 2009.

[43] D. C. Deetz, P. J. Jagielo, T. J. Quinn, P. S. Thorne, S. A. Bleuer, and D. A. Schwartz, "The kinetics of grain dust-induced inflammation of the lower respiratory tract," *American Journal of Respiratory and Critical Care Medicine*, vol. 155, no. 1, pp. 254–259, 1997.

[44] Y. Fong, K. J. Tracey, L. L. Moldawer et al., "Antibodies to cachectin/tumor necrosis factor reduce interleukin 1β and interleukin 6 appearance during lethal bacteremia," *The Journal of Experimental Medicine*, vol. 170, no. 5, pp. 1627–1633, 1989.

[45] G. Arango Duque and A. Descoteaux, "Macrophage cytokines: involvement in immunity and infectious diseases," *Frontiers in Immunology*, vol. 5, article 491, 2014.

[46] G. K. Griffin, G. Newton, M. L. Tarrio et al., "IL-17 and TNF-α sustain neutrophil recruitment during inflammation through synergistic effects on endothelial activation," *Journal of Immunology*, vol. 188, no. 12, pp. 6287–6299, 2012.

[47] S. M. Vieira, H. P. Lemos, R. Grespan et al., "A crucial role for TNF-α in mediating neutrophil influx induced by endogenously generated or exogenous chemokines, KC/CXCL1 and LIX/CXCL5," *British Journal of Pharmacology*, vol. 158, no. 3, pp. 779–789, 2009.

[48] J. J. Liu, X. Li, Y. Yue, J. Li, T. He, and Y. He, "The inhibitory effect of quercetin on IL-6 production by LPS-stimulated neutrophils," *Cellular & Molecular Immunology*, vol. 2, no. 6, pp. 455–460, 2005.

[49] A. B. Troutt and F. Y. Lee, "Tissue distribution of murine hemopoietic growth factor mRNA production," *Journal of Cellular Physiology*, vol. 138, no. 1, pp. 38–44, 1989.

[50] P. Ghezzi, S. Sacco, D. Agnello, A. Marullo, G. Caselli, and R. Bertini, "LPS induces IL-6 in the brain and in serum largely through TNF production," *Cytokine*, vol. 12, no. 8, pp. 1205–1210, 2000.

[51] T. R. Ulich, K. Guo, D. Remick, J. Del Castillo, and S. Yin, "Endotoxin-induced cytokine gene expression in vivo: III. IL-6 mRNA and serum protein expression and the in vivo hematologic effects of IL-6," *Journal of Immunology*, vol. 146, no. 7, pp. 2316–2323, 1991.

[52] Z. Xing, J. Gauldie, G. Cox et al., "IL-6 is an antiinflammatory cytokine required for controlling local or systemic acute inflammatory responses," *The Journal of Clinical Investigation*, vol. 101, no. 2, pp. 311–320, 1998.

[53] T. R. Ulich, S. Yin, K. Guo, E. S. Yi, D. Remick, and J. Del Castillo, "Intratracheal injection of endotoxin and cytokines. II. Interleukin-6 and transforming growth factor beta inhibit acute inflammation," *American Journal of Pathology*, vol. 138, no. 5, pp. 1097–1101, 1991.

[54] H. Saito, C. Patterson, Z. Hu et al., "Expression and self-regulatory function of cardiac interleukin-6 during endotoxemia," *American Journal of Physiology—Heart and Circulatory Physiology*, vol. 279, no. 5, pp. H2241–H2248, 2000.

[55] Y. Zhang, T. Q. Li, G. Wang et al., "Randomized controlled trial of Tanreqing injection in treatment of acute exacerbation of chronic obstructive pulmonary disease (syndrome of retention of phlegm-heat in the lung)," *Chinese Journal of Evidence-Based Medicine*, vol. 4, no. 5, pp. 300–305, 2004.

[56] G. L. Gong and X. Li, "Study of clinical effect on treatment of chronic obstructive pulmonary disease in acute aggravated stage with tanreqing injection and cell factor level," *Zhongguo Zhong Yao Za Zhi*, vol. 34, no. 1, pp. 104–106, 2009.

# 14

# Decoction and Fermentation of Selected Medicinal Herbs Promote Hair Regrowth by Inducing Hair Follicle Growth in Conjunction with Wnts Signaling

**Su Kil Jang,**[1] **Seung Tae Kim,**[1] **Do Ik Lee,**[2] **Jun Sub Park,**[1] **Bo Ram Jo,**[1] **Jung Youl Park,**[3] **Jong Heo,**[4] **and Seong Soo Joo**[1]

[1] *College of Life Science, Gangneung-Wonju National University, 120 Gangneung Daehangno, Gangneung, Gangwon 210-702, Republic of Korea*
[2] *College of Pharmacy, Chung-Ang University, 221 Heukseok-dong, Dongjak-gu, Seoul 156-756, Republic of Korea*
[3] *Industry-Academic Cooperation Foundation, Hanbat National University, Daejeon 305-719, Republic of Korea*
[4] *Heo-jong Oriental Medicine Clinic, Mia-dong, Gangbuk-gu 62-3, Seoul 01205, Republic of Korea*

Correspondence should be addressed to Seong Soo Joo; larryjoo@hanmail.net

Academic Editor: Jian-Li Gao

It is well recognized that regulating the hair follicle cycle in association with Wnt signaling is one of the most interesting targets for promoting hair regrowth. In this study, we examined whether selected herbal medicines processed by decoction and fermentation promote hair growth by upregulating the number and size of hair follicles and Wnt signaling, including activation of $\beta$-catenin and Akt in telogen-synchronized C57BL/6N mice. The results revealed that the fermented extract after decoction (FDE) more effectively promoted hair growth than that of a nonfermented extract (DE). Notably, FDE effectively enhanced formation of hair follicles with clearer differentiation between the inner and outer root sheath, which is observed during the anagen phase. Mechanistic evidence was found for increased $\beta$-catenin and Akt phosphorylation levels in dorsal skin tissue along with elevated expression of hair regrowth-related genes, such as Wnt3/10a/10b, Lef1, and fibroblast growth factor 7. In conclusion, our findings suggest that FDE plays an important role in regulating the hair cycle by increasing expression of hair regrowth-related genes and activating downstream Wnt signaling targets.

## 1. Introduction

Hair is a defining property of mammals that plays important roles in keeping the body warm and dry and protecting against harmful environments. Thus, new hair is required constantly throughout life. In general, new hair is supplied by existing follicles through the anagen (growing phase of follicular epithelium), catagen (apoptosis and regression phase), and telogen phases (resting phase for the epithelium). A hair follicle is a skin organ that generates hair and has been the focus of stem cell studies [1, 2].

Hair follicles may be self-renewed by keratinocyte stem cells (KSCs) located at the bulge region, which contains undifferentiated cells [3, 4]. During the transition from the telogen to the anagen phases, Wnt signaling, which is required to establish the hair follicle and is upregulated only at the end of the telogen phase to promote entry into anagen, plays a key role in activating bulge stem cells to progress toward hair formation, and these signals are relayed in association with $\beta$-catenin and lymphoid enhancer factor 1 (Lef1) [5]. Wnt ligand expression is not detected in telogen phase follicles, and Wnt10a and 10b are only expressed at the onset of the anagen phase in the dermal papilla and secondary hair germ cells, respectively [6]. This is supported by the observation that $\beta$-catenin is generally confined to the membranes of bulge cells through most of the telogen phase and that nuclear $\beta$-catenin only becomes apparent in hair germ cells just before the follicle enters the anagen phase [5, 7].

To date, comprehensively effective highly safe candidate compounds prepared from herbal extracts have been examined for their hair regrowth activities. Among these, we selected eight herbs and derived an optimal extract through decoction and fermentation processes. In this study, we examined the hair regrowth activity of the extract in C57BL6/N mice and its prospective mechanism in conjunction with Wnt signaling.

## 2. Materials and Methods

*2.1. Preparation of the Study Sample.* Eight selected medicinal herbs, such as *Cynanchum wilfordii, Mori Fructus, Schisandrae Fructus, Perillae Herba, Houttuyniae Herba, Ligustri Fructus, Longanae Arillus,* and *Polygonati Rhizoma,* were purchased from Saerom Pharmaceutical Co., Ltd. (Kyunggi, Republic of Korea). The study samples were prepared according to the method developed in our laboratory. In brief, to prepare the decoction, evenly weighed herbs (1:1) were finely ground and primarily immersed in autoclaved distilled water (1:10, w/v) for 30 min, followed by boiling on an electric heater for 2 h. The decoction was filtered using Whatman Grade No. 1 Filter Paper (Whatman International Ltd., Maidstone, UK) and centrifuged at 5000 rpm for 15 min. The supernatant was collected, lyophilized, and stored at 4°C before use. For fermentation, *Bacillus subtilis* was propagated twice in 50 mL MRS broth (Difco, Detroit, MI, USA) at 37°C overnight for fermentation. Then, $10^7$ CFU/mL of *B. subtilis* was inoculated into the decocted extracts and fermented at 37°C for 48 h (FDE). Nonfermented decoction extracts (DE) were used as a normal control. Both samples were serially filtered with a 60 $\mu$m nylon net filter and a 0.22 $\mu$m syringe filter (Millipore, Bedford, MA, USA), precipitated overnight, lyophilized (supernatant), and stored in desiccators at room temperature before use. During fermentation (24 and 48 h), samples of the liquid culture were examined under phase-contrast microscopy to visualize basic cell characteristics.

*2.2. Animals.* Healthy male C57BL6/N mice (7 weeks old) were obtained from Central Lab. Animal Inc. (Seoul, Republic of Korea) and were adapted to laboratory conditions (temperature: 20 ± 2°C, relative humidity: 50%, and light/dark cycle: 12 h) for 1 week. The animals ($n = 3$/group) were maintained at a constant temperature (23 ± 2°C), relative humidity (55 ± 10%), and a 12 h light/dark cycle and fed standard rodent chow and purified water *ad libitum*. Two days before the experiments, all mice (8 weeks of age) were shaved using animal clippers. Telogen-synchronized C57BL/6N mice were divided into six groups, each containing three male mice. The FDE and DE extracts as well as finasteride (FIN; Sigma-Aldrich, St. Louis, MO, USA) were administered daily for 20 consecutive days. The FDE and DE groups were given 64 or 128 mg/kg and 140 or 280 mg/kg, respectively, considering the vaporized solid parts of FDE (3.9 g/100 mL) and DE (8.7 g/mL). FIN (1 mg/kg) was administered as the positive at the same time points. All mice were sacrificed on day 21 and the dorsal hair growth patterns were photographed on days 0, 3, 6, 9, 12, 15, 18, and 20. The back area of each mouse was photographed with a digital camera and the image was inputted to a computer for measurement according to the following formula: [% Hair regrowth = hairy black area ÷ hair removal area] to quantitatively compare the hair regrowth patterns. The animal experiments were approved by the Gangneung-Wonju National University Animal Care and Use Committee (Approval number GWNU-2014-27), and all procedures were conducted in accordance with the Guide for Care and Use of Laboratory Animals published by the US National Institutes of Health.

*2.3. Cell Culture.* Human mesenchymal stem cells (hMSCs) used in this study were provided by Professor Kim (Chungbuk National University, Republic of Korea) [8, 9]. Cells were cultured at a density of $5 \times 10^3$ cells/cm$^2$ in complete medium and Dulbecco's modified Eagle's medium (DMEM, low glucose) was supplemented with 10% fetal bovine serum (FBS; Hyclone, Logan, UT, USA), 2.5 ng/mL hFGF2, 100 U/mL penicillin, and 100 $\mu$g/mL streptomycin (Invitrogen, Carlsbad, CA, USA). Complete medium was changed every 2-3 days, and hMSCs were subcultured when they reach $1 \times 10^4$ cells/cm$^2$. Cultures were maintained under 5% CO$_2$ at 37°C in tissue culture flasks.

*2.4. Cellular Cytotoxicity (Lactate Dehydrogenase, LDH) Assay.* The cytotoxicity induced by the FDE and DE was quantified by measuring LDH release. LDH content was determined using a commercial nonradioactive LDH assay kit, CytoTox 96® (Promega, Madison, WI, USA), which is based on a coupled enzymatic reaction that results in the conversion of a tetrazolium salt into a red formazan product. The increase in the amount of formazan produced in the culture supernatant directly correlates with the increase in the number of lysed cells. The formazan was quantified spectrophotometrically by measuring its absorbance at 490 nm (Spectra Max 340, Molecular Devices, Sunnyvale, CA, USA). Cytotoxicity in experimental samples was determined as % LDH release compared with that in cells treated with 1% Triton X-100.

*2.5. Quantitative Real-Time Polymerase Chain Reaction (PCR) Assay.* Total RNA from C57BL6/N dorsal skin tissues or hMSCs was prepared using the TRIZOL method (Invitrogen). cDNAs were synthesized from RNA by reverse transcription of 1 $\mu$g total RNA using the ImProm-II reverse transcription system (Promega) and oligo dT primers in a total volume of 20 $\mu$L. PCR amplification was performed using the primers described in Table 1 (Bioneer, Daejeon, Republic of Korea). Quantitative real-time PCR (qPCR) reactions were run on a Rotor-Gene 6000 (Corbett Research, Sydney, Australia) using SYBR Green PCR Master Mix (Qiagen, Valencia, CA, USA) in 20 $\mu$L reaction mixtures. Each real-time PCR master mix contained 10 $\mu$L 2x enzyme Mastermix, 7.0 $\mu$L RNase free water, 1 $\mu$L of each primer (10 pmole each), and 1 $\mu$L diluted template. PCR was performed with an initial preincubation step for 10 min at 95°C, followed by 45 cycles of 95°C for 15 s, annealing at 52°C for 15 s, and extension at 72°C for 10 s. A melting curve analysis was used to confirm

TABLE 1: Primer sequences used for the real-time polymerase chain reaction analysis.

| Gene | | Primer | Amino acid sequences | Product size (bp) | Accession number |
|---|---|---|---|---|---|
| **Mouse** | FGF7 | 5′ primer | 5′-TGCTTCCACCTCGTCTGTCT | 212 | NM_008008 |
| | | 3′ primer | 5′-GAGGCAAAGTGAAAGGGACC | | |
| | Wnt3 | 5′ primer | 5′-AGAGACGGGCTCCTTTGGTA | 123 | NM_009521 |
| | | 3′ primer | 5′-TTCTCCTTCCGTTTCTCCGT | | |
| | Wnt10a | 5′ primer | 5′-GTGCGCTCTGGGTAAACTGA | 232 | NM_009518 |
| | | 3′ primer | 5′-AGAGAAGCGTTCTCCGAAGC | | |
| | Wnt10b | 5′ primer | 5′-TCTTGGCTTTGTTCAGTCGG | 124 | NM_011718 |
| | | 3′ primer | 5′-CCCAGCTGTCGCTTACTCAG | | |
| | β-catenin | 5′ primer | 5′-AGGCTTTTCCCAGTCCTTCA | 122 | M90364 |
| | | 3′ primer | 5′-TCTGCATGCCCTCATCTAGC | | |
| | Lef1 | 5′ primer | 5′-CGTCCTCTCAGGAGCCCTAC | 169 | X58636 |
| | | 3′ primer | 5′-GGAGAAAGGGACCCATTTGA | | |
| | β-actin | 5′ primer | 5′-TACAGCTTCACCACCACAGC | 187 | NM_007393 |
| | | 3′ primer | 5′-AAGGAAGGCTGGAAAAGAGC | | |
| **Human** | Wnt3 | 5′ primer | 5′-CACATGCACCTCAAATGCAA | 132 | AB067628 |
| | | 3′ primer | 5′-CGAGGCGCTGTCATACTTGT | | |
| | Wnt10a | 5′ primer | 5′-TTCCACTGGTGCTGCGTAGT | 107 | AB059570 |
| | | 3′ primer | 5′-CTGCGCGAAGTCAGTCTAGC | | |
| | Wnt10b | 5′ primer | 5′-CATACAGGGCATCCAGATCG | 148 | AB059569 |
| | | 3′ primer | 5′-AAAAGCGCTCTCTCGGAAAC | | |
| | GAPDH | 5′ primer | 5′-GGAGCCAAAAGGGTCATCAT | 203 | AK_026525 |
| | | 3′ primer | 5′-GTGATGGCATGGACTGTGGT | | |

formation of the expected PCR product, and products from all assays were tested by 1.2% agarose gel electrophoresis to confirm the correct lengths. An interrun calibrator was used, and a standard curve was created for each gene to obtain PCR efficiencies. Relative sample expression levels were calculated using Rotor-Gene 6000 Series Software 1.7 and were expressed relative to glyceraldehyde 3-phosphate dehydrogenase and corrected for between-run variability. Data are expressed as a percentage of the internal control gene.

*2.6. Western Blot Analysis.* C57BL6/N dorsal skin tissues were homogenized and lysed in 1% RIPA buffer containing protease and phosphatase inhibitors (Roche, Mannheim, Germany), and total proteins were separated on 10% SDS-PAGE. After electrophoresis, the proteins were transferred to polyvinylidene fluoride membranes, and the membranes were blocked with 5% skim milk in Tris-buffered saline solution containing 0.1% Tween-20. The membranes were immunoblotted with primary antibodies, including anti-β-catenin, anti-phospo-Akt, anti-Akt, and anti-actin (Santa Cruz Biotechnology, Santa Cruz, CA, USA), followed by incubation with horseradish peroxidase-conjugated anti-rabbit or anti-mouse secondary antibodies (Stressgen, San Diego, CA, USA). The blots were developed using an enhanced chemiluminescent solution (Thermo, Rockford, IL, USA).

*2.7. Histological Examination and Hair Follicle Count.* Rectangular pieces of central dorsal skin were collected parallel to the vertebral line and fixed in 10% neutral buffered formalin (4 g sodium phosphate, monobasic, 6.5 g sodium phosphate, dibasic, 100 mL of 37% formalin, and 900 mL distilled water) for 5 days. The tissues were then embedded in paraffin, cut into sections (5 $\mu$m), and stained with a hematoxylin-eosin (H&E) solution. The sections were deparaffinized with xylene, hydrated in a descending graded ethanol series, and stained with hematoxylin for 2 min, followed by 2 min washes and eosin staining for 5 s. All tissue samples were examined and imaged in a blinded fashion. Hair follicle counts were performed by using a digital photomicrograph and all of the images were cropped in a fixed area (300 pixels in width). Data were evaluated from representative areas at a fixed magnification of 100x. Images were captured using a Nikon Eclips Ti-S inverted microscope (Nikon, Tokyo, Japan) at 40x magnification.

*2.8. Statistical Analysis.* Statistical comparisons between groups were performed using one-way analysis of variance with Dunnett's post hoc test and SPSS v. 17 software (SPSS Inc., Chicago, IL, USA). A $P < 0.05$ was considered significant.

## 3. Results

*3.1. Hair Growth-Promoting Action in Male C57BL6/N Mice.* Hair growth patterns in the shaved area were compared in all groups. To evaluate the hair growth effect, FIN (1 mg/kg), FDE (low: 64 mg/kg, high: 128 mg/kg), and DE

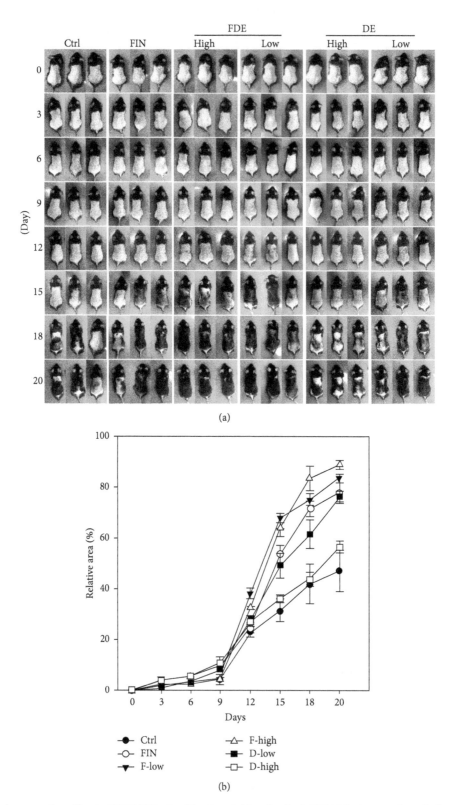

(a)

(b)

FIGURE 1: Hair growth-promoting effect in C57BL/6N mice. The dorsal skin of male C57BL/6N mice was shaved after the mice were orally administered the fermented herbal extract after decoction (FDE), the nonfermented herbal extract after decoction (DE), or finasteride for 20 days. (a) The shaved dorsal skin was photographed at 0, 3, 6, 9, 12, 15, 18, and 20 days. (b) The area of hair regrowth was measured by image software on the indicated day. FIN, finasteride; F, FDE; D, DE.

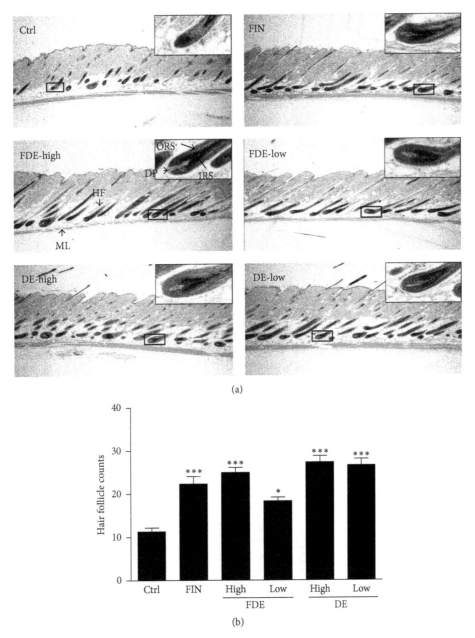

(a)

(b)

Figure 2: Comparison of hair follicle growth in C57BL/6N mice. (a) Hematoxylin-eosin staining of dorsal skin from mice administered the fermented herbal extract after decoction (FDE), the nonfermented herbal extract after decoction (DE), or finasteride for 20 days was analyzed. Arrows are muscle layer (ML), dermal papilla (DP), outer root sheath (ORS), and inner root sheath (IRS). (b) The number of hair follicles in deep subcutis. Values are mean ± standard deviations. $^*P < 0.05$, $^{***}P < 0.001$ versus Ctrl. Ctrl, control group.

(low: 140 mg/kg, high: 280 mg/kg) were administered, and patterns of dorsal hair growth were examined on days 0, 3, 6, 9, 12, 15, 18, and 20 (Figure 1(a)). As shown in Figure 1(a), the FDE and DE caused a gray hair color on day 12 after induction, and the hair shafts were visible on day 15, whereas hair in the control group remained unpigmented until day 15. Interestingly, regrowth of hair in FDE-treated mice was as much as that seen in the FIN positive control, which is a representative oral hair loss drug used worldwide (Figure 1(b)).

3.2. Effects of FDE/DE on Hair Follicle Structure. Hair follicle growth (anagen) between groups was compared in accordance with accepted morphological guidelines [10]. Our results revealed that FDE and DE increased the number and size of hair follicles, which are markers for transition of follicles from the telogen to anagen phase of hair growth, whereas hair in the control group was in the early anagen phase, in which enlarged dermal papilla and the bulb located in the dermis are distinct characteristics (Figure 2(a)). Notably, H&E staining of FDE and DE mice well demonstrated that

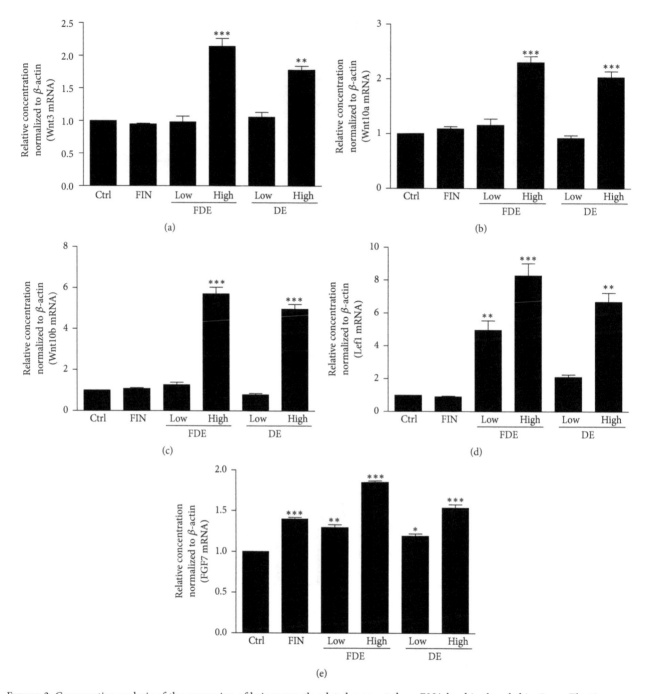

FIGURE 3: Comparative analysis of the expression of hair regrowth-related genes at the mRNA level in dorsal skin tissue. The tissues were collected on day 21, and mRNAs were harvested using TRIZOL. Wnt3/10a/10b, Lef1, and fibroblast growth factor (FGF) 7 genes were compared by real-time quantitative polymerase chain reaction. Results are expressed as means ± standard deviations. $^*P < 0.05$, $^{**}P < 0.01$, and $^{***}P < 0.001$ versus Ctrl. Ctrl, control group.

the hair follicles were at least in the anagen IIIc-IV phase, representing thinner dermal papilla, maximal hair bulb size and volume, and newly formed hair shafts. The number of hair follicles in the longitudinal sections of the FDE-treated mice increased similar to that observed in the positive FIN control (Figure 2(b)).

3.3. Expression of Wnt, Fibroblast Growth Factor (FGF) 7, and Lef1 Genes in C57BL6/N Dorsal Skin. Primary Wnt (Wnt3)

and secondary Wnts (Wnt10a and Wnt10b) are essential for hair follicle initiation, morphogenesis, and development [11] and were examined to determine whether FDE and DE increased expression of dermal Wnt genes implicated in the first signal essential for inducing hair follicles. Figures 3(a)–3(c) indicate that oral administration of FDE and DE contributed largely to differentiation of the hair medulla and regulation of matrix/precortex cells by stimulating Wnt genes (3, 10a, and 10b) at the higher concentration. Moreover,

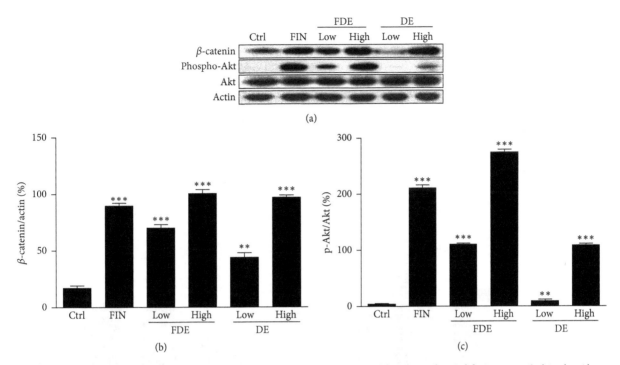

FIGURE 4: Western blot analysis of $\beta$-catenin and Akt phosphorylation. (a) Immunoblotting analysis of $\beta$-catenin and phospho-Akt protein levels was conducted in C57BL6/N dorsal skin tissue sampled on day 21 after treatment. (b) A bar graph shows the quantification of $\beta$-catenin/actin and (c) phospho-Akt/Akt ratio. Finasteride (FIN) was used as the positive control. $^{**}P < 0.01$, $^{***}P < 0.001$ versus Ctrl. Ctrl, control group.

FDE and DE upregulated expression of Lef1, which is an essential regulatory gene in the Wnt signaling pathway that controls cell growth and differentiation through a signaling cascade from Wnts to Lef1 (Figure 3(d)). The FGF7 gene was also overexpressed in the FDE- and DE-treated groups (Figure 3(e)), suggesting a prolonged anagen phase and delayed progression into the catagen phase in dermal papilla cells [12].

### 3.4. Activation of $\beta$-Catenin and Akt Signaling by FDE and DE.

Cytosolic $\beta$-catenin, an essential molecule in the Wnt signaling pathway, translocates into the nucleus where it induces transcription of target genes. Thus, we investigated whether FDE or DE upregulates $\beta$-catenin levels in dorsal skin tissues. $\beta$-catenin level increases during the initial stages of hair regeneration. We also compared the protein level of phosphorylated Akt, a downstream target of phospho-inositide 3-kinase, with that in the FIN group. $\beta$-catenin expression increased in response to the high doses of FDE and DE to levels comparable to those in the FIN group. Moreover, Akt activation, which promotes hair regrowth by regulating dermal papilla cell proliferation in the hair follicle, was upregulated in the presence of FDE and DE, with more upregulation in the FDE than that in the DE (Figures 4(a)–4(c)).

### 3.5. Cytotoxicity and Profiles of Wnts mRNAs in hMSCs.

The cytotoxicity induced by the FDE and DE was quantified by measuring LDH release at varying ranges of concentration (1–1000 $\mu$g/mL). Incubating hMSCs with each of the study samples did not result in cell cytotoxicity except at the highest dose (1000 $\mu$g/mL). Figures 5(a) and 5(b) show that the FDE and DE did not significantly increase LDH release for 1–100 $\mu$g/mL exposure for up to 24 h but a higher concentration (1000 $\mu$g/mL) induced a significant increase in LDH release. Figures 5(c)–5(e) clearly show that FDE significantly increased Wnt3, Wnt10a, and Wnt10b mRNA in hMSCs. As expected, results of this *in vitro* study coincide with the *in vivo* dorsal skin results.

## 4. Discussion

The hair follicle is a mammalian skin organ that produces hair, which is repeatedly renewed through canonical signaling, for proper growth and patterning. Otherwise, the hair cycle is disrupted, and hair is lost from the head or body, which is called alopecia. To date, two representative types of drugs have been prescribed for pattern baldness. FIN, which is a 5 alpha-reductase inhibitor, and minoxidil, which is an antihypertensive vasodilator, are the most frequently prescribed medications for alopecia. The selected herbal medicines used in this study have been reported to have diverse pharmacological activities, such as antihypercholesterolemia, immunoregulation, antiallergy, antibacteria, antioxidation, anticancer, hepatoprotection, and anti-insomnia [13–18].

As C57BL/6N mice have been shown to be in a synchronized telogen stage of the hair cycle at 8 weeks of age,

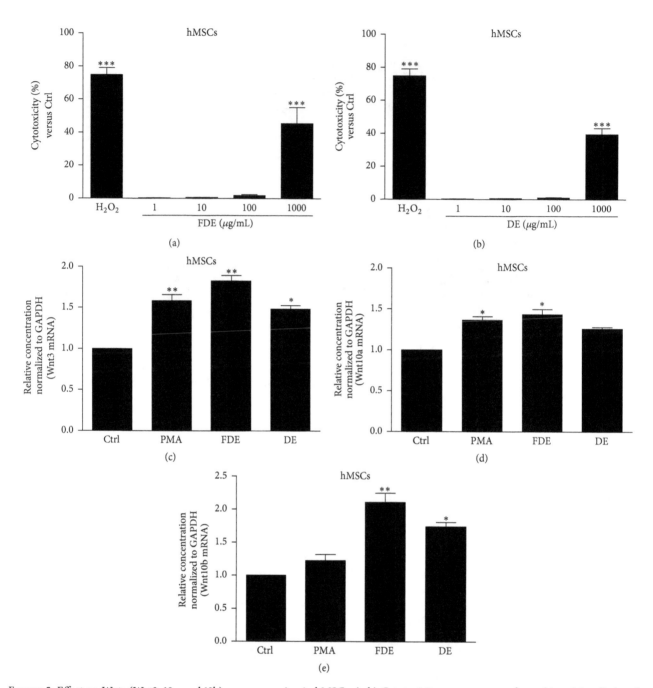

FIGURE 5: Effect on Wnts (Wnt3, 10a, and 10b) gene expression in hMSCs. (a-b) Cytotoxicity assays were performed in a 96-well plate for 24 h, and the results were expressed as the percent cytotoxicity for identical treatments of HDE and DE (1–1000 $\mu$g/mL). For gene expression analysis, cells were seeded on a 6-well plate and treated with the HDE (100 $\mu$g/mL) or DE (100 $\mu$g/mL) in the presence or absence of 50 $\mu$M phorbol myristic acetate (PMA) for 24 h. (c–e) Wnt3, Wnt10a, and Wnt10b mRNA were quantified by fold units using the real-time polymerase chain reaction. Results are expressed as means ± standard deviations from three separate experiments. $^{*}P < 0.05$, $^{**}P < 0.01$, and $^{***}P < 0.001$ versus Ctrl. Ctrl, control group.

their hair follicle regeneration and regrowth have been well described. The high dose of FDE promoted hair regrowth during the 20 consecutive days of administration that was equal to that seen in the positive FIN control. Wnt signaling is required to establish the hair follicle [19] and plays a key role activating bulge stem cells to progress toward hair formation, and this signal is relayed by $\beta$-catenin and Lef1 [5].

In recent studies, a hierarchy of Wnts that control hair follicle development has been introduced. According to the prior reports, among 19 Wnts, Wnts 3, 4, and 6 were considered to mediate hair follicle initiation and Wnts 2, 7b, 10a, and 10b were considered to depend on the epidermal activation [6, 10, 20]. In line with this, Wnt secretion mediates hair follicle development by acting as signaling molecules and they can be classified as primary Wnts (Wnts 3, 4, and 6) and secondary Wnts (Wnts 2, 7b, 10a, and 10b), which are essential for initiating hair follicle growth and are involved in development of the hair follicle, respectively [10, 21]. In particular, matrix and precortex cells express Wnt3 and Wnt10a/b, which send a signaling cascade to Lef1 [22, 23]. Importantly, $\beta$-catenin, which is a key regulator of hair follicle growth, is involved in inducing the transition from telogen to anagen [23]. Thus, it is important that a hair regrowth candidate should be associated with Wnt signaling. H&E staining demonstrated that FDE and DE actively promoted hair follicle regrowth by increasing the number and size of hair follicles, which is an indicator for the transition of hair growth from the telogen to anagen phases at particular times. The hair of FDE-treated mice was more prone to transition into the late anagen phase (i.e., IIIc), in which the dermal papilla reaches the deepest position and rests close to the muscle layer along with the distinguishable inner and outer root sheaths [10].

The increase in Wnt3/10a/10b and Lef1 gene expression in the dorsal skin strongly indicates that hair follicles were actively developing because these genes are predominantly expressed in the hair placode epithelium during induction of the hair follicle [24–26]. Coincident data were obtained from qPCR analysis in hMSCs, which are known to express all of the common stem cell markers and can be differentiated into various types of specialized cells under appropriate growth conditions [27]. Taken together, FDE could play an essential role in the initiation and development of hair follicles, as shown by the H&E staining results. Furthermore, the increase in FGF7 mRNA helps understand how FDE prolongs the anagen phase and delays progression into the catagen phase.

## 5. Conclusion

Our data clearly demonstrate that FDE effectively promotes hair regrowth by enhancing Wnt signaling and activating Akt together with overexpression of hair regrowth-related primary and secondary Wnts (Wnt3/10a/10b), Lef1, and FGF7. Although more in-depth chemical screening studies are required, it is certain that the extract from eight selected herbal medicines could be a promising hair regrowth candidate when fermented after decoction.

## Conflict of Interests

The authors declare that they have no conflict of interests.

## Authors' Contribution

Su Kil Jang and Seung Tae Kim equally contributed to this paper.

## Acknowledgment

This study was supported by a grant from the Korea Healthcare Technology R&D Project, Ministry for Health, Welfare, and Family Affairs, Republic of Korea (A091121).

## References

[1] R. Paus and G. Cotsarelis, "The biology of hair follicles," *The New England Journal of Medicine*, vol. 341, no. 7, pp. 491–497, 1999.

[2] E. Fuchs, B. J. Merrill, C. Jamora, and R. Dasgupta, "At the roots of a never-ending cycle," *Developmental Cell*, vol. 1, no. 1, pp. 13–25, 2001.

[3] S. Claudinot, M. Nicolas, H. Oshima, A. Rochat, and Y. Barrandon, "Long-term renewal of hair follicles from clonogenic multipotent stem cells," *Proceedings of the National Academy of Sciences of the United States of America*, vol. 102, no. 41, pp. 14677–14682, 2005.

[4] M. Ohyama, A. Terunuma, C. L. Tock et al., "Characterization and isolation of stem cell-enriched human hair follicle bulge cells," *The Journal of Clinical Investigation*, vol. 116, no. 1, pp. 249–260, 2006.

[5] W. E. Lowry, C. Blanpain, J. A. Nowak, G. Guasch, L. Lewis, and E. Fuchs, "Defining the impact of $\beta$-catenin/Tcf transactivation on epithelial stem cells," *Genes & Development*, vol. 19, no. 13, pp. 1596–1611, 2005.

[6] S. Reddy, T. Andl, A. Bagasra et al., "Characterization of Wnt gene expression in developing and postnatal hair follicles and identification of Wnt5a as a target of Sonic hedgehog in hair follicle morphogenesis," *Mechanisms of Development*, vol. 107, no. 1-2, pp. 69–82, 2001.

[7] V. Greco, T. Chen, M. Rendl et al., "A two-step mechanism for stem cell activation during hair regeneration," *Cell Stem Cell*, vol. 4, no. 2, pp. 155–169, 2009.

[8] J. C. Ra, I. S. Shin, S. H. Kim et al., "Safety of intravenous infusion of human adipose tissue-derived mesenchymal stem cells in animals and humans," *Stem Cells and Development*, vol. 20, no. 8, pp. 1297–1308, 2011.

[9] D. Park, G. Yang, D. K. Bae et al., "Human adipose tissue-derived mesenchymal stem cells improve cognitive function and physical activity in ageing mice," *Journal of Neuroscience Research*, vol. 91, no. 5, pp. 660–670, 2013.

[10] S. Müller-Röver, B. Handjiski, C. van der Veen et al., "A comprehensive guide for the accurate classification of murine hair follicles in distinct hair cycle stages," *The Journal of Investigative Dermatology*, vol. 117, no. 1, pp. 3–15, 2001.

[11] T. Andl, S. T. Reddy, T. Gaddapara, and S. E. Millar, "WNT signals are required for the initiation of hair follicle development," *Developmental Cell*, vol. 2, no. 5, pp. 643–653, 2002.

[12] D. M. Danilenko, B. D. Ring, D. Yanagihara et al., "Keratinocyte growth factor is an important endogenous mediator of hair follicle growth, development, and differentiation: normalization of the nu/nu follicular differentiation defect and amelioration of chemotherapy-induced alopecia," *American Journal of Pathology*, vol. 147, no. 1, pp. 145–154, 1995.

[13] G. S. Kim, D. H. Kim, J. J. Lim et al., "Biological and antibacterial activities of the natural herb *Houttuynia cordata* water extract against the intracellular bacterial pathogen *Salmonella* within the RAW 264.7 macrophage," *Biological & Pharmaceutical Bulletin*, vol. 31, no. 11, pp. 2012–2017, 2008.

[14] X.-Y. Yang, G.-S. Park, M. H. Lee et al., "Toll-like receptor 4-mediated immunoregulation by the aqueous extract of Mori Fructus," *Phytotherapy Research*, vol. 23, no. 12, pp. 1713–1720, 2009.

[15] H.-S. Lee, J.-H. Choi, Y.-E. Kim, I.-H. Kim, B.-M. Kim, and C.-H. Lee, "Effects of the cynanchum wilfordii ethanol extract on the serum lipid profile in hypercholesterolemic rats," *Preventive Nutrition and Food Science*, vol. 18, no. 3, pp. 157–162, 2013.

[16] X.-Y. Wang, Z.-L. Yu, S.-Y. Pan et al., "Supplementation with the extract of schisandrae fructus pulp, seed, or their combination influences the metabolism of lipids and glucose in mice fed with normal and hypercholesterolemic diet," *Evidence-Based Complementary and Alternative Medicine*, vol. 2014, Article ID 472638, 11 pages, 2014.

[17] Y. Shi, J. Dong, J. Zhao, L. Tang, and J. Zhang, "Herbal insomnia medications that target GABAergic systems: a review of the psychopharmacological evidence," *Current Neuropharmacology*, vol. 12, no. 3, pp. 289–302, 2014.

[18] Z. Pang, Z. Zhi-Yan, W. Wang et al., "The advances in research on the pharmacological effects of *Fructus Ligustri Lucidi*," *BioMed Research International*, vol. 2015, Article ID 281873, 5 pages, 2015.

[19] L. Alonso and E. Fuchs, "Stem cells in the skin: waste not, Wnt not," *Genes & Development*, vol. 17, no. 10, pp. 1189–1200, 2003.

[20] J. Fu and W. Hsu, "Epidermal Wnt controls hair follicle induction by orchestrating dynamic signaling crosstalk between the epidermis and dermis," *Journal of Investigative Dermatology*, vol. 133, no. 4, pp. 890–898, 2013.

[21] Y. Zhang, P. Tomann, T. Andl et al., "Reciprocal requirements for EDA/EDAR/NF-κB and Wnt/β-catenin signaling pathways in hair follicle induction," *Developmental Cell*, vol. 17, no. 1, pp. 49–61, 2009.

[22] S. E. Millar, K. Willert, P. C. Salinas et al., "WNT signaling in the control of hair growth and structure," *Developmental Biology*, vol. 207, no. 1, pp. 133–149, 1999.

[23] A. E. Oro and K. Higgins, "Hair cycle regulation of Hedgehog signal reception," *Developmental Biology*, vol. 255, no. 2, pp. 238–248, 2003.

[24] C. van Genderen, R. M. Okamura, I. Farinas et al., "Development of several organs that require inductive epithelial-mesenchymal interactions is impaired in LEF-1-deficient mice," *Genes & Development*, vol. 8, no. 22, pp. 2691–2703, 1994.

[25] P. Zhou, C. Byrne, J. Jacobs, and E. Fuchs, "Lymphoid enhancer factor 1 directs hair follicle patterning and epithelial cell fate," *Genes & Development*, vol. 9, no. 6, pp. 700–713, 1995.

[26] R. DasGupta and E. Fuchs, "Multiple roles for activated LEF/TCF transcription complexes during hair follicle development and differentiation," *Development*, vol. 126, no. 20, pp. 4557–4568, 1999.

[27] B. A. Bunnell, M. Flaat, C. Gagliardi, B. Patel, and C. Ripoll, "Adipose-derived stem cells: isolation, expansion and differentiation," *Methods*, vol. 45, no. 2, pp. 115–120, 2008.

# 15

# Supercritical Fluid Extract of Spent Coffee Grounds Attenuates Melanogenesis through Downregulation of the PKA, PI3K/Akt, and MAPK Signaling Pathways

**Huey-Chun Huang,[1] Chien-Mei Wei,[2] Jen-Hung Siao,[2] Tsang-Chi Tsai,[3] Wang-Ping Ko,[3] Kuei-Jen Chang,[3] Choon-Hoon Hii,[4] and Tsong-Min Chang[2]**

[1]*Department of Medical Laboratory Science and Biotechnology, China Medical University, No. 91 Hsueh-Shih Road, Taichung 40402, Taiwan*

[2]*Department of Applied Cosmetology and Master Program of Cosmetic Science, Hungkuang University, No. 1018, Section 6, Taiwan Boulevard, Shalu District, Taichung 43302, Taiwan*

[3]*O'right Plant Extract R&D Center, No. 18, Gaoping Section, Jhongfong Road, Longtan District, Taoyuan 32544, Taiwan*

[4]*Department of Emergency Medicine, Kuang Tien General Hospital, No. 321, Jingguo Road, Dajia District, Taichung 43761, Taiwan*

Correspondence should be addressed to Choon-Hoon Hii; choonhoonhii@gmail.com
and Tsong-Min Chang; ctm@sunrise.hk.edu.tw

Academic Editor: Caio P. Fernandes

The mode of action of spent coffee grounds supercritical fluid $CO_2$ extract (SFE) in melanogenesis has never been reported. In the study, the spent coffee grounds were extracted by the supercritical fluid $CO_2$ extraction method; the chemical constituents of the SFE were investigated by gas chromatography-mass spectrometry (GC-MS). The effects of the SFE and its major fatty acid components on melanogenesis were evaluated by mushroom tyrosinase activity assay and determination of intracellular tyrosinase activity and melanin content. The expression level of melanogenesis-related proteins was analyzed by western blotting assay. The results revealed that the SFE of spent coffee grounds (1–10 mg/mL) and its major fatty acids such as linoleic acid and oleic acid (6.25– 50 $\mu$M) effectively suppressed melanogenesis in the B16F10 murine melanoma cells. Furthermore, the SFE decreased the expression of melanocortin 1 receptor (MC1R), microphthalmia-associated transcription factor (MITF), tyrosinase, tyrosinase-related protein-1 (TRP-1), and tyrosinase-related protein-2 (TRP-2). The SFE also decreased the protein expression levels of p-JNK, p-p38, p-ERK, and p-CREB. Our results revealed that the SFE of spent coffee grounds attenuated melanogenesis in B16F10 cells by downregulation of protein kinase A (PKA), phosphatidylinositol-3-kinase (PI3K/Akt), and mitogen-activated protein kinases (MAPK) signaling pathways, which may be due to linoleic acid and oleic acid.

## 1. Introduction

Melanin is produced and secreted by melanocytes that are distributed in the basal layer of the skin epidermis [1]. Melanin is responsible for skin color and also plays an important critical role in protecting the skin against ultraviolet (UV) light damage. It is reported that accumulation of an excessive level of epidermal melanin resulted in various dermatological disorders. Those skin hyperpigmented syndromes include melasma, postinflammatory melanoderma, age spots, freckles, and sites of actinic damage [2]. Recently,

the inhibitors of melanogenesis have been increasingly applied in skin care products for the treatment or prevention of skin hyperpigmented disorders [3]. It is well known that tyrosinase (EC 1.14.18.1) catalyzes the first two steps of melanin synthesis. It first hydroxylates L-tyrosine to L-3, 4-dihydroxyphenylalanine (L-DOPA), and L-DOPA is further oxidized into the corresponding *o*-dopaquinone [4]. There are many factors that participate in the regulation of melanogenesis. For example, the microphthalmia-associated transcription factor (MITF), tyrosinase-related protein-1 (TRP-1), and tyrosinase-related protein-2 (TRP-2) were reported to regulate the production of melanin [5–7]. In addition, the melanocortin 1 receptor (MC1R) also plays a key role in alpha-melanocyte stimulating hormone- ($\alpha$-MSH-) induced melanin synthesis [8]. It is reported that $\alpha$-MSH could elevate cyclic adenine monophosphate (cAMP) level and cAMP is usually used to induce the phosphorylation of cAMP response element-binding protein (CREB) and enhance MITF protein levels [9]. In addition, phosphorylation of mitogen-activated protein kinases (MAPK) and signaling cascades of extracellular responsive kinase (ERK), c-Jun N-terminal kinase (JNK), and p38 also modulate melanin synthesis [10, 11]. Hence, some skin whitening agents can inhibit MITF transcriptional activity by decreasing protein levels of tyrosinase or TRP-1 or TRP-2 through downregulation of MAPK-mediated MITF phosphorylation.

*Coffea arabica* is a plant belonging to the family Rubiaceae. The *Coffea* species are widely distributed in the world. Coffee beans and coffee extract have been used as psychoactive beverages or alternative medicine. It was reported that coffee contains caffeine, several vitamins, minerals, and antioxidants [12]. Caffeine potently blocks an inhibitory neurotransmitter in the brain, leading to a net stimulant effect. In addition, caffeine can improve mood and raises metabolism and increases the oxidation of fatty acids [13]. However, there is relatively little knowledge regarding the modes of action of spent coffee grounds in skin care or dermatology, including the kinds of bioactive components in the spent coffee grounds extract and the effects of the extract or its active components on melanin production [13]. Because of the importance of various compounds present in the coffee waste, the extraction method of the coffee waste appears as an important alternative to increase the aggregated value of the agroindustrial residues. The quality of extracts obtained from a raw material is strongly related to the extraction technique employed, and the quality of the extracts is measured by the chemical profile of the product. Supercritical technology is then a modern technique for extraction that seeks to increase quality by exploiting the selectivity of the process. Hence, the spent coffee grounds were extracted by supercritical technology to get the SFE, and the possible skin care effects of the SFE were further evaluated.

The inhibitory effects of spent coffee grounds SFE on melanogenesis were reported by Sung et al. [14]. However, the action mechanisms of spent coffee grounds for depigmentation still remained to be elucidated. The aim of the current study was to investigate the antimelanogenic activity of the SFE in murine B16F10 melanoma cells. The potential action mechanism of the SFE in melanogenesis was also evaluated by examining the MITF transcription regulators and phosphorylation of regulators of PKA, PI3K/Akt, and MAPK signaling pathways.

## 2. Methods

### 2.1. Chemicals and Reagents.
The antibodies were from Santa Cruz Biotech (Santa Cruz, CA, USA), and the ECL reagent was from Millipore (MA, USA). Protein kinase regulators including GF 109203X (classical PKC inhibitor),

H89 (cAMP-dependent protein kinase inhibitor; PKA inhibitor), 3-isobutyl-1-methyl-xanthine (IBMX), LY294002 (phosphatidylinositol-3-kinase inhibitor; PI3K inhibitor), PD98059 (MEK 1/2-inhibitor), SB203580 (p38 MAPK-inhibitor), SP600125 (c-Jun N-terminal kinase inhibitor; JNK inhibitor), and U0126 (MEK 1-inhibitor) were from Tocris (Ellisville, Missouri, USA). The chemical reagents were purchased from Sigma-Aldrich Chemical Co. (St. Louis, MS, USA).

### 2.2. Preparation of Spent Coffee Grounds Powder.
The spent coffee grounds of *arabica* blends were harvested in 2014 from the coffee shops located in Taoyuan County, Taiwan. The spent coffee grounds were washed completely, exposed to sunlight and air-dried for one day, and then dried at 80°C for 2 h in an oven until the water content of the grounds was less than 5%. The dehydrated coffee grounds were pulverized to a fine powder (#50 mesh) with a committed mill (Retsch Ultra Centrifugal Mill and Sieving Machine, Type ZM1, Haan, Germany). The powder was collected in a sealed glass bottle and stored at 25°C until use.

### 2.3. Supercritical Fluid $CO_2$ Extraction (SFE) of Spent Coffee Grounds Powder.
The pulverized desiccated spent coffee grounds powder (1000 g) was placed in the extraction vessel (2000 mL) of the supercritical fluid $CO_2$ extraction (SFE) apparatus (SFE-400S-2000, Metal Industries Research & Development Centre (MIRDC), Kaohsiung, Taiwan). The extraction was with 10% cosolvent of ethanol in supercritical fluid $CO_2$ (flow rate, 45 mL/min) at 2,900 psi (=200 bar) in combination with temperature at 50°C for 2 h. The extracts were evaporated to dryness on a rotary evaporator at 40°C under reduced pressure. The concentrated SFEs were weighed and stored at 4°C. The yield obtained from the extraction was 13–15% (dry weight basis). In the following experiments, the SFEs were redissolved in dimethyl sulfoxide (DMSO) as indicated.

### 2.4. Gas Chromatography (GC) Analysis of Spent Coffee Grounds SFE.
The fatty acids in the spent coffee grounds SFE were analyzed using a Thermo GC-MS system (GC-MS Trace DSQ-MASS Spectrometer, MSD 201351, Thermo, Minneapolis, MN, USA). An EquityTM-5 capillary column (Supelco, St. Louis, MO, USA) with 100 m length and 0.25 mm inside diameter with a 0.20 $\mu$m thick film was used. The oven temperature gradient was programmed as follows: isothermal heat-treatment in a process at 40°C, followed by a 5°C temperature ramp every minute to 100°C, which was held for 5 min. Subsequently, the temperature was increased 5°C every minute to 250°C and held for 20 min. The carrier gas was helium (1 mL/min). The injection port's and detector's temperatures were 285°C. Ionization of the test sample (1 $\mu$L) was performed in the EI mode (70 eV). The linear retention indices for all compounds were determined by coinjection of the spent coffee extract with a solution containing a homologous series of C8–C22 n-alkanes [15]. The compound was identified by retention indices and compared with compounds known from the literature [16]. Their mass

spectra were also compared with known, previously obtained compounds or from the Trace DSQ-MASS spectral database (Thermo).

*2.5. Cell Viability Assay.* The B16F10 cells (ATCC CRL-6475, BCRC60031) were obtained from the Bioresource Collection and Research Center (BCRC), Taiwan. The cells were maintained in DMEM (Hyclone, Logan, UT) supplemented with 10% fetal bovine serum and 1% antibiotics at 37°C, 5% $CO_2$ in a humidified incubator. The cell viability assay was performed using 3-(4,5-dimethylthiazol-2-yl)-2,5-diphenyltetrazolium bromide (MTT) method [17]. The cells ($5 \times 10^4$ cells/mL) were exposed to various concentrations of spent coffee grounds SFE (1, 5, and 10 mg/mL) or the same volume of DMSO (as negative control) for 24 h, and the MTT solution was then added to the wells. The insoluble derivative of MTT produced by intracellular dehydrogenase was solubilized with ethanol-DMSO (1:1 mixture solution). The absorbance of the wells at 570 nm was read using a microplate reader. Results are expressed as percent viability relative to control and the data are presented as the mean values ± SD from three independent experiments performed in triplicate.

*2.6. Assay of Mushroom Tyrosinase Activity.* The mushroom tyrosinase inhibition experiments were conducted as previously described [18]. In brief, 10 μL of the aqueous solution of mushroom tyrosinase (200 units) was added to a 96-well microplate, for a total volume of a 200 μL mixture containing 5 mM L-DOPA, which was dissolved in 50 mM phosphate buffered saline (PBS) (pH 6.8), spent coffee grounds SFE (1, 5, and 10 mg/mL), or arbutin (2 mM). The assay mixture was incubated at 37°C for 30 min and the absorbance of dopachrome produced was measured at 490 nm. The results are presented as percentages of the control and the data are presented as the mean values ± SD from three independent experiments performed in triplicate.

*2.7. Measurement of Melanin Content.* The intracellular melanin content was measured as described by Tsuboi et al. [19]. The B16F10 melanoma cells ($5 \times 10^4$ cells/mL) were treated with α-MSH (100 nM) for 24 h, and the melanin content was then determined after treatment with either spent coffee grounds SFE (1, 5, and 10 mg/mL) or arbutin (2 mM) for an additional 24 h. After treatment, the cell pellets containing a known number of cells were solubilized in 1 N NaOH at 60°C for 60 min. The melanin content was assayed at 405 nm. The results are presented as percentages of the control and the data are presented as the mean values ± SD from three independent experiments performed in triplicate.

*2.8. Assay of Intracellular Tyrosinase Activity.* The cellular tyrosinase activity was determined as described previously [20]. The B16F10 melanoma cells ($5 \times 10^4$ cells/mL) were treated with α-MSH (100 nM) for 24 h and then with spent coffee grounds SFE (1, 5, and 10 mg/mL) or arbutin (2 mM) for 24 h. After treatments, the cell extracts (100 μL) were mixed with freshly prepared L-DOPA solution (0.1% in PBS) and incubated at 37°C; the absorbance at 490 nm was measured.

The results are presented as percentages of the control and the data are presented as the mean values ± SD from three independent experiments performed in triplicate.

*2.9. Western Blotting Assay.* The cells were treated with spent coffee grounds SFE (1, 5, and 10 mg/mL) or arbutin (2 mM), lysed in proteinase inhibitor containing PBS at 4°C for 20 min. Proteins (50 μg) were resolved by SDS-polyacrylamide gel electrophoresis and electrophoretically transferred to a polyvinylidene fluoride (PVDF) filter. The filter was blocked in 5% fat-free milk in PBST buffer (PBS with 0.05% Tween-20) for 1 h. After a brief wash, the filter was incubated overnight at 4°C with several antibodies; these antibodies included anti-MITF (1:1000), anti-TRP-1 (1:6000), anti-TRP-2 (1:1000), anti-MC1R (1:500), anti-GAPDH (1:1500), anti-tyrosinase (1:2000), anti-p-p38 (1:500), anti-p38 (1:500), anti-p-JNK (1:500), anti-JNK (1:500), anti-p-ERK (1:500), anti-ERK (1:500), anti-p-CERB (1:500), and anti-CERB (1:200). Following incubation, the filter was extensively washed in PBST buffer. Subsequent incubation with goat anti-mouse antibody (1:10000) conjugated with horseradish peroxidase was conducted at room temperature for 2 h. The blot was visualized using an ECL reagent. The relative amounts of expressed proteins compared to total GAPDH were analyzed using Multi Gauge 3.0 software (Fuji, Tokyo).

*2.10. Protein Kinase Regulators Assay.* The cells were treated with α-MSH (100 nM) for 24 h followed by a 1 h addition of 10 μM of different protein kinase regulators, including GF109203X, H89, IBMX, LY294002, PD98059, SB203580, SP600125, and U0126, respectively. After these treatments, spent coffee grounds SFE (10 mg/mL) and 10 μM of the above kinase regulators were added to the cells and incubated for an additional 23 h, respectively. The melanin contents were assayed as described above. The results are presented as percentages of the control and the data are presented as the mean values ± SD from three independent experiments performed in triplicate.

*2.11. Statistical Analysis.* Statistical analysis of the experimental data points was performed by the ANOVA test, which was used for comparison of measured data using SPSS 12.0 statistical software (SPSS Inc., Chicago, USA). Differences were considered as statistically significant at $p \leq 0.05$.

# 3. Results

The average amounts of fatty acids in spent coffee grounds SFE were shown in Table 1. The fatty acid constituents in the spent coffee grounds SFE are linoleic acid (43.26%), palmitic acid (35.23%), oleic acid (8.86%), stearic acid (7.15%), arachidic acid (2.68%), α-linoleic acid (1.26%), behenic acid (0.52%), gadoleic acid (0.34%), lignoceric acid (0.23%), margaric acid (0.11%), myristic acid (0.083%), tricosanoic acid (0.083%), heneicosanoic acid (0.067%), eicosadienoic acid (0.05%), palmitoleic acid (0.047%), and pentadecanoic acid (0.033%) (Table 1). Unsaturated fatty acids like oleic acid

TABLE 1: Fatty acid composition of spent coffee grounds SFE.

| Fatty acid | Carbon number | Content (%) |
|---|---|---|
| Myristic acid | C14:0 | $0.083 \pm 0.0047$ |
| Pentadecanoic acid | C15:0 | $0.033 \pm 0.0047$ |
| Palmitic acid-2 | C16:0 | $35.23 \pm 0.2628$ |
| Palmitoleic acid | C16:1 | $0.047 \pm 0.0170$ |
| Margaric acid-9 | C17:0 | $0.11 \pm 00142$ |
| Stearic acid-4 | C18:0 | $7.15 \pm 0.0712$ |
| Oleic acid-3 | C18:1 | $8.8567 \pm 0.066$ |
| Linoleic acid-1 | C18:2 | $43.2567 \pm 0.296$ |
| $\alpha$-Linoleic acid | C18:3 | $1.2567 \pm 0.017$ |
| Arachidic acid-5 | C20:0 | $2.68 \pm 0.0589$ |
| Gadoleic acid-7 | C20:1 | $0.3367 \pm 0.0047$ |
| Eicosadienoic acid | C20:2 | $0.05 \pm 0.0023$ |
| Heneicosanoic acid | C21:0 | $0.0667 \pm 0.0047$ |
| Behenic acid-6 | C22:0 | $0.52 \pm 0.0356$ |
| Tricosanoic acid | C23:0 | $0.083 \pm 0.0047$ |
| Lignoceric acid-8 | C24:0 | $0.23 \pm 0.0163$ |

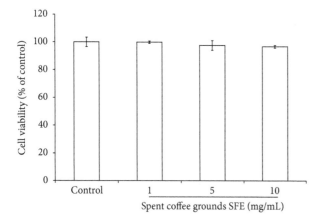

FIGURE 1: Effect of spent coffee grounds SFE on the proliferation of B16F10 cells. Cell viability was measured by MTT assay method after 24 h incubation. Data are expressed as a percentage of the number of viable cells observed with the control and each column was presented as mean values ± SD from three independent experiments performed in triplicate.

and linoleic acid have been reported to lighten ultraviolet-induced hyperpigmentation of the skin [21]. Hence, it is predicted that linoleic acid and oleic acid in the SFE may contribute to their antimelanogenic activities.

The MTT assay was used to assess the effect of spent coffee grounds SFE on B16F10 cells viability. The cells were treated with various concentrations of the SFE (1, 5, and 10 mg/mL) for 24 h and then MTT assay was performed. After treatment, the spent coffee grounds SFE showed no cytotoxic effect on B16F10 cell viability (Figure 1).

The results shown in Figure 2(a) revealed that the remaining mushroom tyrosinase activity was $91.37 \pm 2.45\%$, $85.33 \pm 2.67\%$, and $71.71 \pm 3.54\%$ of the control for the 1, 5, and 10 mg/mL of spent coffee grounds SFE treatments, respectively. In addition, the tyrosinase activity was also

inhibited by arbutin (2 mM), and the residual enzyme activity was $62.74 \pm 2.16\%$ of control (Figure 2(a)).

The results shown in Figure 2(b) indicated that higher concentrations of spent coffee grounds SFE significantly decreased the melanin content in B16F10 melanoma cells. After treatment, the melanin content in the B16F10 cells was $97.87 \pm 1.03\%$, $87.18 \pm 1.71\%$, and $70.82 \pm 1.48\%$ for the 1, 5, and 10 mg/mL of spent coffee grounds SFE treatments, respectively. For the positive standard arbutin (2 mM), the intracellular melanin content was $69.45 \pm 1.15\%$ of the control (Figure 2(b)). The results indicated that 10 mg/mL of spent coffee grounds SFE showed similar effects as arbutin does.

The B16F10 intracellular tyrosinase activity was $96.22 \pm 1.96\%$, $86.99 \pm 1.23\%$, and $69.31 \pm 0.98\%$ for the 1, 5, and 10 mg/mL of spent coffee grounds SFE treatments, respectively. The residual intracellular tyrosinase activity was $69.16 \pm 0.53\%$ of control after the cells were treated with arbutin (2 mM) (Figure 2(c)). The results indicated that higher concentration of spent coffee grounds SFE exhibited similar inhibitory effect on $\alpha$-MSH-induced tyrosinase activity in B16F10 cells than arbutin did.

The expression levels of melanogenesis-related proteins were examined using western blots (Figure 3(a)). The results indicate that 1–10 mg/mL of spent coffee grounds SFE treatment led to a reduced level of MITF, tyrosinase, TRP-1, and TRP-2. The inhibitory effects of the SFE on protein expression were apparent at the concentration of 10 mg/mL. After treatments with the 1, 5, and 10 mg/mL of spent coffee grounds SFE, respectively, the fold changes of protein expression levels were $0.98 \pm 0.09$, $0.87 \pm 0.09$, and $0.74 \pm 0.07$ for MITF; $0.94 \pm 0.08$, $0.89 \pm 0.11$, and $0.77 \pm 0.09$ for tyrosinase; $0.88 \pm 0.07$, $0.83 \pm 0.03$, and $0.79 \pm 0.03$ for MC1R; $0.98 \pm 0.04$, $0.94 \pm 0.09$, and $0.63 \pm 0.08$ for TRP-1; $0.99 \pm 0.07$, $0.89 \pm 0.07$, and $0.79 \pm 0.06$ for TRP-2 (Figure 3(b)).

The protein expression levels of melanogenesis-related signaling proteins were examined using western blots (Figure 3(c)). The results indicate that 1–10 mg/mL of spent coffee grounds SFE treatment led to a reduced level of p-JNK, p-p38, p-ERK, and p-CREB. The inhibitory effects of the SFE on protein expression were apparent at the concentration 10 mg/mL. The fold changes of protein expression levels for p-JNK were $0.96 \pm 0.09$, $0.91 \pm 0.08$, and $0.83 \pm 0.06$; for p-p38 were $0.97 \pm 0.05$, $0.82 \pm 0.11$, and $0.59 \pm 0.08$; for p-ERK were $0.89 \pm 0.04$, $0.77 \pm 0.08$, and $0.69 \pm 0.08$; for p-CREB were $0.99 \pm 0.07$, $0.89 \pm 0.14$, and $0.71 \pm 0.04$ for the 1, 5, and 10 mg/mL of spent coffee grounds SFE treatments, respectively (Figure 3(d)).

The addition of the SFE to H89 treated B16F10 cells significantly decreased the cellular melanin content, which indicated that PKA-mediated signaling pathway was affected by spent coffee grounds SFE (Figure 4(a)). The results shown in Figure 4(b) revealed that the specific inhibitor of PI3K/Akt, LY294002, attenuated $\alpha$-MSH-stimulated melanin synthesis. These results suggest that spent coffee grounds SFE inhibited melanin synthesis by downregulating PI3K/Akt signaling and, subsequently, decreased melanin synthesis in $\alpha$-MSH-stimulated B16F10 cells. The addition of spent coffee grounds SFE in PD98059 treated B16F10 cells also significantly decreased the cellular melanin content. The results

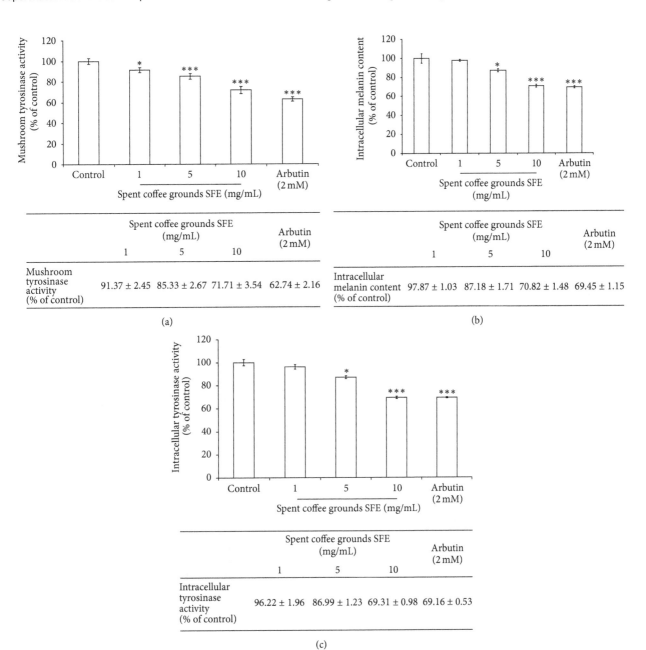

FIGURE 2: The inhibitory effects of spent coffee grounds SFE on melanogenesis. (a) The effects of spent coffee grounds SFE on mushroom tyrosinase activity. (b) The effects of spent coffee grounds SFE on melanin content in B16F10 cells. (c) The effects of spent coffee grounds SFE on tyrosinase activity in B16F10 cells. The results are presented as percentages of the control, and the data are presented as the mean ± SD of three separate experiments. The values are significantly different compared with the control. $^{*}p \leq 0.05$; $^{***}p < 0.001$.

indicate that the ERK-mediated signaling pathway involved in melanin production was affected by spent coffee grounds SFE treatment (Figure 4(c)).

To further investigate the biological activities of the major components of spent coffee grounds SFE, the potential inhibitory effects of linoleic acid, oleic acid, palmitic acid, and stearic acid on cellular melanin content and tyrosinase activity were investigated. After treatment, the melanin content in the B16F10 cells was 88.88 ± 2.11%, 66.53 ± 1.29%, 51.47 ± 2.03%, and 45.49 ± 3.08% for the 6.25, 12.5, 25, and 50 $\mu$M of linoleic acid treatments, respectively (Figure 5(a)).

The melanin content in the cells was 98.48 ± 0.95%, 95.64 ± 1.26%, 89.49 ± 1.03%, and 81.09 ± 1.56% for the 6.25, 12.5, 25, and 50 $\mu$M of oleic acid treatments, respectively (Figure 5(b)). The results shown in Figures 5(a) and 5(b) indicated that linoleic acid and oleic acid significantly decreased intracellular melanin content. The remaining intracellular tyrosinase activity was 89.21 ± 1.94%, 67.42 ± 1.41%, 50.94 ± 1.19%, and 45.94 ± 0.86% for the 6.25, 12.5, 25, and 50 $\mu$M of linoleic acid treatments, respectively (Figure 5(c)). In addition, the intracellular tyrosinase activities were also inhibited by oleic acid. The remaining intracellular tyrosinase

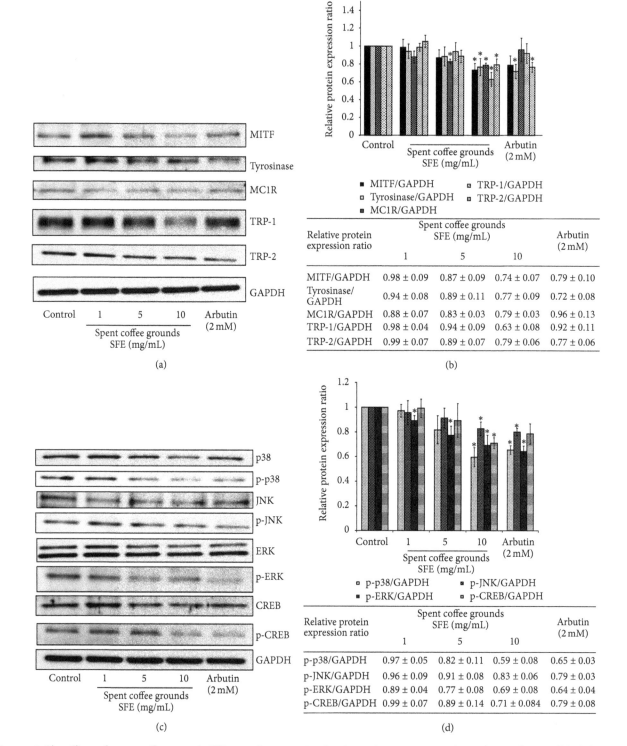

FIGURE 3: The effects of spent coffee grounds SFE on melanogenesis-related protein expression and signaling pathways. ((a), (c)) Western blotting of cellular proteins in B16F10 cells. ((b), (d)) The relative amounts of MITF, tyrosinase, MC1R, TRP-1, and TRP-2 or phosphorylated proteins (p-p38, p-JNK, p-ERK, and p-CREB) compared to the total GAPDH were calculated and analyzed using Multi Gauge 3.0 software, and the values represented the mean of triplicate experiments ± standard deviations. $^*p \leq 0.05$.

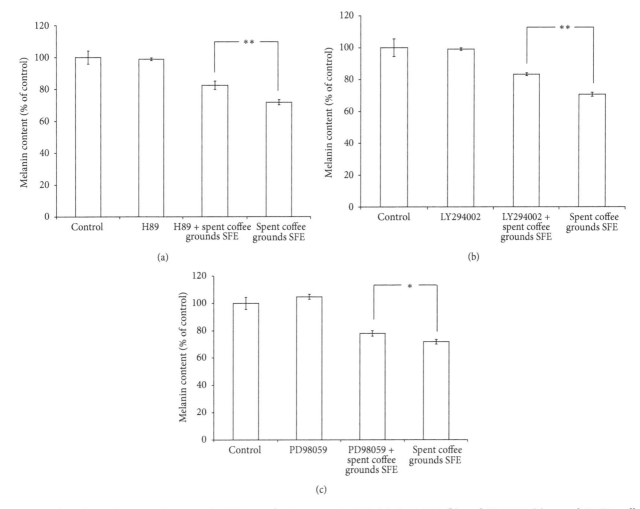

FIGURE 4: The effects of spent coffee grounds SFE on melanin content in H89 (a), Ly294002 (b), and PD98059 (c) treated B16F10 cells, respectively. The results are represented as percentages of the control, and the data are presented as the mean ± SD of three separate experiments. The values are significantly different compared with the control. $^*p \leq 0.05$; $^{**}p < 0.01$.

activity was 98.39 ± 1.13%, 95.43 ± 0.66%, 89.64 ± 1.23%, and 80.71 ± 1.18% for the 6.25, 12.5, 25, and 50 $\mu$M of oleic acid treatments, respectively (Figure 5(d)). However, both palmitic acid and stearic acid showed no inhibitory effects on intracellular tyrosinase activity and melanin content (data not shown). Hence, this study suggests that the antimelanogenic activity of spent coffee grounds SFE was probably due to the inhibitory effects of linoleic acid and oleic acid on intracellular tyrosinase activity and subsequently decreased melanin production.

## 4. Discussion

The MTT assay is a common colorimetric assay to measure the activity of NADH/NADPH-dependent cellular oxidoreductase enzymes that reduce MTT to formazan dyes, giving a purple color. This assay could be used to determine the cytotoxicity of potential medicinal agents and toxic materials, since those agents enhance or inhibit cell viability. The results shown in Figure 1 indicated that the spent coffee grounds SFE showed no cytotoxic effect on B16F10 melanoma cell viability.

Thus, we used 1–10 mg/mL of the spent coffee grounds SFE in the following experiments.

Mushroom tyrosinase is widely applied as the target enzyme in screening potential inhibitors of melanin production. It was first found that the dosage range (1–10 mg/mL) of the spent coffee grounds SFE could inhibit the activity of mushroom tyrosinase. The results shown in Figure 2(a) indicated that the spent coffee grounds SFEs show lower inhibitory effect on mushroom tyrosinase activity than arbutin does. Tyrosinase plays an essential role in the melanin synthesis pathway. To evaluate the inhibitory effect of the spent coffee grounds SFE on melanin production, we measured the B16F10 melanin content and intracellular tyrosinase activity after treatment with the extract. The results shown in Figure 2(b) indicated that the spent coffee grounds SFE (10 mg/mL) exhibits a similar inhibitory effect on melanin formation as arbutin does. The results shown in Figure 2(c) were in accordance with the results indicated in Figure 2(b), which means the spent coffee grounds SFE inhibited B16F10 intracellular tyrosinase activity and decreased the melanin

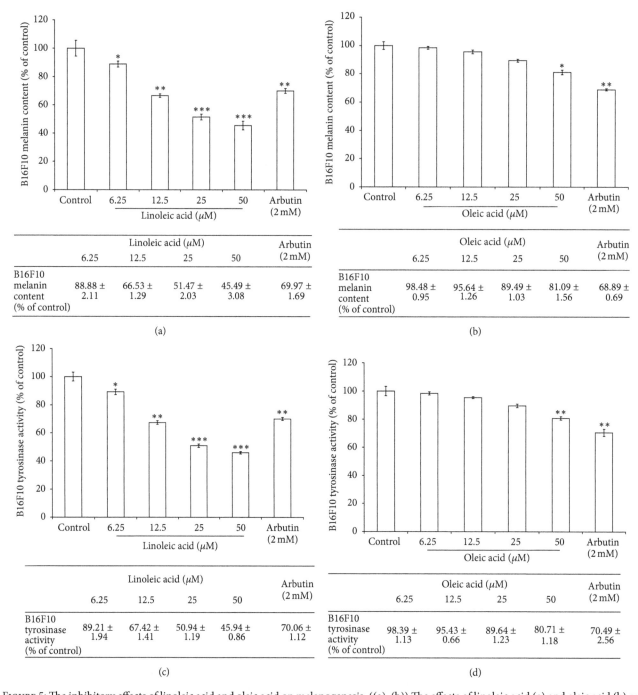

FIGURE 5: The inhibitory effects of linoleic acid and oleic acid on melanogenesis. ((a), (b)) The effects of linoleic acid (a) and oleic acid (b) on melanin content in B16F10 cells. ((c), (d)) The effects of linoleic acid (c) and oleic acid (d) on tyrosinase activity in B16F10 cells. The results are presented as percentages of the control, and the data are presented as the mean ± SD of three separate experiments. The values are significantly different compared with the control. $^{*}p \leq 0.05$; $^{**}p < 0.01$; $^{***}p < 0.001$.

content. The data provided evidence that the spent coffee grounds SFE truly downregulates melanin production in the murine melanoma cells. In those intracellular experiments, we used $\alpha$-MSH as a cAMP inducer to stimulate melanin production. $\alpha$-MSH was reported to bind melanocortin 1 receptor (MC1R) and then activate adenylate cyclase, which in turn catalyzes ATP to cAMP and increases the intracellular

cAMP level [9]. Further, cAMP-mediated PKA signaling pathway was activated and melanogenesis was enhanced. The results indicated that the spent coffee grounds SFE could inhibit melanin synthesis induced by $\alpha$-MSH mediated intracellular cAMP upregulation.

It was found that binding of the human MC1R by its ligands can activate the cAMP-mediated signaling pathway and regulate melanogenesis of human melanocytes [22]. In mammalian cells, melanin synthesis was also regulated by tyrosinase, TRP-1, and TRP-2 [23]. In addition, MITF is the major transcriptional regulator of the tyrosinase, TRP-1, and TRP-2 genes and is the most important regulator of melanocyte differentiation and melanogenesis [24]. The results shown in Figures 3(a) and 3(b) indicated that the spent coffee grounds SFE decreased the protein expression levels of MITF, tyrosinase, MC1R, TRP-1, and TRP-2 and finally decreased melanin content in the B16F10 cells. The results shown in Figure 3(c) indicated that spent coffee grounds SFE decreased MC1R expression and further suggests that spent coffee grounds SFE inhibited melanogenesis induced via $\alpha$-MSH-mediated intracellular cAMP upregulation. Moreover, the results shown in Figure 4(a) further confirm that spent coffee grounds SFE inhibited cAMP-mediated PKA signaling.

It has been reported that MAPK act to modulate melanin synthesis [25–27]. The MAPK family consists of three types of protein kinases, including extracellular responsive kinase (ERK), c-Jun N-terminal kinase (JNK), and p38 MAPK. It was found that the p38 MAPK can activate the cAMP response element-binding protein (CREB) and then CREB activates MITF expression, which contributes to melanin production [28]. The results in Figure 3(c) provide evidence that spent coffee grounds SFE could inactivate ERK, JNK, p38, and CREB, which in turn inhibits MITF expression (Figure 3(a)). Furthermore, the protein kinase A (PKA) signaling is also reported to be involved in melanin production [29]. The $\alpha$-MSH-mediated elevation of cellular cAMP levels could activate PKA. In turn, activated PKA can activate CREB, leading to the activation of MITF transcriptional activity and resulting in the expressions of melanogenesis-related proteins. Our results shown in Figure 4(a) also suggest that spent coffee grounds SFE inhibits melanin synthesis through downregulation of the PKA pathway. Figure 4(b) revealed that the specific inhibitor of PI3K/Akt, LY294002, attenuated $\alpha$-MSH-stimulated melanin production, which suggested that spent coffee grounds SFE inhibited melanin synthesis through downregulating PI3K/Akt signaling and, subsequently, decreased melanin synthesis in $\alpha$-MSH-stimulated B16F10 cells. Figure 4(c) indicated that the addition of spent coffee grounds SFE in PD98059 treated B16F10 cells also decreased the cellular melanin content, which implied that the ERK-mediated signaling pathway involved in melanin production was affected by spent coffee grounds SFE treatment. The results shown in Figure 5 indicated that linoleic acid and oleic acid may contribute to the inhibitory effects of the spent coffee grounds SFE on melanogenesis. Although we carried out the same experiments for palmitic acid and stearic acid, the two kinds of fatty acids exhibited no inhibitory effects on melanin production in B16F10 cells (data not shown).

The previous study has shown that the SFC from spent coffee exhibited significantly high activities in the inhibition of melanin synthesis and tyrosinase activity [14], which is in accordance with our results. The authors concluded that high fatty acid content did not correspond with the capacity to inhibit melanin synthesis or tyrosinase activity. However, our results have found that the unsaturated fatty acids in the spent coffee grounds SFE play an important

role in the inhibition of melanogenesis. The GC-MS analysis results shown in Table 1 revealed that linoleic acid, oleic acid, palmitic acid, and stearic acid were the four major components in the spent coffee grounds SFE. Free fatty acids have been shown to have remarkable regulatory effects on melanogenesis in cultured B16F10 murine melanoma cells. Unsaturated fatty acids, such as oleic acid (C18:1), linoleic acid (C18:2), or $\alpha$-linolenic acid (C18:3), decreased melanin synthesis and tyrosinase activity, while saturated fatty acids, such as palmitic acid (C16:0) or stearic acid (C18:0), increased it [21, 30, 31]. Those reports supported our results shown in Figure 5 that oleic acid and linoleic acid in the spent coffee grounds SFE contributed to the inhibition of melanogenesis in the B16F10 cells. Interestingly, it has been reported that topical application of linoleic acid lightened UV-stimulated hyperpigmented skin of experimental guinea pig [9], which further supported our proposal that linoleic acid existing in the SFE might play an important role in the inhibitory effects on melanogenesis in the melanoma cells. In addition, the regulatory effects of fatty acids on melanin production are probably through proteolytic degradation of tyrosinase [32]. Our results indicated that spent coffee grounds SFE inhibited melanogenesis in B16F10 cells by downregulation of both mitogen-activated protein kinases (MAPK) and protein kinase A (PKA) signaling pathways. Hence, the spent coffee grounds SFE could be used as an effective skin whitening agent.

## 5. Conclusion

This is the first report on the action mechanisms of the inhibitory effect of spent coffee grounds SFE on melanin biosynthesis. The present study concluded that spent coffee grounds SFE inhibits melanin synthesis in B16F10 melanoma cells by downregulation of protein kinase A (PKA), phosphatidylinositol-3-kinase (PI3K/Akt), and mitogen-activated protein kinases (MAPK) signaling pathways. Hence, the spent coffee grounds SFE could be used as a novel dermatological antimelanogenesis agent in skin care products.

## Competing Interests

All authors are in agreement with the content of the paper and do not have any actual or potential conflict of interests, including any financial competing interests, nonfinancial competing interests, or personal or other relationships with other organizations or people within that could inappropriately influence the work.

## Authors' Contributions

Huey-Chun Huang carried out the tyrosinase-related studies, participated in the enzyme assays, and drafted the paper. Chien-Mei Wei performed GC analysis and cell culture experiments. Jen-Hung Siao carried out melanin-related experiments. Tsang-Chi Tsai carried out the supercritical fluid CO$_2$ extraction of spent coffee grounds. Wang-Ping

Ko and Kuei-Jen Chang carried out western blot experiments. Tsong-Min Chang and Choon-Hoon Hii participated in design and coordination of the study, performed the statistical analysis, and drafted the paper. All authors read and approved the final paper.

## Acknowledgments

This study was financially supported by the National Science Council, Taiwan, under Grant nos. MOST 104-2313-B-241-001 and NSC 102-2632-B-241-001-MY3.

## References

[1] R. A. Spritz and V. J. Hearing Jr., "Genetic disorders of pigmentation," *Advances in Human Genetics*, vol. 22, pp. 1–45, 1994.

[2] S. Briganti, E. Camera, and M. Picardo, "Chemical and instrumental approaches to treat hyperpigmentation," *Pigment Cell Research*, vol. 16, no. 2, pp. 101–110, 2003.

[3] Y. Funasaka, M. Komoto, and M. Ichihashi, "Depigmenting effect of α-tocopheryl ferulate on normal human melanocytes," *Pigment Cell Research*, vol. 13, no. 8, pp. 170–174, 2000.

[4] S.-Y. Seo, V. K. Sharma, and N. Sharma, "Mushroom tyrosinase: recent prospects," *Journal of Agricultural and Food Chemistry*, vol. 51, no. 10, pp. 2837–2853, 2003.

[5] V. J. Hearing and M. Jiménez, "Mammalian tyrosinase—the critical regulatory control point in melanocyte pigmentation," *International Journal of Biochemistry*, vol. 19, no. 12, pp. 1141–1147, 1987.

[6] C. Jiménez-Cervantes, F. Solano, T. Kobayashi et al., "A new enzymatic function in the melanogenic pathway: the 5,6-dihydroxyindole-2-carboxylic acid oxidase activity of tyrosinase-related protein-1 (TRP1)," *The Journal of Biological Chemistry*, vol. 269, no. 27, pp. 17993–18000, 1994.

[7] K. Tsukamoto, I. J. Jackson, K. Urabe, P. M. Montague, and V. J. Hearing, "A second tyrosinase-related protein, TRP-2, is a melanogenic enzyme termed DOPAchrome tautomerase," *The EMBO Journal*, vol. 11, no. 2, pp. 519–526, 1992.

[8] J. C. García-Borrón, B. L. Sánchez-Laorden, and C. Jiménez-Cervantes, "Melanocortin-1 receptor structure and functional regulation," *Pigment Cell Research*, vol. 18, no. 6, pp. 393–410, 2005.

[9] R. Buscà and R. Ballotti, "Cyclic AMP a key messenger in the regulation of skin pigmentation," *Pigment Cell Research*, vol. 13, no. 2, pp. 60–69, 2000.

[10] M. Wu, T. J. Hemesath, C. M. Takemoto et al., "c-Kit triggers dual phosphorylations, which couple activation and degradation of the essential melanocyte factor Mi," *Genes & Development*, vol. 14, no. 3, pp. 301–312, 2000.

[11] M. M. Haddad, W. Xu, D. J. Schwahn, F. Liao, and E. E. Medrano, "Activation of a cAMP pathway and induction of melanogenesis correlate with association of p16(INK4) and p27(KIP1) to CDKs, loss of E2F-binding activity, and premature senescence of human melanocytes," *Experimental Cell Research*, vol. 253, no. 2, pp. 561–572, 1999.

[12] J. H. Bae, J. H. Park, S. S. Im, and D. K. Song, "Coffee and health," *Integrative Medicine Research*, vol. 3, no. 4, pp. 189–191, 2014.

[13] C. Fortes, S. Mastroeni, P. Boffetta et al., "The protective effect of coffee consumption on cutaneous melanoma risk and the role of GSTM1 and GSTT1 polymorphisms," *Cancer Causes and Control*, vol. 24, no. 10, pp. 1779–1787, 2013.

[14] H. M. Sung, H. J. Jung, J. S. Sin, K. M. Kim, and J.-H. Wee, "Skin whitening activity of supercritical fluid extract from spent coffee in B16F10 melanoma cell," *Food Science and Biotechnology*, vol. 24, no. 3, pp. 1087–1096, 2015.

[15] R. P. Adama, *Identification of Essential Oil Components by Gas Chromatography/Mass Spectroscopy*, Allured Publishing Co., Carol Stream, Ill, USA, 1995.

[16] H. Vandendool and P. D. Kratz, "A generalization of the retention index system including linear temperature programmed gas—liquid partition chromatography," *Journal of Chromatography A*, vol. 11, pp. 463–471, 1963.

[17] H. Tada, O. Shiho, K.-I. Kuroshima, M. Koyama, and K. Tsukamoto, "An improved colorimetric assay for interleukin 2," *Journal of Immunological Methods*, vol. 93, no. 2, pp. 157–165, 1986.

[18] M. L. Bilodeau, J. D. Greulich, R. L. Hullinger, C. Bertolotto, R. Ballotti, and O. M. Andrisani, "BMP-2 stimulates tyrosinase gene expression and melanogenesis in differentiated melanocytes," *Pigment Cell Research*, vol. 14, no. 5, pp. 328–336, 2001.

[19] T. Tsuboi, H. Kondoh, J. Hiratsuka, and Y. Mishima, "Enhanced melanogenesis induced by tyrosinase gene-transfer increases boron-uptake and killing effect of boron neutron capture therapy for amelanotic melanoma," *Pigment Cell Research*, vol. 11, no. 5, pp. 275–282, 1998.

[20] J.-Y. Yang, J.-H. Koo, Y.-G. Song et al., "Stimulation of melanogenesis by scoparone in B16 melanoma cells," *Acta Pharmacologica Sinica*, vol. 27, no. 11, pp. 1467–1473, 2006.

[21] H. Ando, A. Ryu, A. Hashimoto, M. Oka, and M. Ichihashi, "Linoleic acid and α-linolenic acid lightens ultraviolet-induced hyperpigmentation of the skin," *Archives of Dermatological Research*, vol. 290, no. 7, pp. 375–381, 1998.

[22] Z. Abdel-Malek, V. Swope, C. Collins, R. Boissy, H. Zhao, and J. Nordlund, "Contribution of melanogenic proteins to the heterogeneous pigmentation of human melanocytes," *Journal of Cell Science*, vol. 106, part 4, pp. 1323–1331, 1993.

[23] K. Kameyama, C. Sakai, S. Kuge et al., "The expression of tyrosinase, tyrosinase-related proteins 1 and 2 (TRP1 and TRP2), the silver protein, and a melanogenic inhibitor in human melanoma cells of differing melanogenic activities," *Pigment Cell Research*, vol. 8, no. 2, pp. 97–104, 1995.

[24] C. Levy, M. Khaled, and D. E. Fisher, "MITF: master regulator of melanocyte development and melanoma oncogene," *Trends in Molecular Medicine*, vol. 12, no. 9, pp. 406–414, 2006.

[25] N. Hirata, S. Naruto, K. Ohguchi et al., "Mechanism of the melanogenesis stimulation activity of (−)-cubebin in murine B16 melanoma cells," *Bioorganic and Medicinal Chemistry*, vol. 15, no. 14, pp. 4897–4902, 2007.

[26] D.-S. Kim, Y.-M. Jeong, I.-K. Park et al., "A new 2-imino-1,3-thiazoline derivative, KHG22394, inhibits melanin synthesis in mouse B16 melanoma cells," *Biological and Pharmaceutical Bulletin*, vol. 30, no. 1, pp. 180–183, 2007.

[27] K. Smalley and T. Eisen, "The involvement of p38 mitogen-activated protein kinase in the α-melanocyte stimulating hormone (α-MSH)-induced melanogenic and anti-proliferative effects in B16 murine melanoma cells," *FEBS Letters*, vol. 476, no. 3, pp. 198–202, 2000.

[28] S. K. Singh, C. Sarkar, S. Mallick, B. Saha, R. Bera, and R. Bhadra, "Human placental lipid induces melanogenesis through p38

MAPK in B16F10 mouse melanoma," *Pigment Cell Research*, vol. 18, no. 2, pp. 113–121, 2005.

[29] T. Hirobe, "Basic fibroblast growth factor stimulates the sustained proliferation of mouse epidermal melanoblasts in a serum-free medium in the presence of dibutyryl cyclic AMP and keratinocytes," *Development*, vol. 114, no. 2, pp. 435–445, 1992.

[30] S. Shono and K. Toda, "Phenotypic expression in pigment cells," in *Pigment Cell*, pp. 263–268, University of Tokyo Press, Tokyo, Japan, 1981.

[31] H. Ando, A. Itoh, Y. Mishima, and M. Ichihashi, "Correlation between the number of melanosomes, tyrosinase mRNA levels, and tyrosinase activity in cultured murine melanoma cells in response to various melanogenesis regulatory agents," *Journal of Cellular Physiology*, vol. 163, no. 3, pp. 608–614, 1995.

[32] H. Ando, Y. Funasaka, M. Oka et al., "Possible involvement of proteolytic degradation of tyrosinase in the regulatory effect of fatty acids on melanogenesis," *Journal of Lipid Research*, vol. 40, no. 7, pp. 1312–1316, 1999.

# Permissions

# List of Contributors

**Suzanne Cochrane**
School of Science & Health, Western Sydney University, Locked Bag 1797, Penrith, NSW2751, Australia

**Caroline A. Smith and Alan Bensoussan**
National Institute of Complementary Medicine, Western Sydney University, Locked Bag 1797, Penrith, NSW 2751, Australia

**Alphia Possamai-Inesedy**
School of Social Science & Psychology, Western Sydney University, Locked Bag 1797, Penrith, NSW2751, Australia

**M. Rondanelli, G. Peroni and S. Perna**
Department of Public Health, Experimental and Forensic Medicine, Section of Human Nutrition, Endocrinology and Nutrition Unit, Azienda di Servizi alla Persona, University of Pavia, 27100 Pavia, Italy

**A. Miccono**
Department of Clinical Sciences, Faculty of Medicine and Surgery, University of Milan, Milan, Italy

**F. Guerriero**
Azienda di Servizi alla Persona, Pavia, Italy

**P. Morazzoni and A. Riva**
Research and Development Unit, Indena, 20139 Milan, Italy

**D. Guido**
Department of Public Health, Experimental and Forensic Medicine, Section of Human Nutrition, Endocrinology and Nutrition Unit, Azienda di Servizi alla Persona, University of Pavia, 27100 Pavia, Italy
Department of Brain and Behavioral Sciences, Medical and Genomic Statistics Unit, University of Pavia, 27100 Pavia, Italy
Department of Public Health, Experimental and Forensic Medicine, Biostatistics and Clinical Epidemiology Unit, University of Pavia, 27100 Pavia, Italy

**Li Han, Xiaojuan Guo, Hua Bian, Lei Yang and Wenhua Zang**
Zhang Zhongjing College of Chinese Medicine, Nanyang Institute of Technology, 80 Changjiang Road, Nanyang 473004, China

**Zhong Chen**
College of Pharmaceutical Science, Soochow University, 199 Ren-ai Road, Suzhou 215123, China

**Jingke Yang**
Affiliated CancerHospital, ZhengzhouUniversity, Dongming Road 127, Zhengzhou 450008, China

**Mei-Ling Hou and Chia-Ming Lu**
Institute of TraditionalMedicine, National Yang-MingUniversity, No. 155, Section 2, Li-Nong Street, Taipei 112, Taiwan

**Tung-Hu Tsai**
Institute of TraditionalMedicine, National Yang-MingUniversity, No. 155, Section 2, Li-Nong Street, Taipei 112, Taiwan
Graduate Institute of Acupuncture Science, China Medical University, No. 91, Hsueh-Shih Road, Taichung 404, Taiwan
School of Pharmacy, College of Pharmacy, KaohsiungMedical University,No. 100, Shih-Chuan 1st Road, Kaohsiung 807, Taiwan
Department of Education and Research, Taipei City Hospital,No. 145, Zhengzhou Road, Datong District, Taipei 103, Taiwan

**Sher Zaman Safi, Kalaivani Batumalaie, Rajes Qvist and Ikram Shah Ismail**
Faculty of Medicine, Department of Medicine, University of Malaya, 50603 Kuala Lumpur, Malaysia

**Kamaruddin Mohd Yusof**
Department of Molecular Biology and Genetics, Faculty of Arts and Science, Canik Basari University, Samsun, Turkey

**M. FawziMahomoodally and A. Mootoosamy**
Department of Health Sciences, Faculty of Science, University of Mauritius, 230 R´eduit, Mauritius

**S. Wambugu**
Department of Veterinary Anatomy and Physiology, University of Nairobi, Nairobi 30197 00100, Kenya

**Wei-An Mao**
Department of Dermatology, Seventh People's Hospital, Shanghai University of Traditional Chinese Medicine, Shanghai 200137, China

**Yuan-Yuan Sun**
Department of Graduate, Bengbu Medical College, Bengbu 233000, China

**Jing-Yi Mao**
Yueyang Hospital, Shanghai University of Traditional Chinese Medicine, Shanghai 200437, China

**Li Wang, Jian Zhang and Jie Zhou**
Department of Dermatology, Seventh People's Hospital, Shanghai University of Traditional Chinese Medicine, Shanghai 200137, China

**Khalid Rahman and Ying Ye**
School of Pharmacy and Biomolecular Sciences, Faculty of Science, Liverpool John Moores University, Liverpool L3 3AF, UK
5Central Laboratory, Seventh People's Hospital, Shanghai University of Traditional Chinese Medicine, Shanghai 200137, China

**Tao Wang and Renli Deng**
The Fifth Affiliated (Zhuhai) Hospital of Zunyi Medical University, No. 1439, Zhufeng Road, Zhuhai, Guangdong 519100, China

**Jing-Yu Tan**
School of Nursing, Fujian University of Traditional Chinese Medicine, No. 1, Qiuyang Road, Fuzhou, Fujian 350122, China

**Feng-Guang Guan**
The Second Affiliated People's Hospital, Fujian University of Traditional Chinese Medicine, No. 282, Wusi Road, Fuzhou, Fujian 350003, China

**Pawe B Olczyk**
Department of Community Pharmacy, School of Pharmacy and Division of Laboratory Medicine in Sosnowiec, Medical University of Silesia in Katowice, Kasztanowa 3, 41-200 Sosnowiec, Poland

**Robert Koprowski**
Department of Biomedical Computer Systems, Faculty of Computer Science and Materials Science, Institute of Computer Science, University of Silesia, Bedzinska 39, 41-200 Sosnowiec, Poland

**Justyna Kafmierczak, Lukasz Mencner, Krystyna Olczyk and Katarzyna Komosinska-Vassev**
Department of Clinical Chemistry and Laboratory Diagnostics, School of Pharmacy and Division of Laboratory Medicine in Sosnowiec, Medical University of Silesia in Katowice, Jednosci 8, 41-200 Sosnowiec, Poland

**Robert Wojtyczka**
Department and Institute of Microbiology and Virology, School of Pharmacy and Division of Laboratory Medicine in Sosnowiec, Medical University of Silesia in Katowice, Jagiellonska 4, 41-200 Sosnowiec, Poland

**Jerzy Stojko**
Center of Experimental Medicine, Medics 4, Faculty of Medicine in Katowice, Medical University of Silesia in Katowice, 40-752 Katowice, Poland

**Hyo-Seon Kim, Hyeong-Geug Kim, Sung-Bae Lee, Jin-Seok Lee, Hwi-Jin Im, Won-Yong Kim and Chang-Gue Son**
Liver and Immunology Research Center, Daejeon Oriental Hospital, Oriental Medical College, Daejeon University, 176-9 Daeheung-ro, Jung-gu, Daejeon 34929, Republic of Korea

**Hye-Won Lee**
TKM-Based Herbal Drug Research Group, Korea Institute of Oriental Medicine, Daejeon 34054, Republic of Korea

**Dong-Soo Lee**
Department of Internal Medicine, Daejeon St. Mary's Hospital, The Catholic University of Korea, 64 Daeheung-ro, Jung-gu, Daejeon 34943, Republic of Korea

**Cailan Li, Zhizhun Mo, Lieqiang Xu, Lihua Tan, Dandan Luo, Hanbin Chen, Hongmei Yang, Yucui Li and Ziren Su**
School of Chinese Materia Medica, Guangzhou University of Chinese Medicine, Guangzhou 510006, China

**Jianhui Xie**
Guangdong Provincial Key Laboratory of Clinical Research on Traditional Chinese Medicine Syndrome, The Second Affiliated Hospital, Guangzhou University of Chinese Medicine, Guangzhou 510120, China

**Zuqing Su**
The Second Affiliated Hospital, Guangzhou University of Chinese Medicine, Guangzhou 510120, China

**Gunver S. Kienle**
Institute for Applied Epistemology and Medical Methodology, University ofWitten/Herdecke, Zechenweg 6, 79111 Freiburg, Germany
Center for Complementary Medicine, Institute for Environmental Health Sciences and Hospital Infection Control, University Medical Center Freiburg, Breisacher Strasse 115B, 79106 Freiburg, Germany

**Milena Mussler and Helmut Kiene**
Institute for Applied Epistemology and Medical Methodology, University of Witten/Herdecke, Zechenweg 6, 79111 Freiburg, Germany

**Dieter Fuchs**
Department of Theology, Caritas Sciences, University of Freiburg, Werthmannplatz 3, 79098 Freiburg, Germany

**Wei Liu, Hong-li Jiang, Lin-li Cai,Min Yan, Shou-jin Dong and Bing Mao**
Pneumology Group, Department of Integrated Traditional Chinese andWestern Medicine,West China Hospital, Sichuan University, Chengdu 610041, China

**Su Kil Jang, Seung Tae Kim, Jun Sub Park, Bo Ram Jo and Seong Soo Joo**
College of Life Science, Gangneung-Wonju National University, 120 Gangneung Daehangno, Gangneung, Gangwon 210-702, Republic of Korea

**Do Ik Lee**
College of Pharmacy, Chung-Ang University, 221 Heukseok-dong, Dongjak-gu, Seoul 156-756, Republic of Korea

**Jung Youl Park**
Industry-Academic Cooperation Foundation, Hanbat National University, Daejeon 305-719, Republic of Korea

**Jong Heo**
Heo-jong Oriental Medicine Clinic, Mia-dong, Gangbuk-gu 62-3, Seoul 01205, Republic of Korea

**Huey-Chun Huang**
Department of Medical Laboratory Science and Biotechnology, China Medical University, No. 91 Hsueh-Shih Road, Taichung 40402, Taiwan

**Chien-MeiWei, Jen-Hung Siao and Tsong-Min Chang**
Department of Applied Cosmetology and Master Program of Cosmetic Science, Hungkuang University, No. 1018, Section 6, Taiwan Boulevard, Shalu District, Taichung 43302, Taiwan

**Tsang-Chi Tsai, Wang-Ping Ko and Kuei-Jen Chang**
O'right Plant Extract R&D Center, No. 18, Gaoping Section, Jhongfong Road, Longtan District, Taoyuan 32544, Taiwan

**Choon-Hoon Hii**
Department of Emergency Medicine, Kuang Tien General Hospital, No. 321, Jingguo Road, Dajia District, Taichung 43761, Taiwan

# Index

CPSIA information can be obtained
at www.ICGtesting.com
Printed in the USA
BVHW02*0448020218
506942BV00003B/35/P

9 781632 398826